MEMORIAL HOSPITAL
PERINATAL/GENETIC CENTER

OBSTETRICAL MEASUREMENTS IN ULTRASOUND
A Reference Manual

Obstetrical Measurements in Ultrasound

A Reference Manual

ALFRED B. KURTZ, M.D.
Professor of Radiology and of Obstetrics and Gynecology
Associate Director
Division of Diagnostic Ultrasound
Department of Radiology
Thomas Jefferson University
Philadelphia, Pennsylvania

BARRY B. GOLDBERG, M.D.
Professor of Radiology
Director, Division of Diagnostic Ultrasound
Department of Radiology
Thomas Jefferson University
Philadelphia, Pennsylvania

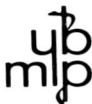

YEAR BOOK MEDICAL PUBLISHERS, INC.
Chicago • London • Boca Raton

Copyright © 1988 by Year Book Medical Publishers, Inc. All rights reserved. No part of this publication may be reproduced, stored in a retrieval system, or transmitted, in any form or by any means—electronic, mechanical, photocopying, recording, or otherwise—without prior written permission from the publisher. Printed in the United States of America.

1 2 3 4 5 6 7 8 9 0 R K 92 91 90 89 88

Library of Congress Cataloging-in-Publication Data
Kurtz, Alfred B.
  Obstetrical measurements in ultrasound : A reference manual /
Alfred B. Kurtz, Barry B. Goldberg.
    p. cm.
  Includes bibliographies and index.
  ISBN 0-8151-5222-1
  1. Gestational age—°Nomograms. 2. Fetus—°Nomograms.
3. Ultrasonics in obstetrics. I. Goldberg, Barry B., 1937-   .
II. Title.
  [DNLM: 1. Gestational Age. 2. Ultrasonic Diagnosis—in pregnancy.
WQ 210.5 K96o]
RG613.5.K87   1988   87-34517
618.2'07543—dc19   CIP
DNLM/DLC

Sponsoring Editor: Daniel J. Doody/James D. Ryan, Jr.
Associate Managing Editor, Manuscript Services: Deborah Thorp
Production Project Manager: Gayle Paprocki
Proofroom Supervisor: Shirley E. Taylor

To our families, without whose support and encouragement this book would not have been written.

PREFACE

Ultrasound has been used extensively to analyze the pregnant uterus. To date, hundreds of articles have been published in both the radiologic and obstetrical literature detailing numerous ultrasonically measurable parameters of the uterus and fetus. While many of these articles contain tables with specific numbers, some present their information in only graph or equation form. In this manual, whenever possible, tables with specific numbers will be used. Extrapolation of graphs back to numbers and using equations to calculate the numbers may not be completely accurate and may thus introduce errors.

Ideally, a specific fetal measurement should be regarded as corresponding to a range of gestational ages. Tables giving a single or mean gestational age without a range were thought to be incomplete and therefore were avoided whenever possible. Still other tables gave a range of fetal measurements for each gestational age. This type of table was excluded as impractical, since in everyday practice a specific measurement is obtained and then related to a range of gestational ages. Also, many published tables and graphs do not meet appropriate standards of scientific rigor. The chosen tables were thought to best meet scientific and statistical standards for number of patients, methods of statistical analysis, r^2 and F values, and range of standard deviation.

The tables presented come directly from published articles. The numbers have not been changed but have been reorganized, whenever possible, to obtain a consistent format with the measured variable (in millimeters) on the left, the mean gestational age (in weeks, including tenths of a week) in the middle, and gestational age range, when available, on the right. When known, it will be stated if the mean gestational age is the true statistical number or is "predicted" from an equation.

All fetal dating commences from the woman's last menstrual period. While some articles do not specifically state this, it can be assumed that the last menstrual period is being used, since no other reference point has been proposed. Ideally, the date of conception would be optimal for measurement accuracy, but could be used only in certain specific instances such as in vitro fertilization. Therefore, the last menstrual period, which begins approximately 2 weeks earlier and is not as accurate, is still a clinically useful method of dating the gestation. In patients with optimal menstrual histories, almost 85% of women deliver within 2 weeks.[1] This number decreases to 70% in women with uncertain menstrual dates.[1]

This review divides the pregnancy into the first trimester and the second and third trimesters. In the first trimester, the gestational sac and fetal crown-rump length can be routinely imaged. Specific fetal anatomy, however, cannot be consistently demonstrated. In the second and third trimesters, the fetal head, body, extremities, and internal structures are routinely seen. In addition, the uterine contents, including the amniotic fluid and the placenta, can be more accurately evaluated.

In most sections, after evaluating multiple articles, one was found to be clearly superior and was therefore recommended. Occasionally, two articles had equal validity so that both were recommended. There were instances, however, where one of two problems arose: either a type of measurement was of questionable value, or no article could be established as the best. In these cases, our own judgment had to suffice as to whether a table could be recommended.

Alfred B. Kurtz, M.D.
Barry B. Goldberg, M.D.

REFERENCE

1. Campbell S, Warsof SL, Little D, et al: Routine ultrasound screening for the prediction of gestational age. *Obstet Gynecol* 1985; 65:613–620.

ACKNOWLEDGMENTS

The authors wish to thank the following individuals for their efforts in making this book possible: Mrs. Emily N. Pompetti, Mrs. Joann Gardner, and Ms. Diane Hokans for their assistance in typing the manuscript; Mr. Larry Kradle and Mr. Fred Ross for preparing the illustrations; and Mr. Steven Mervis and Mrs. Phyllis Goldberg for researching the articles.

Alfred B. Kurtz, M.D.
Barry B. Goldberg, M.D.

CONTENTS

Preface   vii

PART I   FIRST TRIMESTER OBSTETRICAL MEASUREMENTS   *1*

1 / Uterine Length   2

2 / Gestational Sac   3

3 / Crown-Rump Length   12

4 / Trunk Circumference   19

PART II   SECOND AND THIRD TRIMESTER OBSTETRICAL MEASUREMENTS   *21*

5 / Fetal Head Measurements   22
   Biparietal Diameter   22
   Unusual Head Shape: Detection and Correction Factors   29
   Head Circumference   32
   Head Area   35
   Head Volume   35
   Ventricular Size   38
   Ocular Dimensions   44
   Orbital Dimensions   45
   The Cerebellar Dimensions   51
   Subarachnoid Cisterns   51

6 / Fetal Body Measurements   63
   Thoracic Diameter   63
   Thoracic Circumference   63
   Thoracic Area   64
   Abdominal Diameter   64
   Abdominal Circumference   66
   Abdominal Area   71
   Body Volume   74
   Total Fetal Volumes   74
   Total Fetal Length   74
   Fetal Body Organ Measurements   77
   Fetal Extremity Measurements   95
   Other Osseous Structures   115
   Soft Tissue Measurements: Arms, Leg, Neck   115

xii *Contents*

7 / Combined Fetal Head and Body Measurements   *125*
  Fetal Measurement Comparisons   125
  Multiple Parameters   137
  Interval Growth   141
  Fetal Weight   146

8 / Uterine Measurements   *181*
  Uterine Volume   181
  Placenta   182
  Amniotic Fluid   187
  Umbilical Cord and Umbilical Vein   190
  The Cervix   193

9 / Mathematical Growth Models   *199*

PART III MULTIPLE GESTATIONS   *201*

10 / Twins   *202*

Index   *211*

PART 1

First Trimester Obstetrical Measurements

Chapter 1

Uterine Length

Articles have been published describing the increase in size of the overall uterine length and the greatest anterior-posterior diameter of the uterine fundus from 6 to 20 gestational weeks.[1-4] The measurements were performed on bistable equipment. Although the exact measurement points were not discussed, in general the uterine length increased from 8.5 cm at 6 weeks to 11 cm at 10 weeks to 13 cm at 12 weeks, while the anterior-posterior diameter increased from 5 cm at 6 weeks to 6 cm at 10 weeks, to 7 cm at 12 weeks.

The articles proposed that these measurements provided an accurate evaluation of the early gestational period with a variation of plus or minus slightly more than 1 week.[4] Two other first trimester measurements, the gestational sac and crown-rump length, however, have been more extensively evaluated and have been shown to have the same or greater accuracy. Uterine size measurements are therefore not necessary. In addition, measurements of the uterus are only an indirect evaluation of the growing fetus and could be very inaccurate if uterine masses are present.

REFERENCES

1. Hellman LF, Kobayashi M, Fillisti L, et al: Growth and development of the human fetus prior to the 20th week of gestation. *Am J Obstet Gynecol* 1969; 103:784–800.
2. Hoffbauer H: The importance of ultrasonic diagnosis in early pregnancy. *Electromedia* 1970; 3:227–230.
3. Piiroinen O: Studies in diagnostic ultrasound. *Acta Obstet Gynecol Scand [Suppl]* 1975; 55:1–60.
4. Jouppila PC: Length and depth of the uterus and the diameter of the gestation sac in normal gravidas during early pregnancy. *Acta Obstet Gynecol Scand* 1971; 50(suppl. 15):29–31.

Chapter 2

Gestational Sac

The gestational sac from 5 to 13 gestational weeks has been evaluated in six articles.[1-6] Five articles used linear measurements, two with actual numbers[2,4] and three in graph form.[1,3,5] The sixth article[6] gave gestational sac volumes in numerical form, with the volume obtained by taking parallel scans at 0.5– to 1– cm intervals. A planimeter was used to calculate the area of each scan, with the areas then added together to obtain a volume. No article adequately stated the landmarks used in measuring the gestational sac. In addition, the linear measurement articles failed to state whether an average diameter or the longest diameter of the gestational sac was used. This is important, since the linear measurement articles do not take into account the potential effect that a distended urinary bladder would have on the shape of the sac, usually changing its shape from round to ovoid or, less commonly, tear-drop (Figs 2–1 to 2–4). Only an average linear or a volume measurement would compensate for this distortion.

The overall accuracy of this method has been studied by one group and found to be approximately ± 1 week.[4] While not substantiated, if correct, it would be slightly better than uterine size but inferior to crown-rump length measurements. The measurement is still valuable, however, particularly in the early part of the first trimester. By transabdominal approach, the gestational sac can be routinely imaged by 5 weeks, while the crown-rump length is frequently not seen until the 7th. Although not completely studied, it seems that endovaginal imaging will permit routine identification of the gestational sac and crown-rump length at least one week earlier (Fig 2–5).

An average linear measurement seems to be as accurate as a volume measurement and is therefore preferable, since it is less cumbersome to obtain. It is recommended that this measurement be performed from inner to inner edge. If the sac is round, only one measurement is needed (see Fig 2–1). If ovoid or tear-drop shaped, three measurements are obtained and averaged (see Figs 2–2 to 2–4). Two of these measurements are taken from the long axis of the uterus, the length and the anteroposterior (AP) dimension perpendicular to the length. By turning into a transaxial projection at the point of the AP dimension, the

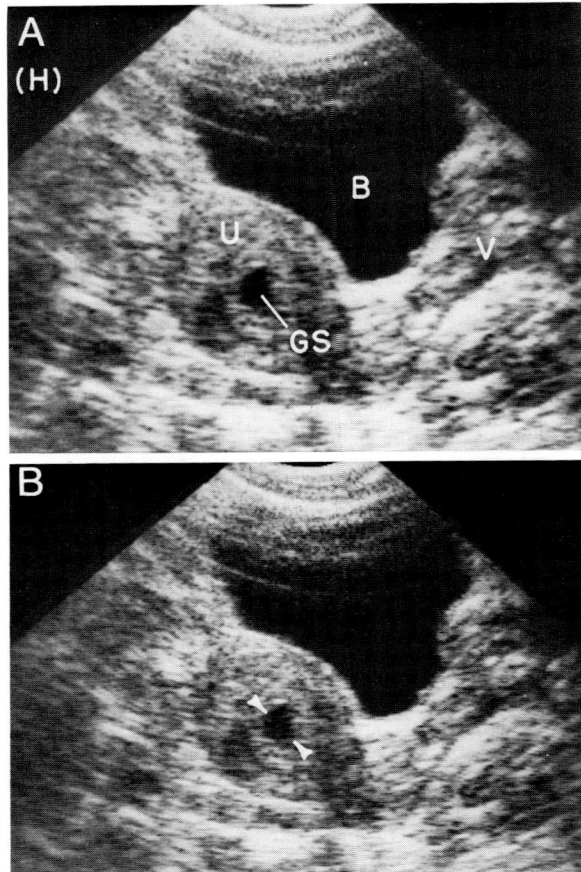

FIG 2–1.
A, long-axis ultrasound image of a round gestational sac *(GS)* within the uterus *(U)* at 5 weeks. Since the sac is round, only one measurement is needed. **B,** same image as **A.** *Arrowheads* denote inner edges of rounded sac to be measured. *V* indicates vagina; *B,* maternal bladder; *(H),* toward patient's head.

width measurement is obtained. It is recommended that the measurements obtained from the endovaginal approach, while oriented differently, be similarly performed (Figs 2–5 and 2–6).

The gestational sac measurement tables will require further evaluation to elevate them to the standards of other obstetrical ultrasound measurements. Nevertheless, we recommend the use of the graph and equation by Hellman and co-workers,[1] since we have had more clinical experience with this article and have found it to be accurate, particularly in evaluating the early gestational sac prior to the imaging of the crown-rump length (Table 2–1). The numbers from this chart are, however, slightly lower than measurements from the other linear charts. On average, at 6 weeks the numbers are 7.5 mm below those of other charts, decreasing to 5 mm below by 8 weeks, and equivalent by 10–12 weeks. No obvious reasons for these discrepancies can be found. While the number of patients included in each study was not routinely provided, one study involved only 25 patients[1] and another only 70 patients.[4] It is, therefore, possible that all of these numbers are within statistical error.

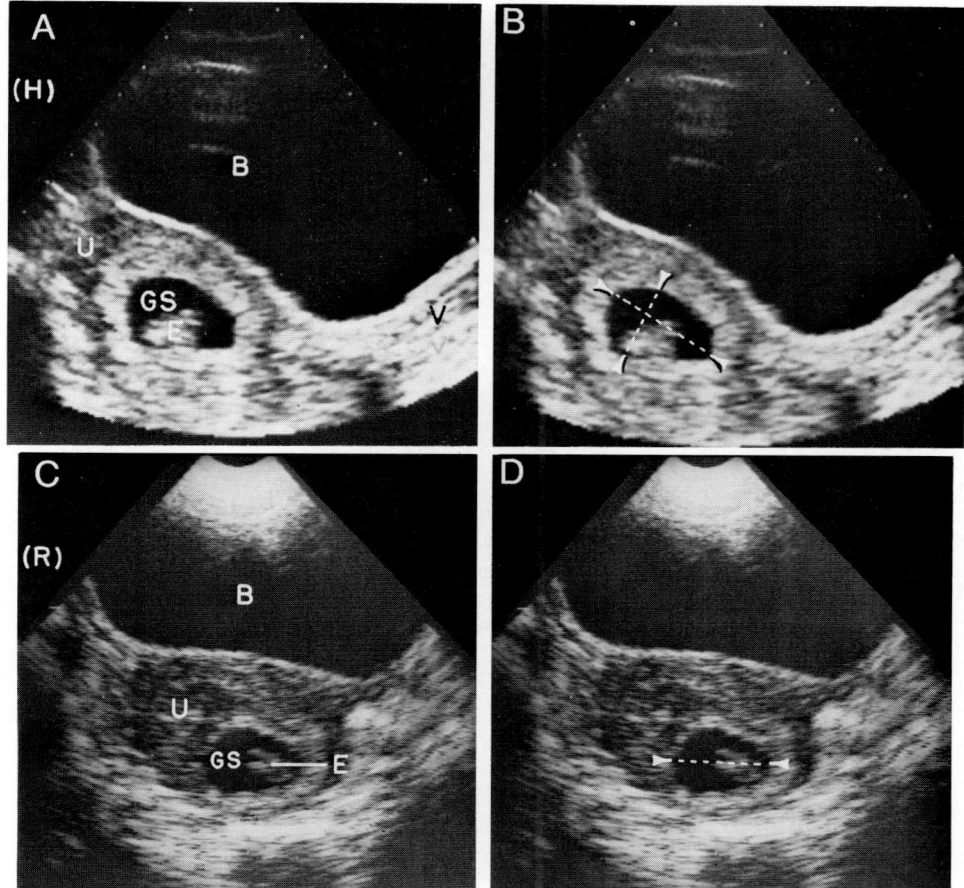

FIG 2–2.
Ultrasound images of an 8-week pregnancy within an ovoid gestational sac *(GS)*. **A,** long-axis scan showing the uterus *(U)* with a living embryo *(E)* within the gestational sac. **B,** same image as **A** showing the length measurement *(arrowheads* and *dotted line* along the long axis of the uterus) and the AP measurement *(arrowheads* and *dotted line* perpendicular to the length). **C,** transaxial scan taken perpendicular to the point at which the AP measurement was obtained. Within the uterus *(U)* is the gestational sac *(GS)* containing the living embryo *(E)*. **D,** same image as **C** showing the width measurement *(arrowheads* and *dotted line)*. B indicates maternal bladder; *V,* vagina; *(H),* toward patient's head; *(R),* toward patient's right.

6 First Trimester Obstetrical Measurements

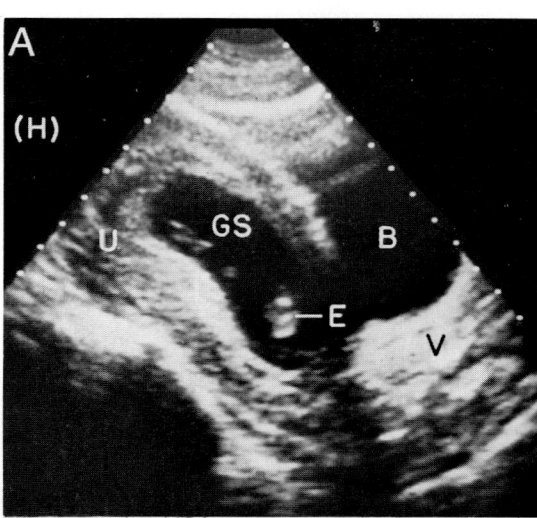

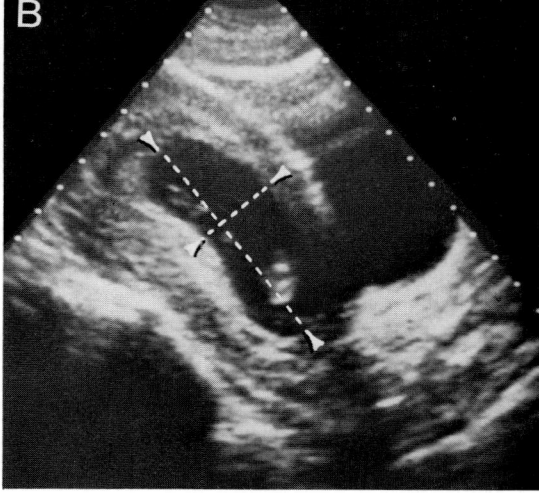

FIG 2–3.
A, long-axis ultrasound image of a 10-week pregnancy showing a markedly ovoid gestational sac *(GS)* within the uterus *(U)*. A partially seen embryo *(E)* is identified. **B,** same image as **A** showing the length and AP (perpendicular to the length) measurements, both denoted by *arrowheads* and *dotted lines*. V indicates vagina; B, maternal bladder; *(H)*, toward patient's head.

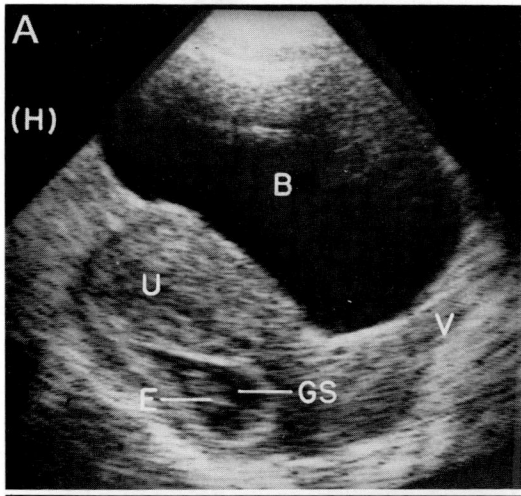
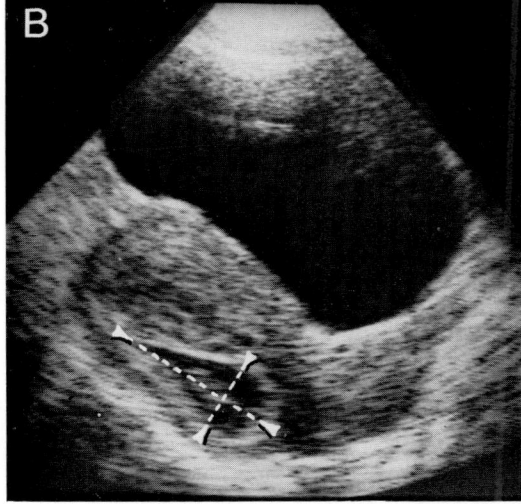

FIG 2–4.
A, long-axis ultrasound image of an 8-week pregnancy showing a tear-drop shaped gestational sac *(GS)* within the uterus *(U)*. B, same image as **A** showing the length and AP (perpendicular to the length) measurements, both denoted by *arrowheads* and *dotted lines*. *V* indicates vagina; *B*, maternal bladder; *E*, embryo; *(H)*, toward patient's head.

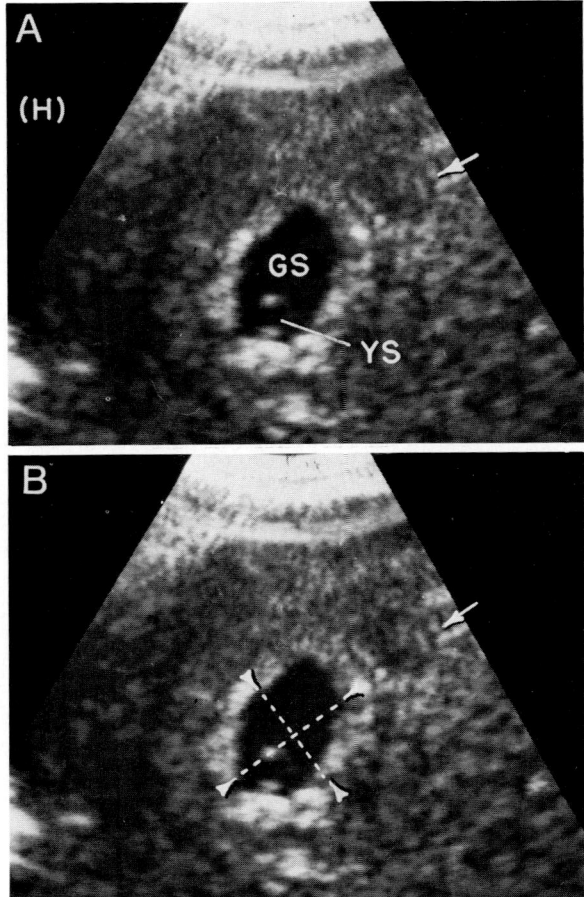

FIG 2–5.
Endovaginal ultrasound. **A,** magnified long-axis image of an anteverted uterus in a less than 5-week pregnancy. The slightly ovoid gestational sac *(GS)* measures less than 8 mm. *YS,* yolk sac. *Arrow* points toward the uterine fundus and denotes endometrial canal. **B,** same image as **A**. The length of the sac (along the same line as the endometrial canal) and the AP diameter (perpendicular to the length) are denoted by *arrowheads* and *dotted lines*. *(H),* toward patient's head.

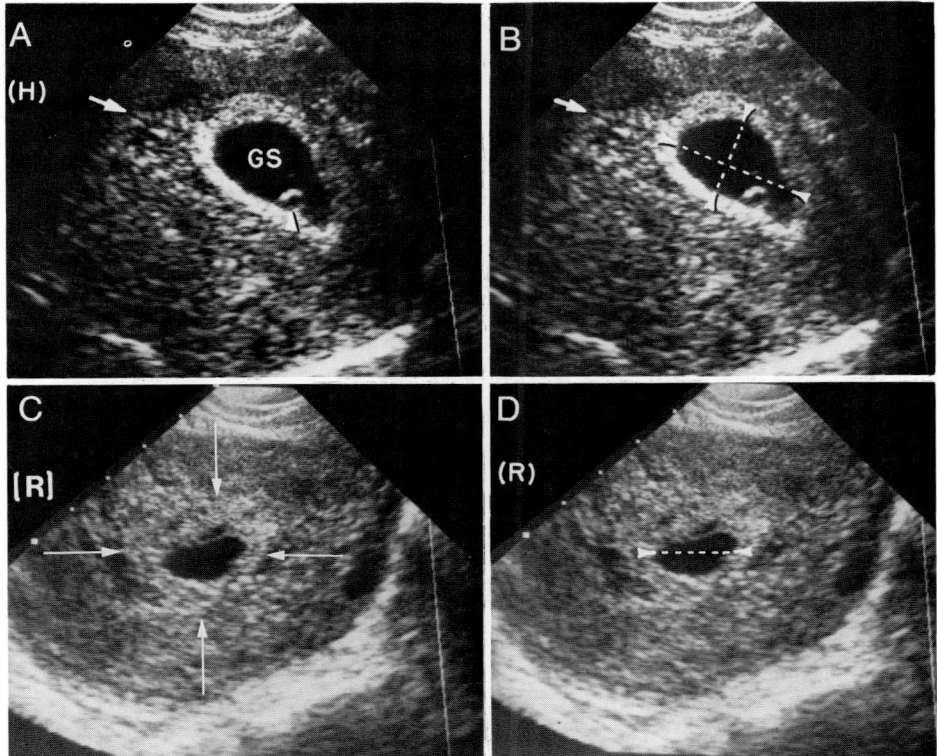

FIG 2–6.
Endovaginal ultrasound of a 6-week pregnancy. **A,** long-axis image of a retroverted uterus showing a tear-drop shaped gestational sac *(GS)*. *Arrow* points from fundus toward cervix and denotes endometrial canal. *Arrowhead,* yolk sac. **B,** same image as **A** showing the length (along the line of the endometrial canal) and AP diameter (perpendicular to the length), both denoted by *arrowheads* and *dotted lines*. **C,** transaxial scan taken perpendicular to the point where the AP measurement was obtained. *Arrows* denote anechoic gestational sac and surrounding normal hyperechoic trophoblastic reaction. **D,** same image as **C** showing the width measurement *(arrowheads* and *dotted line)*. (H) indicates toward patient's head; *(R),* toward patient's right.

TABLE 2–1.
Gestational Sac Measurement Table*

Mean Predicted Gestational Sac, mm	Gestational Age, wk	Mean Predicted Gestational Sac, mm	Gestational Age, wk
10.0	5.0		
11.0	5.2	36.0	8.8
12.0	5.3	37.0	8.9
13.0	5.5	38.0	9.0
14.0	5.6	39.0	9.2
15.0	5.8	40.0	9.3
16.0	5.9	41.0	9.5
17.0	6.0	42.0	9.6
18.0	6.2	43.0	9.7
19.0	6.3	44.0	9.9
20.0	6.5	45.0	10.0
21.0	6.6	46.0	10.2
22.0	6.8	47.0	10.3
23.0	6.9	48.0	10.5
24.0	7.0	49.0	10.6
25.0	7.2	50.0	10.7
26.0	7.3	51.0	10.9
27.0	7.5	52.0	11.0
28.0	7.6	53.0	11.2
29.0	7.8	54.0	11.3
30.0	7.9	55.0	11.5
31.0	8.0	56.0	11.6
32.0	8.2	57.0	11.7
33.0	8.3	58.0	11.9
34.0	8.5	59.0	12.0
35.0	8.6	60.0	12.2

Equation[†]: $\text{Gestational Age (wk)} = \dfrac{\text{Gestational Sac (mm)} + 25.43}{7.02}$

*From Hellman LM, Kobayashi M, Fillisti L, et al: Growth and development of the human fetus prior to the 20th week of gestation. *Am J Obstet Gynecol* 1969; 103:784–800. Used with permission.
†This formula was expressed in centimeters in its original form.

REFERENCES

1. Hellman LF, Kobayashi M, Fillisti L, et al: Growth and development of the human fetus prior to the 20th week of gestation. *Am J Obstet Gynecol* 1969; 103:784–800.
2. Hoffbauer H: The importance of ultrasonic diagnosis in early pregnancy. *Electromedia* 1970; 3:227–230.
3. Piiroinen O: Studies in diagnostic ultrasound. *Acta Obstet Gynecol Scand [Suppl]* 1975; 55:1–60.
4. Jouppila PC: Length and depth of the uterus and the diameter of the gestation sac in normal gravidas during early pregnancy. *Acta Obstet Gynecol Scand* 1971; 50(suppl 15):29–31.
5. Kossoff G, Garrett WJ, Radovanovich G: Grey scale echography in obstetrics and gynaecology. *Austr Radiol* 1974; 18:63–111.
6. Robinson HP: "Gestational sac" volumes as determined by sonar in the first trimester of pregnancy. *Br J Obstet Gynaecol* 1975; 82:100–107.

Chapter 3

Crown-Rump Length

Initial work in 1975 by Robinson[1] described using the longest length of the fetus to evaluate fetal age in the first trimester. The fetal measurements taken from 6 to 14 gestational weeks were compared to the estimated dates of confinement in women with known menstrual histories and in 20 aborted fetuses. A high degree of correlation was found with an error of less than 3 days. This work was expanded by Robinson and Fleming[2] and corroborated by additional examiners.[3-7] Numbers were given in five of the six articles,[2,3,5-7] all showing similar measurements. Robinson and Fleming obtained their measurements with a static scanner, and only the longest axis of the fetus was accepted as the true length.[2] Their smoothed corrected "regression analysis" was initially thought to be most accurate, since it eliminated random errors associated with measurement technique, biologic differences in fetal size, and errors in fetal age.[2]

All of the earlier studies were performed using static scanners.[1-8] Because of the small fetal size and its continual movements during scanning, however, it was found that a high degree of expertise was needed to obtain the longest fetal length during static scanning. To avoid this time-consuming and technically difficult process, one study[9] proposed that multiple static scans in transverse and longitudinal planes be obtained without regard for the lie of the fetus. The authors observed that the "maximum" fetal measurement, even if not the longest length, would be accurate to within 1 week in 75% of fetuses.

More recent studies have found that real-time evaluation[6,7,10-15] is equal in accuracy, easier to perform, and is not affected by the type of real-time scanning array used. Static images could systematically underestimate the size of the fetus, particularly when an inexperienced examiner is performing the examination, while real-time scanning facilitates localization of the fetal long axis and improves reproducibility of measurements. Two of these studies[15,16] suggested that the measurements obtained from real-time evaluation should be analyzed on the Robinson and Fleming curve.[2] They thought that the uncorrected regression analysis rather than the corrected "regression analysis" should be used, since the intercept was closer to 0[15] and the accuracy of fetal dating more accurate.[16] While the differences are small, the uncorrected regression analysis is therefore

TABLE 3–1.
Crown-Rump Length Measurement Table*†

Mean Predicted Crown-Rump Length, mm	Gestational Age, wk	Mean Predicted Crown-Rump Length, mm	Gestational Age, wk
		34.0	10.1
6.7	6.3	35.5	10.3
7.4	6.4	36.9	10.4
8.0	6.6	38.4	10.6
8.7	6.7	39.9	10.7
9.5	6.9	41.4	10.9
10.2	7.0	43.0	11.0
11.0	7.1	44.6	11.1
11.8	7.3	46.2	11.3
12.6	7.4	47.8	11.4
13.5	7.6	49.5	11.6
14.4	7.7	51.2	11.7
15.3	7.9	52.9	11.9
16.3	8.0	54.7	12.0
17.3	8.1	56.5	12.1
18.3	8.3	58.3	12.3
19.3	8.4	60.1	12.4
20.4	8.6	62.0	12.6
21.5	8.7	63.9	12.7
22.6	8.9	65.9	12.9
23.8	9.0	67.8	13.0
25.0	9.1	69.3	13.1
26.2	9.3	71.8	13.3
27.4	9.4	73.9	13.4
28.7	9.6	76.0	13.6
30.0	9.7	78.1	13.7
31.3	9.9	80.2	13.9
32.7	10.0	82.4	14.0

*From Robinson HP, Fleming JEE: A critical evaluation of sonar "crown-rump length" measurements. Br J Obstet Gynaecol 1975; 82:702–710. Used by permission.
†Values derived from "regression analysis."

recommended (Table 3–1). By transabdominal approach, the crown-rump length can be routinely imaged after 7 gestational weeks and occasionally earlier. Initially, the embryo appears as an ill-defined area with heart motion (Fig 3–1). Distinction of the head from the body can be routinely made by 9–10 weeks (Fig 3–2). Although not yet fully studied, endovaginally imaging seems to permit routine embryonic identification at least 1 week earlier (Fig 3–3). All measure-

14 *First Trimester Obstetrical Measurements*

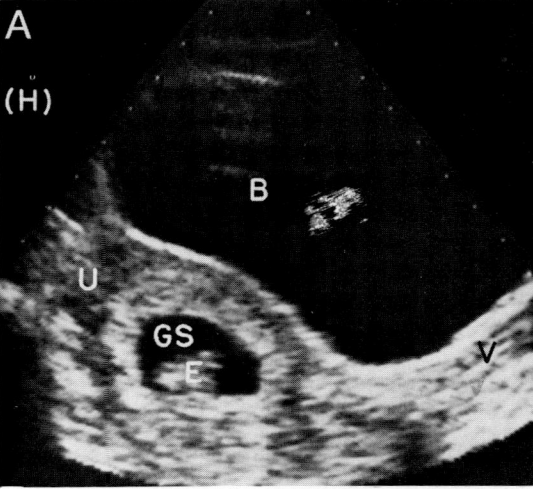

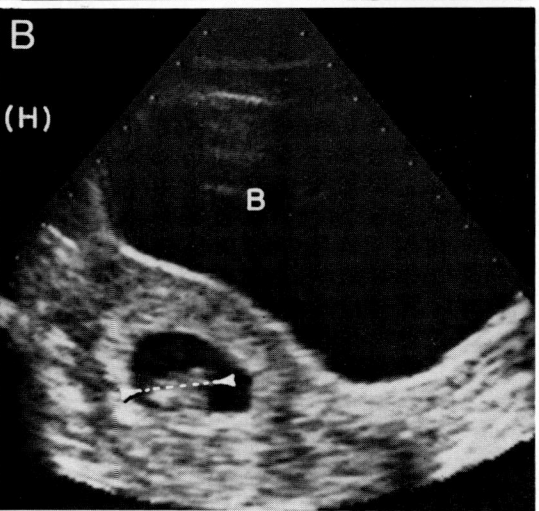

FIG 3–1.
Real-time ultrasound images of a living embryo at 8 gestational weeks. **A,** long-axis scan of the uterus *(U)*. A well-defined gestational sac *(GS)* is identified containing an embryo *(E)*. **B,** same image as **A**. This is the longest axis of this embryo, measured as a crown-rump length *(arrowheads* and *dotted line)*. V indicates vagina; B, maternal bladder; *(H)*, toward patient's head.

ments are obtained along the long axis of the embryo from the top of the head (crown) to the bottom of the trunk (rump).

The accuracy of the crown-rump length measurement has been well studied. Robinson and Fleming[2] found that the error in fetal measurement was ±4.7 days with a 95% probability on the basis of a single measurement. This observation has been corroborated by most other observers, with the accuracy of a crown-rump length measurement found to be ±6 days or to be within 7 to 10 days.[6, 8, 17–20] The observation by Robinson and Fleming[2] that three separate crown-rump length measurements increased its accuracy to ±2.7 days, however, has not been substantiated.

A study evaluated first trimester crown-rump lengths and first trimester biparietal diameters and found both to be accurate to within ±4½ to 5 days.[21] When combined, their accuracy increased to ±3.9 days. The overall combined accuracy, however, is no better, and may be less, than the crown-rump length measurement alone. Therefore, the combination of crown-rump length and biparietal diameter in the first trimester is not recommended.

Studies of different ethnic and racial groups[7, 22] and of different sexes[6, 23] have shown the crown-rump length measurements to be very closely grouped. Only Pedersen[6, 24] thought that an average difference of 2 mm with the male larger than the female was statistically different. The 2–mm difference is, however, within measurement error and probably not significant.

It has been well established that fetuses of diabetic mothers are at increased risk for congenital malformations.[25] This is particularly true in mothers who have had long-standing diabetes with or without additional vascular complications. In these cases, it may be possible to predict which fetuses will be abnormal by evaluating early fetal growth. This has been a preliminary finding in a study by Tchobrovtsky et al.[26] A significant number of fetuses with anomalies, whether from diabetic mothers or not, and fetuses of diabetic mothers without anomalies were smaller than expected in the first trimester. The number of cases in this series is too few to draw definitive conclusions. However, if abnormal first

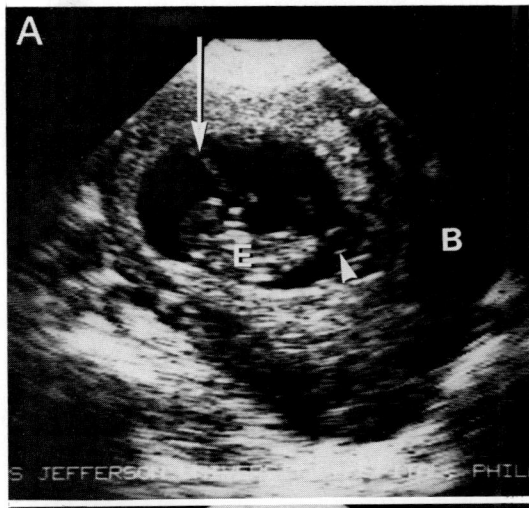
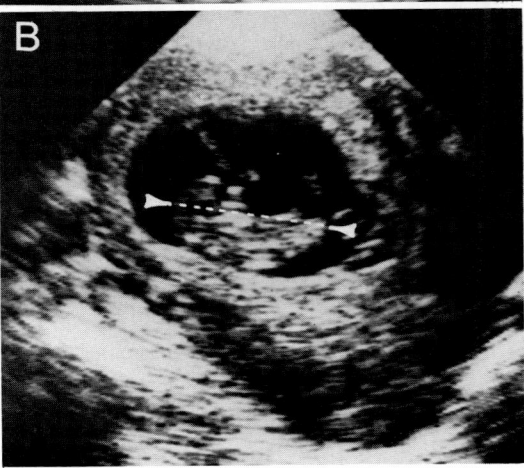

FIG 3–2.
Real-time ultrasound image of a living embryo *(E)* at 10 gestational weeks. **A,** oblique scan showing the long axis of the embryo, yolk sac *(arrowhead)*, and umbilical cord *(arrow)*. Note that the distinction of head and body is now possible with the body, in this case, closer to the yolk sac. **B,** same image as **A** showing the crown-rump length measurement *(arrowheads* and *dotted line)*. B indicates maternal bladder.

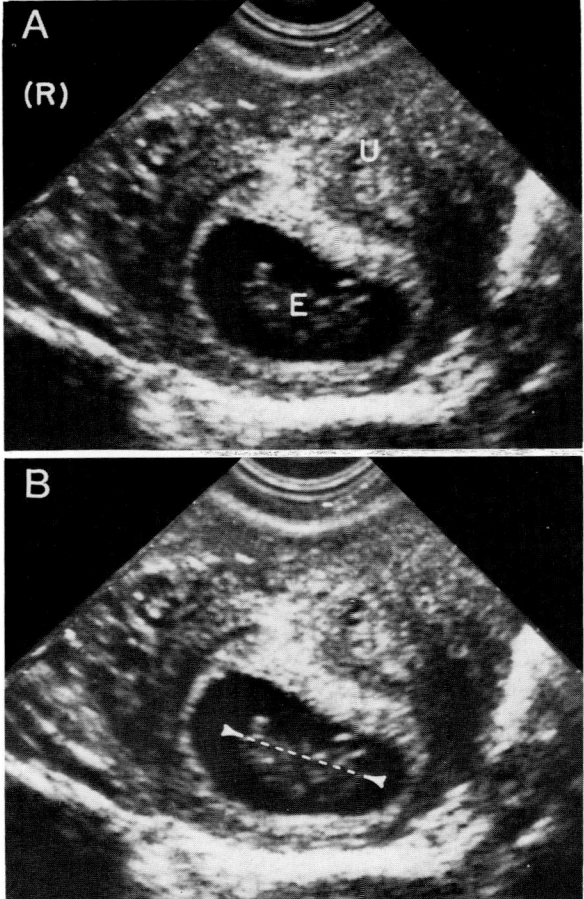

FIG 3–3.
Endovaginal ultrasound transaxial image. **A,** magnified long-axis image of a living embryo *(E)* at 6 weeks. **B,** same image as **A** showing the crown-rump length measurement *(arrowheads* and *dotted line)*. U indicates uterus; *(R),* toward patient's right.

trimester growth could be detected by measuring the crown-rump length, it could become an important clinical tool.

There has been an ongoing debate about whether the crown-rump length or biparietal diameter is a more accurate indicator of fetal age. Drumm[8] found that 100% of fetuses were born within ±10 days by first trimester crown-rump length predictions, while only 82% of fetuses were born within ±12 days by second trimester biparietal diameter predictions. This evaluation was marred by the statement that crown-rump length measurements were obtained on women with both accurate and inaccurate menstrual histories, while biparietal diameter measurements were taken on women with only inaccurate fetal dating. In contradistinction, Berger et al.[27] stated that the crown-rump length was less accurate than the biparietal diameter, with variations of ±3 and ±2 weeks, respectively. Campbell et al.[28] also found a second trimester biparietal diameter, taken between 12 and 18 weeks, to be statistically more accurate than a crown-rump length measurement in predicting date of confinement to within ±2 weeks,

89.4% to 84.6%, respectively ($p<.001$). Two recent articles[17,18] have shown that the crown-rump length in the first trimester and a biparietal diameter at 20 to 24 weeks (in the late second trimester) to be equally accurate in the prediction of gestational age, with equal numbers of overestimations and underestimations. These two articles found both measurements to be accurate to within ± 5 to 7 days, both as accurate as an accurate menstrual history. Since a first trimester crown-rump length and a second trimester biparietal diameter up to 24 weeks are equally accurate, it is recommended that a crown-rump length be used until 11 to 12 weeks. After that time, the fetus is more likely to flex and extend, thus making the crown-rump length less accurate, so that the second trimester biparietal diameter should be used instead.

REFERENCES

1. Robinson HP: Sonar measurement of fetal crown-rump length as means of assessing maturity of first trimester of pregnancy. *Br Med J* 1973; 4:28–31.
2. Robinson HP, Fleming JEE: A critical evaluation of sonar "crown-rump length" measurements. *Br J Obstet Gynaecol* 1975; 82:702–710.
3. Drumm JE, Clinch J, MacKenzie G: The ultrasonic measurement of fetal crown-rump length as a method of assessing gestational age. *Br J Obstet Gynaecol* 1976; 83:417–421.
4. Kurjak A, Cecuk S, Breyer B: Prediction of maturity in first trimester of pregnancy by ultrasonic measurement of fetal crown-rump length. *J Clin Ultrasound* 1976; 4:83–84.
5. Hoffbauer H, Pachaly J, Arabin B, et al: Control of fetal development with multiple ultrasonic body measures. *Contrib Gynecol Obstet* 1979; 6:147–156.
6. Pedersen JF: Fetal crown-rump length measurement by ultrasound in normal pregnancy. *Br J Obstet Gynaecol* 1982; 89:926–930.
7. Parker AJ: Assessment of gestational age of the Asian fetus by the sonar measurement of crown-rump length and biparietal diameter. *Br J Obstet Gynaecol* 1982; 89:836–838.
8. Drumm JE: The prediction of delivery date by ultrasonic measurement of fetal crown-rump length. *Br J Obstet Gynaecol* 1977; 84:1–5.
9. Higginbottom J, Slater J, Porter G: Assessment of gestational age in the first trimester of pregnancy by maximum fetal diameter. *Ultrasound Med Biol* 1977; 3:47–51.
10. Parker AJ, Docker MF, Davies P, et al: The reproducibility of fetal crown rump length measurements obtained with real time ultrasound systems compared with those of a conventional B-scanner. *Br J Obstet Gynaecol* 1981; 88:734–738.
11. Sande HA, Reiertsen O: Crown rump length: A comparison of real time scanning and conventional compound scanning the interindividual measuring variation between two operators. *Ultrasound Med Biol* 1979; 5:279–281.
12. Adam AH, Robinson HP, Dunlop C: A comparison of crown-rump length measurements using a real-time scanner in an antenatal clinic and a conventional B-scanner. *Br J Obstet Gynaecol* 1979; 86:521–524.
13. Deter RL, Harrist RB, Hadlock FP, et al: Longitudinal studies of fetal growth with the use of dynamic image ultrasonography. *Am J Obstet Gynecol* 1982; 143:545–554.
14. Deter RL, Harrist RB, Hadlock FP, et al: The use of ultrasound in the assessment of normal fetal growth: A review. *J Clin Ultrasound* 1981; 9:481–493.
15. Nelson LH: Comparison of methods for determining crown-rump measurement by real-time ultrasound. *J Clin Ultrasound* 1981; 9:67–70.

16. Chervenak FA, Brightman RC, Thornton J, et al: Crown-rump length and serum human chorionic gonadotropin as predictors of gestational age. *Obstet Gynecol* 1986; 67:210–213.
17. Smazal SF, Weisman LE, Hoppler KD, et al: Comparative analysis of ultrasonographic methods of gestational age assessment. *J Ultrasound Med* 1983; 2:147–150.
18. Kopta MM, May RR, Crane JP: A comparison of the reliability of the estimated date of confinement predicted by crown-rump length and biparietal diameter. *Am J Obstet Gynecol* 1983; 145:562–565.
19. Selbing A, Fjallbrant B: Accuracy of conceptual age estimation from fetal crown-rump length. *J Clin Ultrasound* 1984; 12:343–346.
20. van de Velde EHE, Broeders GHB, Horbach JGM, et al: Estimation of pregnancy duration by means of ultrasonic measurements of the fetal crown-rump length. *Eur J Obstet Gynecol Reprod Biol* 1980; 10:225–230.
21. Bovicelli L, Orsini LF, Rizzo N, et al: Estimation of gestational age during the first trimester by real-time measurement of fetal crown-rump length and biparietal diameter. *J Clin Ultrasound* 1981; 9:71–75.
22. Selbing A: Ultrasound in first trimester shows no difference in fetal size between the sexes. *Br Med J* 1985; 290:750.
23. Dubowitz LMS, Goldberg C: Assessment of gestation by ultrasound in various stages of pregnancy in infants differing in size and ethnic origin. *Br J Obstet Gynaecol* 1981; 88:255–259.
24. Pedersen JF; Ultrasound evidence of sexual difference in fetal size in first trimester. *Br Med J* 1980; 281:1253.
25. Pedersen LM, Tygstrup I, Pedersen J: Congenital malformations in newborn infants of diabetic women. *Lancet* 1964; 1:1124–1126.
26. Tchobrovtsky C, Breart GL, Rambaud DC, et al: Correlation between fetal defects and early growth delay observed by ultrasound. *Lancet* 1985; 1:706–707.
27. Berger GS, Edelman DA, Kerenyi TD: Fetal crown-rump length and biparietal diameter in the second trimester of pregnancy. *Am J Obstet Gynecol* 1975; 122:9–12.
28. Campbell, S, Warsof SL, Little D, et al: Routine ultrasound screening for the prediction of gestational age. *Obstet Gynecol* 1985; 65:613–620.

Chapter 4

Trunk Circumference

Recently Reece et al.[1] measured the circumference of the fetal trunk from 7 to 12 weeks in both number and graph form using real-time ultrasound. The trunk circumference was obtained from the transaxial image at a point just caudad to the cardiac pulsation by taking the average abdominal diameter $\times$ π. Comparison was then made to crown-rump lengths obtained in the same study. Both were similar in their prediction of gestational age. When combined, the accuracy did not increase. Therefore, while this is a new and interesting first trimester measurement, the much more thoroughly studied crown-rump length is still recommended.

REFERENCE

1. Reece EA, Scioscia AL, Green J, et al: Embryonic trunk circumference: A new biometric parametric for estimation of gestational age. *Am J Obstet Gynecol* 1987; 156:713–715.

PART 2

Second and Third Trimester Obstetrical Measurements

Chapter 5

Fetal Head Measurements

BIPARIETAL DIAMETER

The biparietal diameter is one of the most discussed and documented obstetrical ultrasound measurements. Starting as far back as 1964, in utero biparietal diameters were compared to caliper measurements of the newborn head. Similar results were obtained.[1-7] These studies were performed using A-mode alone,[1-4] a combination of A-mode and bistable B-mode,[5,6] and gray scale B-mode alone.[7] While there were slight discrepancies, all modalities showed equal accuracy, with no method superior. In general, more than 90% of the cases were only ±2 mm apart, with some variations approaching 4 to 5 mm. Ultrasound and caliper measurements of the heads of aborted fetuses were also compared and found to be less than 3 mm different.[8] There were inherent errors, however, in scanning aborted fetuses, including the collapse of the fetal skull.

Despite the close correlation of fetal to newborn head measurements, inaccuracies exist between in utero ultrasound studies. These inaccuracies can be subdivided into those created by inability of observers to measure consistently, errors caused by failure to image the head in the correct anatomical plane, and errors in instrumentation. Several articles have discussed the observers' inability to measure consistently.[5,9-14] These studies were performed using A-mode, a combination of A-mode and bistable B-mode, and gray-scale B-mode including real-time. The smallest measurement error found in any series was by Campbell[5] where a standard deviation (SD) of ±0.25 mm was obtained between scans. This is surprisingly low. Cooperberg et al.[13] showed an SD of ±0.69–0.91 mm. The remainder of the SDs were higher, errors approaching 2% per reading,[12] and ultrasound "experts" having a smaller error than trainees.[14] The two best controlled studies[9,10] found that paired readings (two readings 15 minutes apart) had an average error of 1.53 mm. When three biparietal diameter readings were taken during any one examination, a SD of ±1.21 mm was obtained. If the measurements were taken either 24 hours or 4 weeks apart, the SD increased to ±2.54 mm. Real-time ultrasound equipment was determined to be easier to use and as accurate as static scanners.[11,13] When a single observer performed all the measurements, accuracy seemed better than when measurements were performed by different observers.[10,11] From these articles it can be appreciated that an error is introduced every time a measurement is taken. While this error is minimized if the observer is skilled, and also if the same observer performs

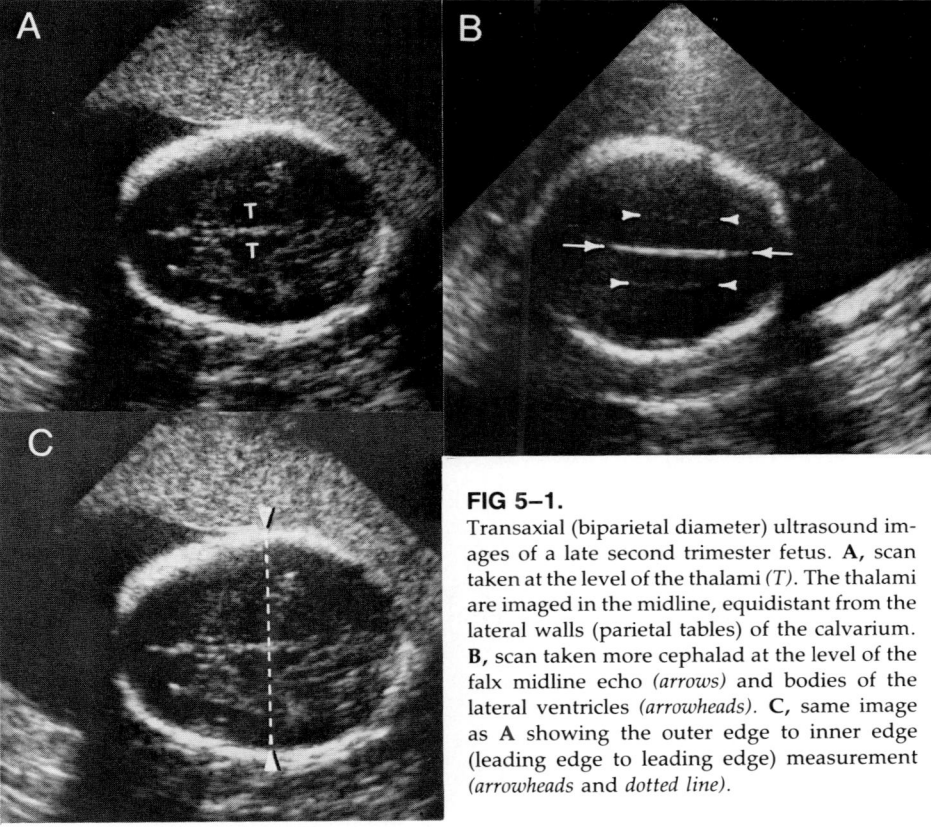

FIG 5–1.
Transaxial (biparietal diameter) ultrasound images of a late second trimester fetus. **A,** scan taken at the level of the thalami *(T)*. The thalami are imaged in the midline, equidistant from the lateral walls (parietal tables) of the calvarium. **B,** scan taken more cephalad at the level of the falx midline echo *(arrows)* and bodies of the lateral ventricles *(arrowheads)*. **C,** same image as **A** showing the outer edge to inner edge (leading edge to leading edge) measurement *(arrowheads* and *dotted line).*

all of the measurements, an error of as little as 1 mm and as much as 2 mm occurs with each examination. When interval measurements are taken, the error could double and approach 4 mm.

Technical factors involved in measuring the fetal head in the correct anatomical plane were also evaluated with static and real-time equipment. Using both A-mode and B-mode on aborted fetuses, Watmough et al.[15] showed that the imaging of a midline echo alone was not sufficient to obtain an accurate biparietal diameter measurement. Instead they showed that scanning at various angles, even if a midline echo was still imaged, caused the biparietal diameter to vary by as much as 19 mm. Therefore, Johnson et al.,[16] using gray-scale equipment, recommended that transaxial scans (biparietal diameters) be performed at the thalamus at the level of the thalamobasal ganglia (Fig 5–1,A). If scans were taken at a slightly more cephalad level, at the bodies of the lateral ventricles, the biparietal diameters were found to be smaller on an average of 3 mm, with a range of 0 to 9 mm (Fig 5–1,B). Shepard and Filly[17] further refined the anatomical positions at the thalamus and brain stem to take the optimum biparietal diameter measurements. They found that an image taken at either the level of the third ventricle with the quadrigeminal cisterns or at the top third ventricle (with visualization of the cavum septi pellucidi) were highly consistent, with correlation coefficients to the maternal age of greater than .99 (Fig 5–2).

Similarly, Hadlock et al.[18] found that the maximum measurements of biparietal diameter, fronto-occipital diameter, and head circumference all should be obtained at the same level, at the level of the thalamus and the cavum septi pellucidi. More cephalad images decreased the biparietal diameter measurement from 0 to 9 mm, while more caudad images gave a decreased measurement of 0 to 10 mm.

Errors in instrumentation include the machine calibration for velocity of sound, the amplification settings (power or gain), and the type of B-mode ultrasound imager; i.e., bistable or gray-scale, static or real-time. The calibrated velocity of sound to which the machine is set varies in different countries. It

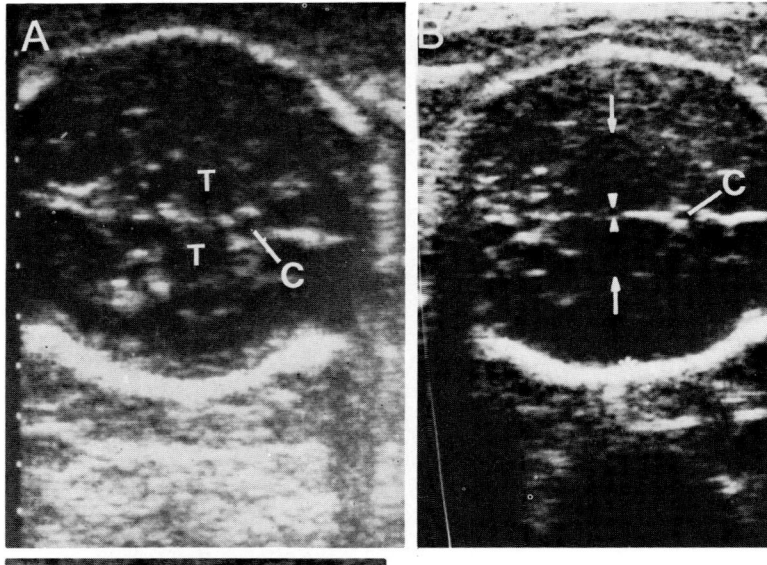

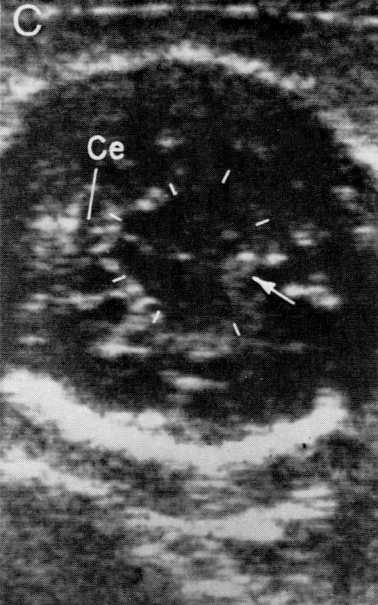

FIG 5–2.
Transaxial (biparietal diameter) ultrasound images of a mid–third trimester fetus. These three levels are all acceptable for obtaining a correct measurement, provided that the thalami or midbrain structures are imaged equidistant from the lateral walls (parietal tables) of the calvarium. **A,** at the level of the upper thalami *(T)*. **B,** at the level of the mid to lower thalami *(arrows)*. Arrowheads indicate slitlike third ventricle. **C,** at the level of the midbrain *(lines)*. Note the heart- or arrow-shaped appearance, with point aimed posteriorly toward the cerebellum *(Ce)*. *Arrow* indicates anterior surface of midbrain; C, cavum septi pellucidi.

can be corrected by a simple ratio of that velocity divided by the standard (1,540 m/sec) used in most countries, including the United States and Canada. The machine amplification settings are also important.[19] As the amplification is increased, the calvarial echoes artifactually widen, increasing from 1 to 2 mm at low settings, to 3 to 5 mm at medium settings, to 6 to 10 mm at high settings. This is of particular importance if outer to outer biparietal diameter measurements are used, since the widening of both calvarial echoes will increase the measurement. Most tables, however, use outer to inner measurements (leading edge to leading edge) which avoids this error (see Figs 5–1,A and C). Nevertheless, medium amplification settings are still recommended, since it is difficult to find the exact points to measure when high amplification is used, and the medium amplification settings correlated best with the true biparietal diameter measurements of neonates.[19] Last, the evaluation of different types of ultrasound imagers, B-mode, bistable or gray-scale, static or real-time, has been studied.[11, 13, 19] All have been found to be equally accurate. It is recommended, however, that real-time gray-scale B-mode equipment be used because of the ability of even inexperienced observers to obtain accurate reproducible results, comparable to those of the expert examiner.[11]

The accuracy of biparietal diameter measurements in predicting gestational age continues to be of major importance. While it had been stated that a crown-rump length measurement obtained from 7 to 13 weeks was the most accurate for establishing fetal age,[20] recent articles have shown that the biparietal diameter measurement between 20 and 24 weeks has comparable accuracy.[21–23] Therefore, the first and second trimester measurements taken from an early crown-rump length at 7 weeks to a biparietal diameter at 24 weeks are of equal accuracy, equivalent to ± 5 to 7 days with close correlation to maternal dating when accurate menstrual history is known.[22, 23] Campbell[24] and Sabbagha et al.[25] even thought that this accuracy could be extended to 30 gestational weeks.

Later on in the pregnancy, in the third trimester, the biparietal diameter becomes more inaccurate in predicting gestational age. Some observers have stated that these inaccuracies approach $\pm 3-3^{1}/_{2}$ weeks at term.[17, 26, 27] If these stated inaccuracies at term are correct, potential errors would be quite extensive, resulting in an equal probability that a fetus at 37 weeks could be either 34 or 40 weeks. This observation of inaccuracy at term is not currently substantiated by all observers. In an article by Weiner et al.[28] the SD of the biparietal diameter was evaluated from 15 weeks to term in 6 works (five previous articles and their own). In two of these studies, the SD increased toward term. In two others, however, the SD did not significantly increase, and in the last two, the SD significantly decreased toward term. Similarly, another article showed that while the biparietal diameter variation was greater in the third trimester, a variation of only ± 2 weeks was observed up to 33 weeks.[22] Although not exactly comparable, this variation of ± 2 weeks continued to term when a range of 90% of the average measurements was compared in 17 tables.[29] In addition, despite all these reported inaccuracies in the use of the biparietal diameter, two articles analyzing multiple fetal parameters in the second and third trimesters found that the head measurements, and in particular the biparietal diameter, were the most reliable indicators of gestational age.[30, 31]

To date, there have been 60 published comparisons of biparietal diameter to gestational age. Of these, 31 compared a single biparietal diameter measurement in millimeters to a single gestational age in weeks.[12, 26, 32–60] (Two of these presented only graphs in their original articles, i.e., Hellman et al.[32] and Garrett and Robinson,[52] with the numbers subsequently published by Kurtz et al.[29]). An additional article by Wladimiroff et al.[38] presented a graph that appeared identical to the graph that accompanied the numbers by Wladimiroff et al.[37] and therefore will not be discussed further.

Of the 30 remaining articles,[12, 26, 32–37, 39–60] all the articles showed an increase in the biparietal diameter as the gestation progressed toward term (17 of these studies are shown in Figure 1 of reference 29). Twenty-six evaluated the second and third trimesters, with two[33, 34] analyzing only the second trimester and two[42, 43] evaluating only the third. There was an equal distribution of the biparietal diameter, evaluated by A-mode, B-mode, or a combination of the two. The calculated velocity of the sound of the ultrasound machine was known in 26 and not discussed in the other four.[48–50, 57] The outer to inner diameter was used to measure the fetal head in 25 articles, and the outer to outer diameter used in only four,[33, 35, 41, 52] with no discussion of where the measurements were taken in one.[57]

Twenty-four of the 60 articles compared the biparietal diameter to gestational age in graph form.[3, 8, 24, 25, 31, 61–79] Seventeen of these 24 studies evaluated the biparietal diameter in both the second and third trimesters, with the other 7 analyzing the third trimester only. While it is difficult to accurately extrapolate curves back to their original numbers and to compare these numbers to the previous 30 articles in table form, 17 of the graphs were within the range of these 30 articles, 5 were consistently high,[3, 24, 31, 64, 65] and 2 were consistently low.[63, 73]

Four of the above articles in graph form evaluated pregnant diabetic women.[71–74] Two of these,[71, 72] while not specifically stating the severity of the diabetes, found no difference in biparietal diameter growth throughout the second and third trimesters. The other two articles,[73, 74] one evaluating class A to C diabetes and the other class A to D diabetes, found no difference in biparietal diameter growth from 13 to 38 weeks. After that time, the biparietal diameter was observed to increase more than the normal nondiabetic group.

At least part of the variation in biparietal diameter measurements is due to biologic growth that occurs normally in any single population group.[80] Studies on different ethnic and racial groups and between the sexes are limited, but in general do not show marked differences. Two studies suggested that female fetuses were only slightly smaller than male fetuses, with the difference increasing toward term both in biparietal diameter[77, 81] and in head circumference.[77] While most of the information was in graph form, numbers given at 36 weeks for males and females revealed a minimal difference, with overlap in biparietal diameter measurements of 90.6 mm ± 3.1 mm vs. 88.2 mm ± 4.0 mm, respectively.[77] Ethnic and racial studies have shown varied results. Four studies found no significant difference in head size either of black vs. white fetuses[58] or of mixed groups,[82–84] although Dubowitz and Goldberg[83] and Okupe et al.[85] did show a slight shift of blacks toward the upper end of the normal curve after 34 and 38 weeks, respectively. Munoz et al.[86] showed the reverse, a decrease in biparietal diameter of blacks (Zulus) after 34 weeks when compared to whites. This study is suspect, however, since the authors failed to take into account fetal head shape, even though the newborn head circumference and birth weight of both groups were similar. Others have found small differences. Walton[78] compared Polynesian to Caucasian fetuses in New Zealand and found a slight but consistent difference. On average, the Polynesian biparietal diameters measured 1.89 mm greater throughout the second and third trimester. Osefo and Chukedebelu[56] compared biparietal diameter measurements of Nigerian fetuses to measurements from previous articles and found them to have, on average, 4 mm smaller biparietal diameters from 20 weeks to term. While more work is clearly needed in this area, it is surprising how close the biparietal diameter measurements are in different racial and ethnic groups.

A newer approach to correlating biparietal diameter with gestational age has been proposed. Because of the variations outlined above, it would be unlikely that a specific biparietal diameter could ever be anticipated to equal a specific gestational age. Rather, a biparietal diameter number would be expected to encompass a range of gestational ages. Although the midpoint would be slightly more probable, the fetus would be equally likely to be anywhere within that range. This has been termed a range table where a biparietal diameter represents a range in days or weeks. This type of study was performed in the remaining 5 of the 60 articles.[17, 23, 28, 29, 87] Of these, Kurtz et al.[29] is a compilation of 17 previous articles comprising greater than 10,000 patients and 27,000 measurements. This table evaluated the average numbers from other tables and included 90% of their variation. The other four range tables used much smaller numbers and were compiled in their home institutions. One of these, Kopta et al.,[23] did not state their confidence limits, while the other three used limits of 95% in two series,[17, 28] and 66% in one series.[87]

In comparing these range tables, the range would be expected to be narrower in the table with the larger number of measurements. The Kurtz et al. table[29] therefore should have the narrowest range. This was found to be true with all except the comparison to the Kopta et al. article[23] between 40 and 80 mm in diameters. Since the confidence limits were not shown on this latter table, it is difficult to make an adequate evaluation. In addition, the ranges of two of the other three tables did not entirely overlap. While Shepard and Filly's[17] upper limits were always outside those of Kurtz et al. (as would be expected, since fewer measurements were used), their lower limits were slightly above those of Kurtz et al.[29] from a BPD of 46 to 88. Similarly, while the Sabbagha range table[87] had a larger range, the range was uniformly lower from 85 mm to term. Despite these discrepancies, it is thought that the Kurtz et al. range table should be used when comparing biparietal diameter to gestational age (Table 5–1). In addition to the range, the average number of weeks was calculated from the equation and is also included for each biparietal diameter measurement.

The most frequent use of the biparietal diameter measurement is in gestational age estimation. The biparietal diameter can also be used to evaluate whether the head is too large or too small. If another fetal measurement (independent of the biparietal diameter) or the last menstrual period is known, the head can be established as normal, large, or small for gestational age. When fetal head enlargement is present, it is almost always secondary to hydrocephalus. This is a relatively straightforward diagnosis, since dilated lateral ventricles can be easily imaged in utero. A small fetal head, termed microcephaly, however, is a much more complicated topic and will be discussed under ratios of the head and body.

TABLE 5–1.
Composite Biparietal Diameter Table*

Biparietal Diameter, mm	Gestational Age, wk		Biparietal Diameter, mm	Gestational Age, wk	
	Mean†	Range, 90% Variation‡		Mean†	Range, 90% Variation‡
20	12.0	12.0			
21	12.0	12.0	61	24.2	22.6–25.8
22	12.7	12.2–13.2	62	24.6	23.1–26.1
23	13.0	12.4–13.6	63	24.9	23.4–26.4
24	13.2	12.6–13.8	64	25.3	23.8–26.8
25	13.5	12.9–14.1	65	25.6	24.1–27.1
26	13.7	13.1–14.3	66	26.0	24.5–27.5
27	14.0	13.4–14.6	67	26.4	25.0–27.8
28	14.3	13.6–15.0	68	26.7	25.3–28.1
29	14.5	13.9–15.2	69	27.1	25.8–28.4
30	14.8	14.1–15.5	70	27.5	26.3–28.7
31	15.1	14.3–15.9	71	27.9	26.7–29.1
32	15.3	14.5–16.1	72	28.3	27.2–29.4
33	15.6	14.7–16.5	73	28.7	27.6–29.8
34	15.9	15.0–16.8	74	29.1	28.1–30.1
35	16.2	15.2–17.2	75	29.5	28.5–30.5
36	16.4	15.4–17.4	76	30.0	29.0–31.0
37	16.7	15.6–17.8	77	30.3	29.2–31.4
38	17.0	15.9–18.1	78	30.8	29.6–32.0
39	17.3	16.1–18.5	79	31.1	29.9–32.5
40	17.6	16.4–18.8	80	31.6	30.2–33.0
41	17.9	16.5–19.3	81	32.1	30.7–33.5
42	18.1	16.6–19.8	82	32.6	31.2–34.0
43	18.4	16.8–20.2	83	33.0	31.5–34.5
44	18.8	16.9–20.7	84	33.4	31.9–35.1
45	19.1	17.0–21.2	85	34.0	32.3–35.7
46	19.4	17.4–21.4	86	34.3	32.8–36.2
47	19.7	17.8–21.6	87	35.0	33.4–36.6
48	20.0	18.2–21.8	88	35.4	33.9–37.1
49	20.3	18.6–22.0	89	36.1	34.6–37.6
50	20.6	19.0–22.2	90	36.6	35.1–38.1
51	20.9	19.3–22.5	91	37.2	35.9–38.5
52	21.2	19.5–22.9	92	37.8	36.7–38.9
53	21.5	19.8–23.2	93	38.8	37.3–39.3
54	21.9	20.1–23.7	94	39.0	37.9–40.1
55	22.2	20.4–24.0	95	39.7	38.5–40.9
56	22.5	20.7–24.3	96	40.6	39.1–41.5
57	22.8	21.1–24.5	97	41.0	39.9–42.1
58	23.2	21.5–24.9	98	41.8	40.5–43.1
59	23.5	21.9–25.1			
60	23.8	22.3–25.5			

*From Kurtz AB, Wapner RJ, Kurtz RJ, et al: Analysis of biparietal diameter as an accurate indicator of gestational age. J Clin Ultrasound 1980; 8:319–326. Used by permission.
†From weighted least mean square fit equation: $Y = -3.45701 + 0.50157x - 0.00441x^2$.
‡For each biparietal diameter, 90% of gestational age data points fell within this range.

UNUSUAL HEAD SHAPE: DETECTION AND CORRECTION FACTORS

The following are measurements used to evaluate and correct unusual head shapes: fronto-occipital diameter, cephalic index, "corrected" biparietal diameter

The distance from the frontal to the occipital bone, termed the fronto-occipital diameter (FOD), is another measurement of the fetal head. It is measured in transaxial view, on the same image that is used to obtain the biparietal diameter.[88] Nine articles have been published comparing the fronto-occipital diameter to the biparietal diameter,[89-97] with one additional article comparing the fronto-occipital diameter to menstrual age.[98] Since this latter article did not compare the FOD to the biparietal diameter, it will not be discussed further. Of the remaining nine, 5 were performed on static scanners, 3 giving actual numbers,[90, 91, 97] with the other 2 in graph form.[89, 93] The other 4 were obtained with real-time images, all giving numbers.[92, 94-96] While one article evaluated the fronto-occipital diameter only in the second trimester,[93] the others evaluated it in both the second and third trimesters. There are two shortcomings to these articles: 1. Although the articles described whether the biparietal diameter was obtained by an outer-to-outer or outer-to-inner measurement, only three articles stated where to measure the fronto-occipital diameter, one using outer-to-outer measurements,[91] one outer-to-inner,[96] and the other middle-to-middle.[95] 2. Only three articles[91, 92, 96] described the internal head landmarks used to define the plane of section necessary to obtain these measurements, with one[91] using a plane of section at the level of the falx echo, slightly higher than the accepted level of the thalamus to obtain the measurements.

Despite these shortcomings, the main reason for obtaining the fronto-occipital measurement is to determine if the fetal head is correctly shaped. If it is, then a biparietal diameter is a valid measurement. If not, then another measurement of the fetal head should be substituted. The correct transaxial head shape can be computed from the biparietal diameter (BPD) and the fronto-occipital diameter (FOD) by using the formula called the cephalic index (CI) (Table 5–2). An equally useful reason for obtaining the fronto-occipital diameter is that the BPD and FOD can be used to calculate the "corrected" biparietal diameter (discussed in this section) and the head circumference (discussed in the next section).

This cephalic index has been previously employed to evaluate the shape of the newborn head. In transaxial view, the head is usually ovoid. However, on occasion, it may be more rounded ("brachycephaly") or more elongated ("dolichocephaly" or "scaphocephaly"). *Dorland's Illustrated Medical Dictionary* defines a normal cephalic index as being between 75.9 and 81.[99] When the CI is below 75.9, the head is dolichocephalic. When the CI is greater than 81, the head is brachycephalic. Two studies on neonates using direct caliper measurements, one after cesarean section and the other two days after vaginal delivery, revealed comparable numbers with a normal mean CI of 80 and a range of 75.6 to 85.0 at ±2 SD.[100, 101] The CI from radiographic evaluation of infants less than 4 weeks of age was somewhat higher, however, with a mean of 81.5 and a range of 79.4 to 85.7,[102] a finding attributed by the author to radiographic distortion of the breadth more than the length measurement.

TABLE 5–2.
Cephalic Index Formula*†

$$\text{Cephalic index} = \frac{\text{short axis (biparietal diameter)}}{\text{long axis (fronto-occipital diameter)}} \times 100 = 78.3$$

Normal range
 At 1 SD = 74 to 83
 At 2 SD = 70 to 86

*Data from Hadlock FP, Deter RL, Carpenter RJ, et al: Estimating fetal age: Effect of head shape on BPD. *AJR* 1981; 137:83–85.
†Measurements of short and long axis taken from outer to outer margins of head.

Using real-time ultrasound, this same CI has been measured on fetuses in two articles between 14 and 42 gestational weeks.[103, 104] The measurements were taken in transaxial view from the widest transverse and longitudinal dimension of the calvarium.[88, 103] In three articles, the optimum place to measure was at the level used to obtain the biparietal diameter, at the thalamus or upper part of the brain stem, in the region of the cavum septi pellucidi (incorrectly labeled as the third ventricle in reference 97).[88, 92, 97] While the measurements are supposed to be taken from the outer margins of the calvarium for both the biparietal diameter and the fronto-occipital diameter[103] (Fig 5–3), it is not certain that all observers adhered to this standard.[104] Instead, they may have used the standard BPD measurement of leading edge to leading edge, which makes the BPD approximately 2 to 3 mm smaller. This minor difference probably has no clinical significance.

The biparietal diameter, termed the "short axis," divided by the fronto-occipital diameter, termed the "long axis," times 100 was found to be equal to 78.3 (see Table 5–2).[103] The range at 1 SD was 74 to 83 and at 2 SD was 70 to 86.[103] Almost identical results obtained by Shields et al.[104] showed a CI range of 59.3 to 89.5. The median was 78.8 with a 2 SD range of 68.4 to 89.2. These numbers are very similar to the neonatal measurements.[100, 101] It should be stressed that an abnormal CI does not, by itself, imply the head is abnormal. An "abnormal" shape only means that a correction measurement of the fetal head is needed and that careful evaluation of the internal fetal head anatomy should be performed (Fig 5–4). It has been found that fetal heads in normal breech presentation and following premature rupture of membranes with oligohydramnios are more likely to be dolichocephalic.[105, 106]

When the CIs were computed from the biparietal diameter and fronto-occipital diameters in the 9 articles on FOD,[89–97] the numbers varied considerably. Levi and Erbsman[91] obtained a mean CI of 72 at 18 gestational weeks, gradually increasing to 77.8 by 38 weeks. Fescina et al.[92] and Jeanty et al.[94] detected a CI of 100 at 10 to 30 weeks, gradually decreasing to 79–80 by term. Hoffbauer et al.,[90] Hannsman,[97] Chevernak et al.,[95] and Persson and Weldner[96] obtained in-

Fetal Head Measurements 31

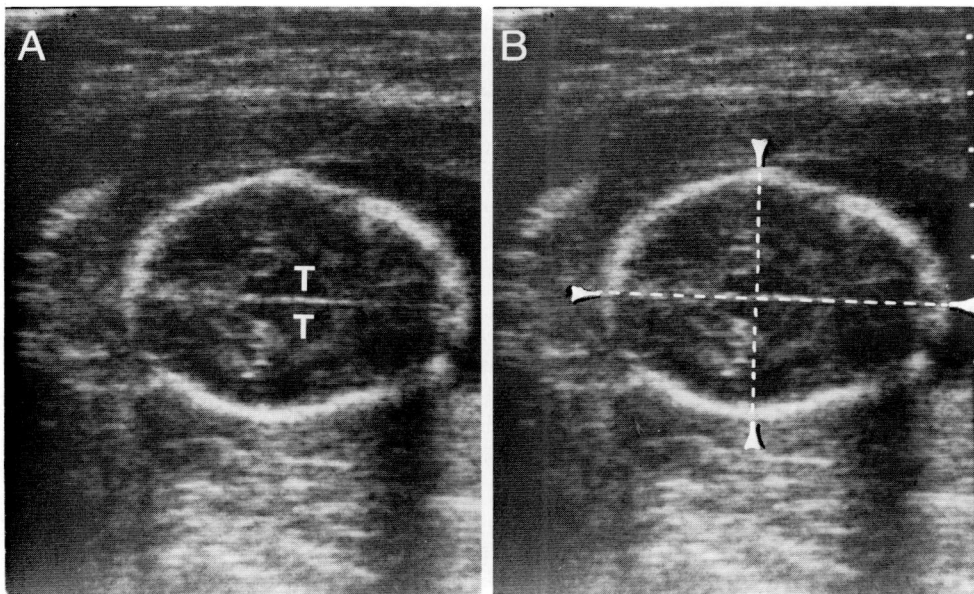

FIG 5–3.
Transaxial ultrasound image of a 32 week fetus. **A,** scan taken at the level of the thalami *(T),* the same level used to measure the biparietal diameter. **B,** same image as **A** showing the outer to outer measurements for both the short axis (biparietal diameter) and long axis (fronto-occipital diameter). Measurements denoted by *arrowheads* and *dotted lines.*

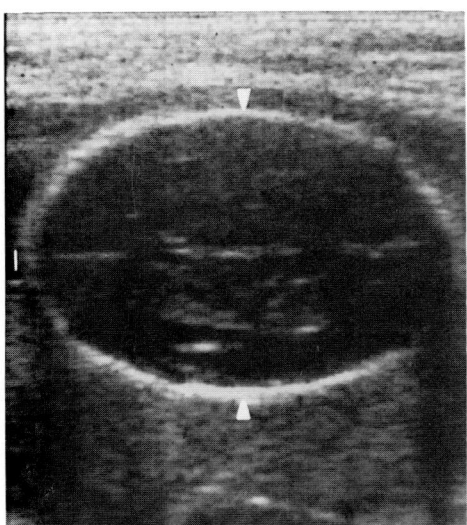

FIG 5–4.
Transaxial ultrasound image of an unusually ovoid fetal head at 30 gestational weeks. When the outer to outer dimension of the short axis *(arrowheads)* was compared to the same dimension of the long axis *(lines),* the cephalic index was low at 68. The internal head anatomy was normal.

termediate CIs varying from 79 to 88 throughout gestation, while the mean CIs from the graphs[89, 93] ranged from 75 to 82.5.

The Hadlock et al.[103] CI numbers are recommended because of their close correlation to the newborn CI. The numbers by Shields et al.[104] would also be acceptable. The only question that remains is whether to use 1 SD between 74 and 83 or enlarge the range to encompass 2 SD between 70 and 86 (see Table 5–2). Their article[104] gave both but recommended using only 1 SD, so that only two thirds of normal fetal heads would be contained within the normal range. While many normal cases (34%) fell outside the normal head shape range, it assured that few if any abnormal head shapes would be overlooked. To make the ratio more clinically useful, however, it is recommended that 2 SD, encompassing 95% of normal cases, be used instead.

A possible new approach to the problem of unusual head shape has been recently proposed. When the FOD and BPD do not have the correct ratio, rather than employing a different head measurement such as circumference,[103] the head shape can be "corrected" so that each biparietal diameter is ideal for CI of 78.3.[107] The formula proposed is termed the area-corrected BPD (Table 5–3). While this approach has theoretical appeal, further work will be necessary to prove its practical usefulness.

HEAD CIRCUMFERENCE

In the prediction of third trimester fetal age, the in utero measurement of head circumference has been found to be accurate to ±2 to 3 weeks.[108] Head circumference measurements have also been found to correlate closely with the true gestational age (±1 week) based on the menstrual history and postnatal evaluation.[109–111] In particular, the head circumference of premature infants has been found to correlate with, but be consistently higher by 1 cm than, the third trimester ultrasound examinations.[109–111] This overestimation is probably caused by the incorporation of the newborn soft tissues surrounding the calvarium into the circumference measurements. Ultrasound disregards these soft tissues and measures only the outer edge of the bone.

While a digitizer or map reader can be employed as the standard way of tracing the outer part of the calvarium to obtain a circumference (Fig 5–5), work had been performed using equations.[112–115] Initially, it was thought that multiplying the biparietal diameter by a factor of 3.5 would give fairly accurate head circumference measurements.[112] Later, two well-controlled studies compared the

TABLE 5–3.
Corrected Biparietal Diameter (BPD)*

Area-corrected BPD (BPDa)

$$BPDa = \sqrt{(BPD \times FOD)/1.265}$$

*Data from Doubilet PM, Greenes RA: Improved prediction of gestational age from fetal head measurements. AJR 1984; 142:797–800.

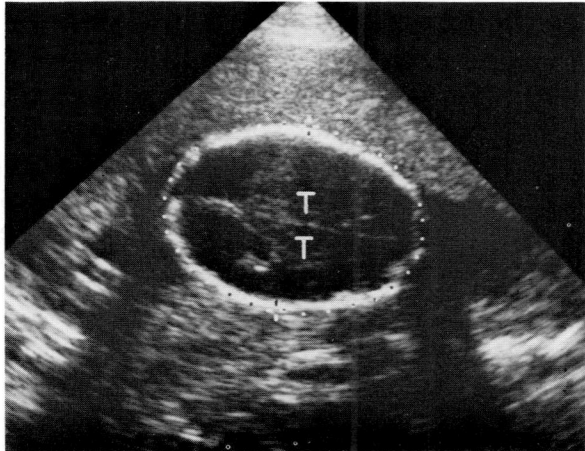

FIG 5–5.
Transaxial ultrasound image of a 28-week fetus. Scan taken at the level of the thalami *(T)*, the same level used to measure the biparietal diameter. *Dotted line* denotes outer margin of calvarium used to calculate the head circumference with a digitizer or map reader.

TABLE 5–4.
Circumference Computations

1. Planimetry
2. Equation for a circle

$$\left(\frac{BPD + FOD}{2}\right) \pi = (BPD + FOD) \times 1.57$$

head circumferences obtained by tracing the margins of the head with an electronic digitizer to those computed by the equation for a circumference (the average of the biparietal and fronto-occipital diameter, taken from the outer rims, multiplied by 1.57) (Table 5–4). One study found an insignificant mean error of, at most, 6% between these two methods at 2 SD.[113] The other found a small but constant overestimation in the head circumference, which was also not significant.[114]

DeVore and Platt[115] and Birnholz[116] pointed out that this formula was really a circumference measurement of a circle. They thought that this equation was not always accurate in obtaining measurements of ovoid fetal heads and compared it to equations which they claimed to be the true equations for an elliptical circumference. While the authors were correct in their statements that an equation of a circumference of a circle may not be precise, the equations chosen[115, 116] were not true circumference equations of ellipses but only approximations and were not more accurate than the circle circumference equation.[114] However, DeVore and Platt[115] correctly recommended that a circle circumference equation be used until the CI fell below 70. Since the CI is unlikely to be below 70, the circle circumference equation will suffice in most instances and has been found to be as accurate as other proposed equation.[114, 117]

There are 16 articles evaluating head circumference to gestational age.[118–133] Ten gave specific numbers,[118, 121, 123–125, 128–130, 132, 133] two performed with static scanners,[118, 121] and the rest with real-time scanners. The other six articles were given in graph form only[119, 120, 126, 127, 131] or as an equation only[122] and will not be discussed further. Since reference 128 is preliminary work by Athey and Hadlock, with the more definitive work in reference 129, 128 will also not be discussed further. Since van Egmond-Linden et al.[133] gave numbers from 16 to 28 weeks without third trimester measurements, this article too will not be discussed further.

The remaining eight articles[118, 121, 123–125, 129, 130, 132] presented measurements obtained throughout the second and third trimesters from 10 weeks until term. For proper selection of the measurement plane, the midline echo was used in one,[121] the midline echo and third ventricle in 4,[123, 129, 130, 132] with the remaining articles not stating a specific anatomical plane. In comparing 6 of the most recent articles,[123–125, 128, 130, 132] all except Ott[132] were fairly closely grouped with the numbers from Ott[132] close at 15 weeks, becoming progressively smaller, 35 mm less at term. Hoffbauer et al.[118] had numbers smaller before 17 weeks and much larger after 38 weeks, and Levi and Erbsman[121] had uniformly larger numbers until 40 weeks by as much as 22 mm. These latter two articles[118, 121] will not be discussed further.

These six recent articles[123–125, 129, 130, 132] appear to have good technique, although the technique was stated in only four.[123, 129, 130, 132] The articles not only had a mean head circumference for menstrual age but also a 95% or greater confidence limits. The major difference among these studies is that only one[129] gave its data in a clinical useful form, with a variation in weeks for each head circumference. The remaining articles present a range of head circumferences in centimeters for each gestational week, a method which has little practicality. It is recommended that the table by Hadlock et al.[129] (Table 5–5) be used.

The reproducibility of the head circumference measurements has been analyzed. The intraobserver error has been found to be insignificant except if technical factors, particularly the use of different measuring devices, are considered. Measuring devices gave varied results, and, in addition, investigators used these devices differently.[134] The interobserver error was found in one study[129] to be approximately 1% with a mean error by three independent readings in the third trimester of only 1.8 mm (less than 0.75%). Another study,[134] however, showed the interobserver error to be larger, with a mean of 1.2% and a range of ±4.3% at 1 SD with no systematic differences between prenatal and postnatal measurements.

The overall accuracy of head circumference measurements, in comparison to the biparietal diameter measurements, has also been evaluated. Hadlock et al.[129] stated that the head circumference was a good predictor of gestational age but not as good as the biparietal diameter. They thought that it still should be used, however, particularly with unusual head shapes. Three other observers[132, 135, 136] stated that the head circumference was more accurate in predicting gestational age, probably secondary to changes in head shape caused by pressure of the uterine wall or external forces on the pliable skull. While an article by Law and MacRae[136] showed strong statistical evidence that the head circumference was more accurate than the biparietal diameter, especially in the third trimester, a major flaw in this work was the omission of the CI to determine if the heads were unusually shaped.

HEAD AREA

Eight articles have been published comparing the area of the head to the gestational age,[137-144] with actual numbers given in three.[138, 140, 142] Six articles utilized static scanners from the late second through the third trimesters, two giving numbers,[138, 142] three in graph form,[137, 141, 143] and one as an equation.[139] The last article[140] analyzed the head area with real-time throughout the second and third trimesters. The intraobserver error was found to be larger than that for head circumferences, ±2.6 weeks.[141] In addition, while all articles showed an expected increase in head area as the gestation progressed, the four articles in graph form[137, 141, 143, 144] had much lower numbers for head areas than the three in number form.[138, 140, 142] Of interest is the article by Wladmirioff et al.,[142] in which head areas were calculated by squaring the biparietal diameter rather than by using a planimeter tracing. Despite this unusual approach, the numbers were quite close to the numbers of Levi and Ebsman[138] and Fescina et al.[140]

The reasons for the discrepancies between studies cannot be ascertained. Since, however, the accuracy is not better than either the biparietal diameter or the head circumference measurements, and since the variation may be greater, it is thought that the head area is not a useful or proven method.

HEAD VOLUME

Four articles have been published calculating the volume of the fetal head.[145-149] In one[145] the volume was obtained by considering the head as an ellipsoid volume and calculating it in the transaxial view by multiplying the fronto-occipital diameter (FOD) × biparietal diameter (BPD) × a constant. The volumes increased from 30 cc at 18 weeks to 514 cc at term. In two other articles,[146, 147] the volume was computed from the cube of an average transaxial diameter, the average diameter calculated as a square root of FOD × BPD. The head volume increased from 16 cc at 12 weeks to 1,191 cc at term. Last, DuBose[148] calculated the head volume by three parameters, the BPD, FOD, and vertical calvarial diameter. The last was measured from the interpetrosal portion of the base of the skull to the vertex in coronal view. It is this measurement that makes the calculated head volumes theoretically more accurate. By using an equation for a sphere, head volumes increased from 10 to 350 cc throughout the second and third trimester.

Despite the theoretical probability that a volume measurement is better for evaluating brain mass and overall head size, this method has not as yet been proved. It should, therefore, at present not be considered in the routine examination of the fetal head. It may have a place in future analysis if it can be shown to be more accurate than the biparietal diameter and head circumference measurements. A problem that head volume might have been able to solve became apparent in a recent article in fetuses with premature rupture of the membranes and oligohydramnios.[149] While the biparietal diameter was unreliable, the fronto-occipital diameter and cephalic index were only able to predict which fetal heads were abnormally shaped in 45% of cases. It is possible that the fetal head had been misshapen by the oligohydramnios primarily in the craniocaudal dimension.

TABLE 5–5.
Head Circumference Measurement Table*

Head Circumference, mm	Gestational Age, wk		Head Circumference, mm	Gestational Age, wk	
	Predicted Mean Values†	95% Confidence Limits‡		Predicted Mean Values†	95% Confidence Limits‡
80	13.4	12.1–14.7	230	24.9	22.6–27.2
85	13.7	12.4–15.0	235	25.4	23.1–27.7
90	14.0	12.7–15.3	240	25.9	23.6–28.2
95	14.3	13.0–15.6	245	26.4	24.1–28.7
100	14.6	13.3–15.9	250	26.9	24.6–29.2
105	15.0	13.7–16.3	255	27.5	25.2–29.8
110	15.3	14.0–16.6	260	28.0	25.7–30.3
115	15.6	14.3–16.9	265	28.1	25.8–30.4
120	15.9	14.6–17.2	270	29.2	26.9–31.5
125	16.3	15.0–17.6	275	29.8	27.5–32.1
130	16.6	15.3–17.9	280	30.3	27.6–33.0
135	17.0	15.7–18.3	285	31.0	28.3–33.7
140	17.3	16.0–18.6	290	31.6	28.9–34.3
145	17.7	16.4–19.0	295	32.2	29.5–34.8
150	18.1	16.5–19.7	300	32.8	30.1–35.5
155	18.4	16.8–20.0	305	33.5	30.7–36.2
160	18.8	17.2–20.4	310	34.2	31.5–36.9
165	19.2	17.6–20.8	315	34.9	32.2–37.6
170	19.6	18.0–21.2	320	35.5	32.8–38.2
175	20.0	18.4–21.6	325	36.3	32.9–39.7

180	20.4	18.8–22.0	330	37.0	33.6–40.4
185	20.8	19.2–22.4	335	37.7	34.3–41.1
190	21.2	19.8–22.8	340	38.5	35.1–41.9
195	21.6	20.0–23.2	345	39.2	35.8–42.6
200	22.1	20.5–23.7	350	40.0	36.6–43.4
205	22.5	20.9–24.1	355	40.8	37.4–44.2
210	23.0	21.4–24.6	360	41.6	38.2–45.0
215	23.4	21.8–25.0			
220	23.9	22.3–25.5			
225	24.4	22.1–26.7			

*From Hadlock FP, Deter RL, Harrist RB, et al: Fetal head circumference: Relation to menstrual age. *AJR* 1982; 139:367–370. Used by permission.
†Data from Table 3 of original article.
‡Data from Table 4 of original article.

VENTRICULAR SIZE

Ultrasound has been shown to be accurate in the evaluation of lateral ventricular size in both children and adults. In infants, a comparison of computed tomography (CT) to real-time ultrasound revealed close correlation.[150, 151] To date there have been eight ultrasound articles analyzing the in utero size of the lateral ventricles.[152–159] Four measured the bodies of the lateral ventricles,[152, 154, 155, 159] three in number[152, 155, 159] and one in graph and equation form.[154] All used real-time equipment, two from 12 weeks to term,[152, 154] one from 15 to 25 weeks[159] and one from 27 weeks to term.[155]

In addition to obtaining linear measurements, a ratio of the lateral ventricle bodies to intracranial hemidiameter was also obtained. The lateral ventricle is measured from the falx midline echo to the widest part of the lateral wall of the body of the lateral ventricle and the intracranial hemidiameter measured on the same side, parallel to the first line, from the falx midline echo to widest part of the inner surface of the calvarium[152] (Fig 5–6). Recently there has been some controversy about the echo produced at the lateral wall of the body of the lateral ventricle. Some observers have suggested that the echo is actually created by interfaces from neural elements in the surrounding tissue rather than from the wall itself. Regardless, the echo is reproducible, and the validity of this ratio has been confirmed in newborn infants, 25 term and 41 preterm.[160] For the term infants, the ratio was found to be 28%, with a range of 24% to 30%, while the ratio in the preterm infants was slightly larger at 31% with a range of 24% to 34%, both comparable to the in utero ratios of Johnson et al.[152] and Jeanty et al.[154]

The Hadlock et al.[155] work is confined solely to the third trimester and has consistently larger ventricular numbers and wider ratio ranges than Johnson et al.[152] and Jeanty et al.[154] The authors[155] attributed these larger numbers to the way that their measurements were obtained, measuring the bodies of the lateral ventricles from the outer margin of the falx echo to the outer border of the body of the lateral ventricle, rather than from the middle of the falx echo to the inner border of the body of the lateral ventricular. Since these margins are thin structures, it does not seem that such small measurement changes alone should be responsible for such large differences in the ventricular numbers or in their ratios. Therefore, this article will not be considered further.

The Johnson et al.[152] and Jeanty et al[154] articles closely correlate in both lateral ventricle measurements and in ratios from the early gestation period until term. Only the work by Johnson et al.[152] is recommended, because its results are in numerical form. The main weakness in the Johnson et al.[152] data, however, is in the early second trimester. There were not even enough data points to calculate a ventricular width or a ratio at 19 weeks. Pretorius et al.[159] from the same institution, reevaluated the second trimester with 122 normal fetuses and directly analyzed her work against that of Johnson et al.[152] Since the two compare closely, a combined table using the original work by Johnson et al.[152] from 26 weeks to term and the later work by Pretorius et al.[159] from 15 to 25 weeks is recommended (Table 5–6).

In the early second trimester, the lateral ventricles are very prominent and take up most of the inner area of the calvarium, as much as 74% of the head at 15 weeks. At this stage of gestation, approximately 12 to 18 weeks, the hyper-

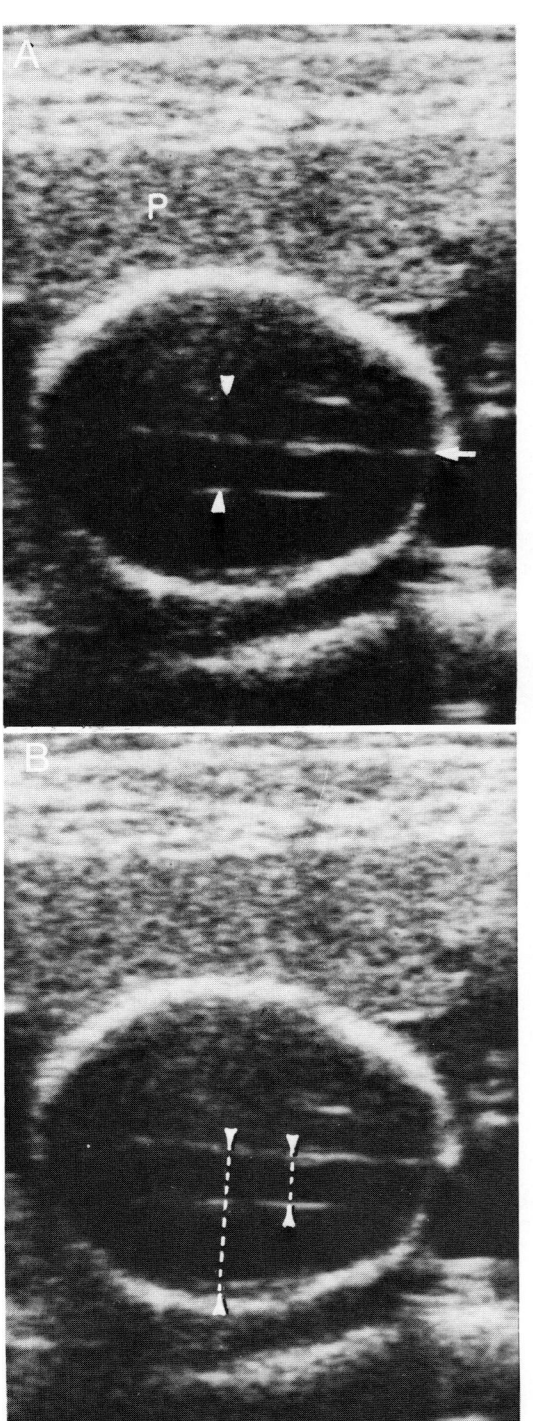

FIG 5–6.
Transaxial scan of the fetal head near term at the region of the bodies of the lateral ventricles. **A,** the two linear lines *(arrowheads),* of the lateral ventricular bodies are parallel to the falx midline echo *(arrow).* **B,** same image as **A** showing the measurements of the bodies of the lateral ventricles (LV) on the right and the intracranial hemidiameter (ICHD) on the left, both denoted by *arrowheads* and *dotted lines.* The LV and the ICHD measurements should be taken at their widest points, parallel to each other. Note that the LV/ICHD ratio is small near term, only 33%. *P* indicates placenta.

TABLE 5–6.
Lateral Ventricular Measurement Table*

Menstrual Age, wk	Measurements in Millimeters		Lateral Ventricular Width
	Lateral Ventricular Width, 2 SD	Hemispheric Width, 2 SD	Hemispheric Width Ratio (LVW/HW), 2 SD
15	8 (6–10)	15 (12–18)	56 (38–74)
16	9 (7–11)	15 (13–17)	57 (46–68)
17	9 (8–10)	15 (14–16)	58 (49–67)
18	9 (8–10)	18 (17–19)	51 (41–61)
19	9 (7–11)	20 (19–21)	49 (41–57)
20	9 (7–11)	19 (17–20)	46 (38–54)
21	9 (7–11)	21 (20–22)	42 (31–53)
22	9 (7–11)	23 (21–25)	40 (29–51)
23	8 (7–9)	24 (22–26)	34 (26–42)
24	9 (8–10)	25 (23–27)	35 (27–43)
25	9 (8–10)	28 (25–31)	33 (29–37)
26	9	30	30 (24–36)
27	9	30	28 (23–34)
28	11	33	31 (18–45)
29	10	34	29 (22–37)
30	10	34	30 (26–34)
31	10	34	29 (23–36)
32	11	36	31 (26–36)
33	11	34	31 (25–37)
34	11	38	28 (23–33)
35	11	38	29 (26–31)
36	11	39	28 (23–34)
37	12	41	29 (24–34)
Term	12	43	28 (22–33)

*Combined table of two articles from the same group: Fifteen to 25 gestational weeks: Pretorius DH, Drose JA, Manco-Johnson ML: Fetal lateral ventricular ratio determined during the second trimester. J Ultrasound Med 1986; 5:121–124. Used by permission. Twenty-six gestational weeks to term: Johnson ML, Dunne MC, Mack LA, et al: Evaluation of fetal intracranial anatomy by static and realtime ultrasound. J Clin Ultrasound 1980; 8:311–318. Used by permission.

echoic choroid plexus almost completely fills the lateral ventricular bodies (Fig 5–7). As the pregnancy progresses toward term, the cerebral cortex grows, causing the head to enlarge and the choroid plexus and the lateral ventricles to become relatively less prominent. By 21 weeks, the bodies of the lateral ventricles have decreased to a maximum of 53% (Fig 5–8), further decreasing to 33% by term (see Fig 5–6).

The atria of the lateral ventricles have also been evaluated.[155, 156] A measurement in this region could be more clinically useful, since early hydrocephalus has been shown to enlarge the atrial regions prior to affecting either the bodies or frontal horns of the lateral ventricles.[156] McGahan and Phillips[156] stated that a ratio of the diameter of the hippocampal-trigone region divided by the trigone-midline was fairly constant from 29 to 44 weeks at 35%, with a range of 29% to 40% (Fig 5–9,A and B), the trigone denoting the lateral margin of the lateral ventricle at the atria-occipital region. Hadlock et al.[155] calculated the ratio of the atria of the lateral ventricles to the calvarial hemidiameter and found it to be slightly more prominent than the ratio taken at the bodies of the lateral ventricles (Fig 5–9,C). At 27 to 28 weeks this atrial region ratio was 56%, with a range of 53% to 60%, decreasing at term to 51%, with a range of 47% to 55%.[155] Of these two approaches, the ratio of McGahan and Phillips[156] is more compelling, since it is constant throughout the third trimester. The atria of the lateral ventricles, however, are more difficult to image than the bodies and cannot be consistently

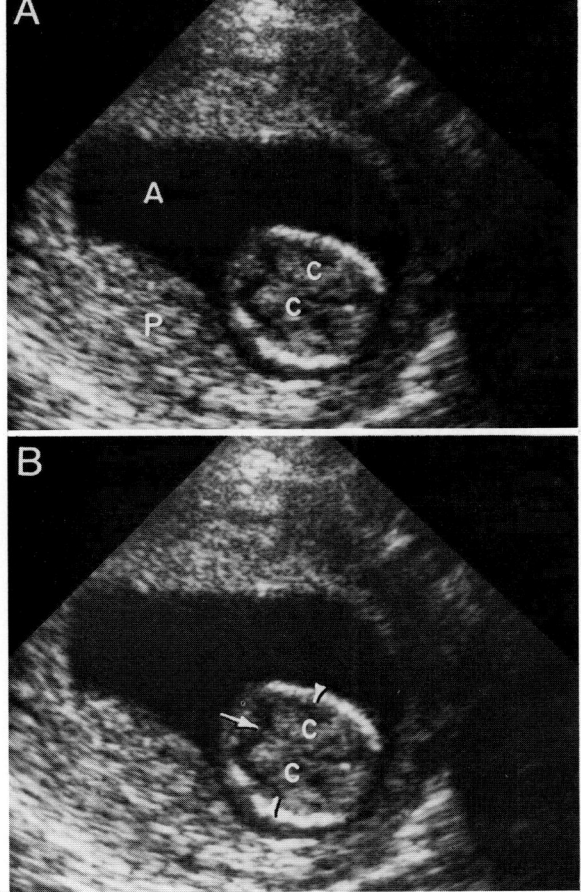

FIG 5–7.
Transaxial scan of the fetal head at 15 weeks. **A,** the choroid plexus (C) are hyperechoic and almost completely fill the prominent lateral ventricles. **B,** same image as **A** showing the falx midline echo *(arrow)* and lateral margins of the bodies of the lateral ventricles *(arrowheads)*. In the early third trimester, the lateral ventricles are so prominent that the ratio of the lateral ventricle to intracranial hemidiameter can normally approach 70%. *A* indicates amniotic fluid; *P,* placenta.

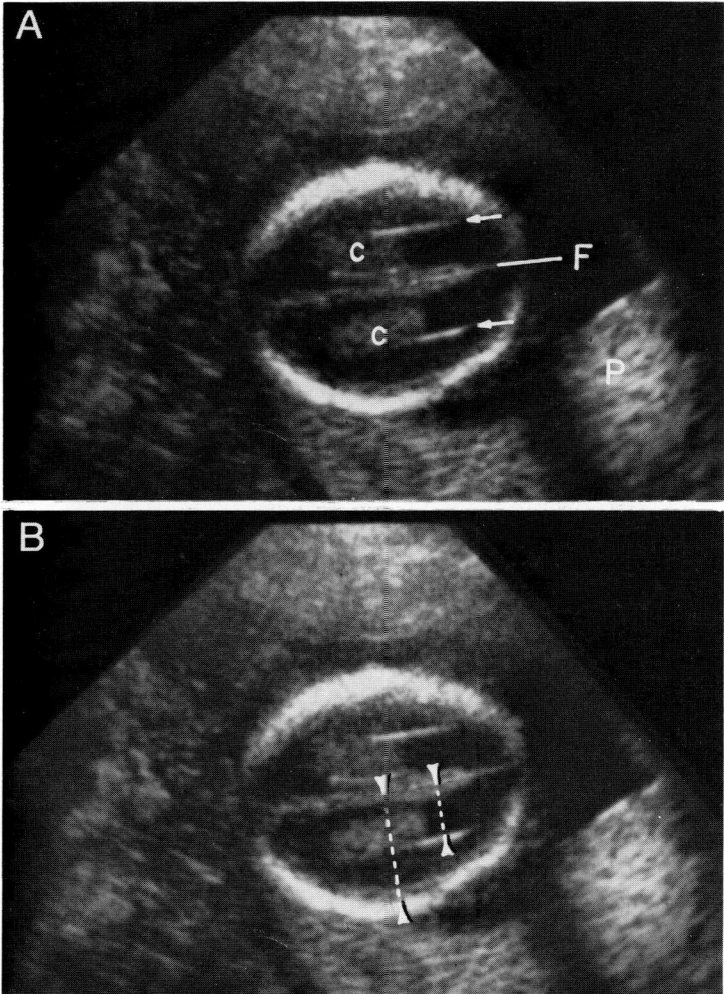

FIG 5–8.
Transaxial scan of the fetal head at 21 weeks. **A**, at the bodies of the lateral ventricles *(arrows)*, the falx midline echo *(F)* and the choroid plexus *(C)* are seen. **B**, same image as **A** showing the measurements of the bodies of the lateral ventricles (LV) on the right and intracranial hemidiameter (ICHD) on the left, both denoted by *arrowheads* and *dotted lines*. The LV and ICHD measurements should be taken at their widest points, parallel to each other. Note the LV/ICHD ratio is approximately 50%. *P* indicates placenta.

identified. For this reason, despite its appeal, no measurement or ratio is recommended.

The lateral ventricles have been measured at the frontal horns,[153, 157, 158] all in number form (Fig 5–9,C). Denkhaus and Winsberg[157] evaluated the entire second and third trimester, while vanEgmond-Linden et al.[153] analyzed the second and Jorgensen et al.[158] the third trimesters. Denkhaus and Winsberg[157] did not use the intracranial hemidiameter but rather the biparietal diameter, which is larger because it encompasses the parietal bone of the calvarium. Their ratio numbers would, therefore, be expected to be uniformly smaller than the other two, but this was not found to be consistently true. In general, combining all three articles, the frontal horn to intracranial hemidiameter decreased from 48% at 13 weeks to 25% at term. At 17 weeks the ratio varied among the three articles from 37% to 46%, while at term the two remaining articles[157, 158] had ratios that were very close, 26% and 28%. Consistent imaging of this part of the fetal head can at times be difficult. Since these articles are discrepant, no measurement from this region is recommended.

The third ventricle has also been evaluated.[155, 156] Hadlock et al.[155] thought that after 34 weeks the third ventricle could be correctly defined between the thalami, measuring no greater than 2–5 mm in its widest diameter (Fig 5–10). Denkhaus and Winsberg,[157] however thought that the third ventricle could be routinely imaged from 13 weeks to term, increasing from 2.5 mm at 13 weeks to 8.2 mm at term. These latter measurements are quite prominent, and analysis of one of their images suggests that at least some of their measurements were taken of the prominent cavum septi pellucidi instead of the third ventricle, a

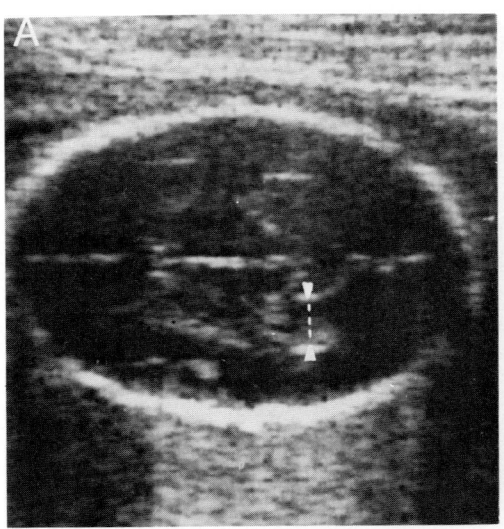
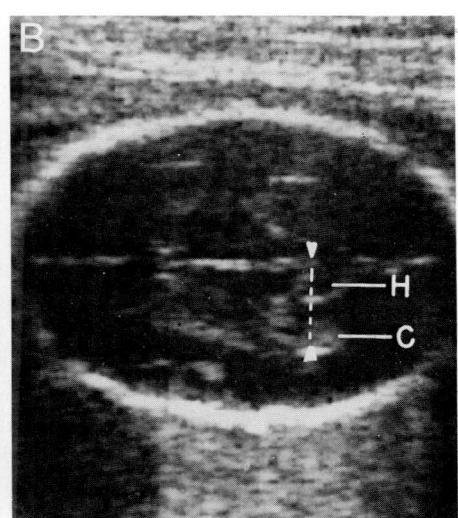
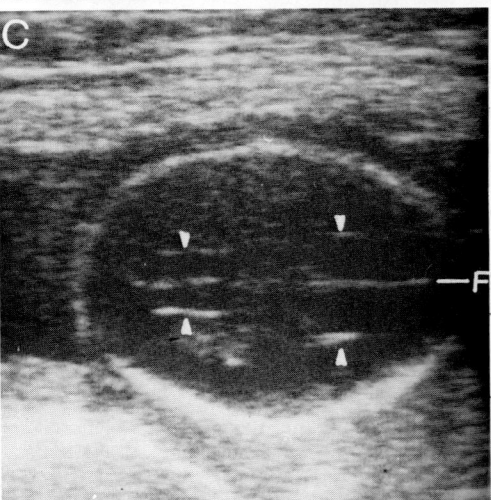

FIG 5–9.
Transaxial scan of the fetal head at 25 weeks. **A** and **B**, at the region of the atria of the lateral ventricles, the measurement of the trigone to the midline *(A)* divided into the measurement of the hippocampus to the trigone *(B)*, both denoted by *arrowheads* and *dotted lines*, is constant at 29% to 40%. *H* indicates hippocampus; *C*, choroid plexus. **C**, image showing the larger atria-occipital horns *(arrowheads on the right)* and smaller frontal horns *(arrowheads on left)* of the lateral ventricles. *F* indicates falx midline echo.

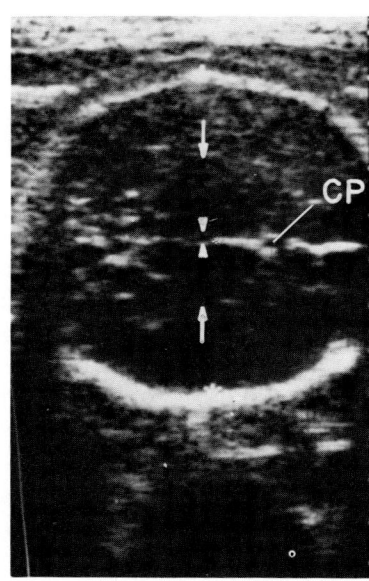

FIG 5–10.
Transaxial scan of the fetal head at 36 weeks. Note the third ventricle *(arrowheads)* between the thalami *(arrows)*. The cavum septi pellucidi *(CP)* is anteriorly located.

structure which is actually anterior to the brain stem and third ventricle[157] (see Fig 5–10).

The diagnosis of enlarged ventricles can be made when the lateral ventricles measure larger than would be expected for any particular gestational age. Prominent or enlarged ventricles do not necessarily imply hydrocephalus. Occasionally prominent ventricles can be caused by atrophy of the brain with passive expansion of the ventricles to fill the empty space. The size of both the choroid plexuses and the fetal head are helpful in making the distinction between atrophy and obstructive hydrocephalus. Since the choroid plexuses are hyperechoic and normally completely fill the prominent lateral ventricles in the early second trimester, from the time the fetal head is imaged at 12 weeks until approximately 18 weeks (see Fig 5–7), if the choroid plexuses are not present or are too small, early hydrocephalus should be considered.[161] Later in the pregnancy, if the lateral ventricles are enlarged, and particularly if the head is also larger than expected for a particular gestational age, the diagnosis of obstructive hydrocephalus should be considered. If the ventricles are prominent but the fetal head is smaller than expected, cerebral atrophy and diagnosis of microcephaly must be considered. If the ventricles are enlarged and head is normal in size, while hydrocephalus is more common, either hydrocephalus or cerebral atrophy may be present.

OCULAR DIMENSIONS

The fetal eye can be routinely imaged.[162–164] Two articles have evaluated the eye[163, 164] throughout the second and third trimester, one in number form[163] and one in equation and graph form.[164] In the second and third trimesters, a view of one or both eyes could be obtained in 96% of cases and the eyeball (globe), lens, iris, pupil, and cornea routinely identified.[163] While the hyaloid artery, between the lens and posterior choroid, could be identified prior to 20 weeks, it is generally absent after 25 weeks.[163]

The globe appears as a rounded structure with less than a 5% variation between the major diameters in two views, sagittal and base.[163] The globe is surrounded by hyperechoic retrobulbar fat so that its measurement can easily be taken from its anechoic borders (Fig 5–11). By examining 157 normal fetuses, it was found that the average diameter increased continually throughout the second and third trimester with periods of accelerated growth, between 12 and 20, 28 and 32, and at term.[163] In contradistinction, Jeanty et al.[164] showed a more asymptotic growth near term. Numerical measurements were presented in one article, comparing favorably to a previous pathologic series referenced within the article.[163] While these values are slightly lower than those shown by Jeanty et al.,[164] approximately 1–2 mm after 20 weeks, the measurements are considered close enough that a table is recommended[163] (Table 5–7). Further work is needed to confirm these measurements.

ORBITAL DIMENSIONS

Three articles have evaluated orbital diameters.[165–167] Jeanty et al.[165] measured the outer orbital diameter (outer to outer orbital distance) and the inner orbital diameter (inner to inner orbital distance) in both equation and graph form. Jeanty et al.[166] measured the outer orbital diameter, also termed binocular distance, in number and equation form. Mayden et al.[167] measured the outer

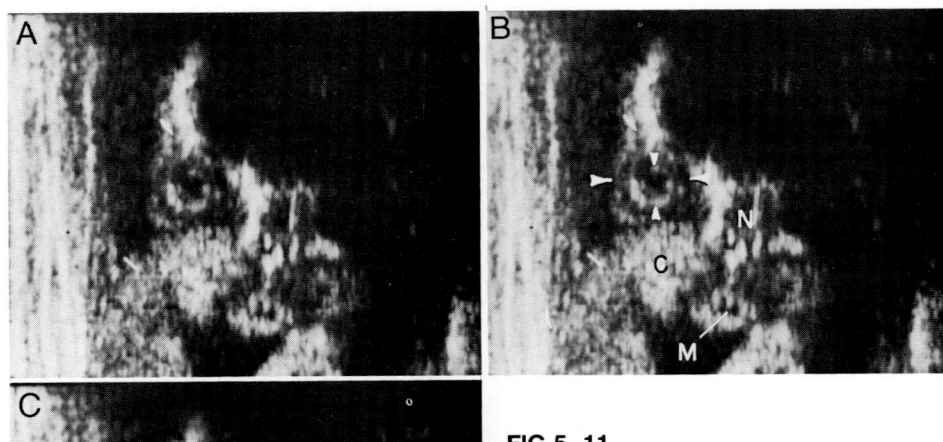

FIG 5–11.
Coronal view of fetal face and globe (eyeball). **A,** image without labels, oriented with transducer on the left. **B,** same image with labels. *Larger arrowheads* denote orbit and *small arrowheads* hyperechoic retrobulbar fat surrounding the globe. *M* indicates mouth; *N,* nasal cavity; *C,* cheek. **C,** same image with measured globe *(arrowheads* and *dotted line).*

and inner orbital diameters in number and graph form. In the same article,[167] aborted fetuses were evaluated in a water bath and their orbital diameters correlated well with in utero measurements obtained on live fetuses of the same gestational age.

All articles used real-time equipment, and Mayden et al.[167] also evaluated the fetal orbits with a static scanner. All used greater than 180 normal subjects from 12 to 42 weeks. The criteria used for all the studies were comparable: the sections had to have both orbits imaged symmetrically with each orbit of largest possible diameter (Fig 5–12). Of the three, two[156, 167] demonstrated the outer margins used to obtain the outer orbital diameter taken at the inner margins of the bone. Only one[167] showed the margins for the inner orbital diameter.

There are technical difficulties in obtaining the precise landmarks to make outer orbital diameter measurements. The globe is surrounded by hyperechoic fat and the hyperechoic orbital rim. These tend to blend together, especially when the fetus is face up or occiput up, causing indistinct margins (Fig 5–13). Nevertheless, when the numbers in these articles were compared, all three demonstrated an outer orbital diameter increase from 13 mm at 12 weeks to 59 mm or greater by term. Their numbers were closely grouped, varying from 0 to 3 mm at each stage of gestation. The outer orbital diameter was shown to closely parallel the increase in biparietal diameter as gestation progressed, and therefore, to be a useful means of verifying fetal age. In addition, the outer orbital diameter was found to be a good indicator of hypotelorism[167] and perhaps could also be used to diagnose hypertelorism, although no cases were observed. The inner orbital diameter varied very little throughout gestation, 5 mm at 12 weeks to 19 mm at term, did not correlate well with either the biparietal diameter or the gestational age,[165, 167] and will not be discussed further.

There are two reasons to obtain an outer orbital (binocular) diameter. First, it is a good method of confirming gestational age and obtaining valid measurements of the face, even when the head may be in a difficult position to obtain an accurate biparietal diameter. This latter circumstance can be a particular problem near term, especially when the head is in vertex presentation. In this instance, a table comparing the outer orbital diameter to gestational age is needed[166] (Table 5–8). Second, there are circumstances in which a facial to

TABLE 5–7.
Fetal Globe (Eyeball) Diameter Measurement Table*

Globe Diameter, mm		Gestational Age, wk	
Mean Diameter	Range of 16%–84%, 1SD	Mean Age	Range of 16%–84%, 1 SD
4.7	4.0–5.5	14.5	12.5–16.5
7.4	6.2–8.6	17.9	16.5–19.3
9.9	9.6–10.2	22.4	21.4–23.5
11.2	10.3–12.1	25.7	24.6–26.8
13.4	12.5–14.4	30.4	29.2–31.6
14.9	14.5–15.3	33.6	32.6–34.7
16.0	15.1–16.9	38.2	36.8–39.2

*From Birnholz JC: Ultrasonic fetal ophthalmology. *Early Fetal Dev* 1985; 12:199–209. Used by permission.

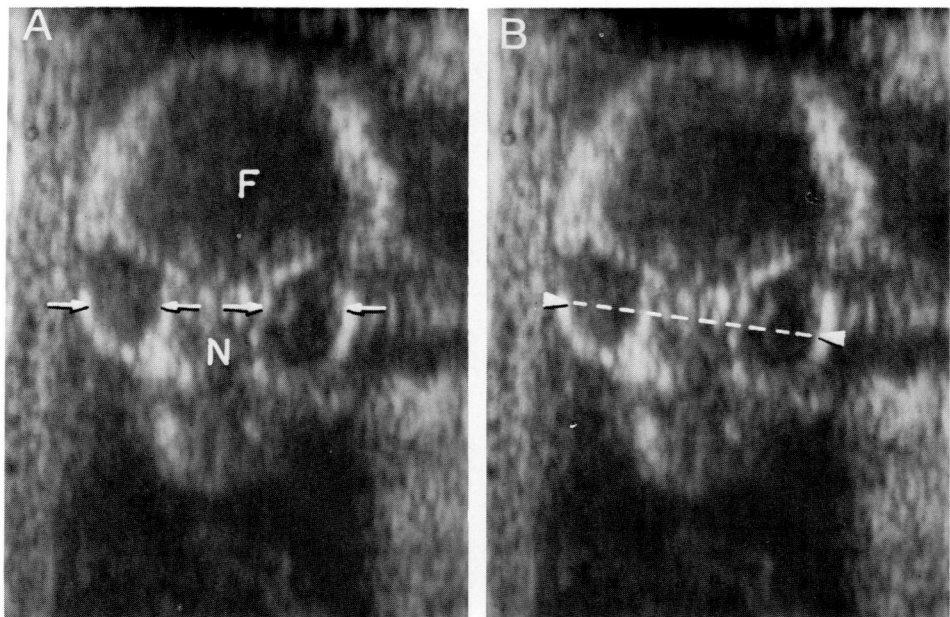

FIG 5–12.
Coronal scan of the face in a 30 week fetus. **A,** image oriented with transducer on the left showing the two orbits *(arrows)*. N indicates nasal cavity; F, frontal bone. **B,** same image as **A** showing outer to outer orbital (binocular distance) measurement *(arrowheads and dotted line)*. Margins of the orbits are distinct and separable from the hyperechoic bone outside the orbits.

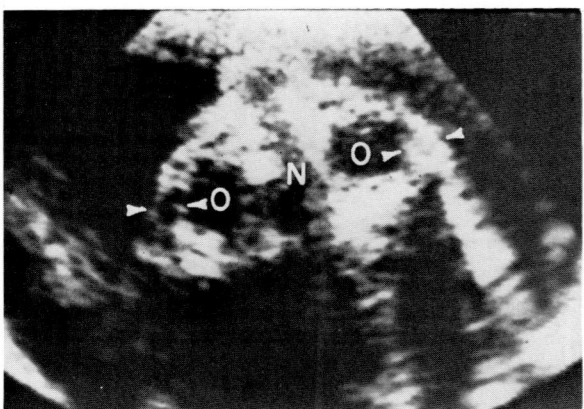

FIG 5–13.
Face-up magnified image of the fetal orbits. While the globes *(O)* can be clearly identified, a combination of hyperechoic retrobulbar fat, bone, and overlying subcutaneous tissue *(arrowheads)* make the outer borders indistinct. N indicates nasal cavity.

calvarial disproportion is suspected. When this is considered, a table comparing the outer orbital diameter to the biparietal diameter is needed[167] (Table 5–9). While ideally one table could have all these parameters—i.e., the outer orbital diameter, biparietal diameter, and gestational age (including range)—the articles published had only 2 of the 3, and therefore two tables are recommended.

TABLE 5–8.
Outer Orbital Diameter (Binocular Distance) Measurement Table*

Outer Orbital Diameter, mm	Gestational Age, wk		Outer Orbital Diameter, mm	Gestational Age, wk	
	Predicted Mean Values	Range from 5th to 95th Percentile		Predicted Mean Values	Range from 5th to 95th Percentile
15	10.4	7.1–13.9	41	25.9	22.6–29.1
16	11.0	7.7–14.4	42	26.6	23.1–29.9
17	11.6	8.3–15.0	43	27.1	23.9–30.4
18	12.1	8.9–15.6	44	27.7	24.4–31.0
19	12.9	9.6–16.1			
20	13.4	10.1–16.7	45	28.3	25.0–31.6
21	14.0	10.7–17.3	46	28.9	25.6–32.1
22	14.6	11.3–17.9	47	29.6	26.1–32.9
23	15.1	11.9–18.6	48	30.1	26.9–33.4
24	15.9	12.6–19.1	49	30.7	27.3–34.0
25	16.4	13.1–19.7	50	31.3	27.9–34.6
26	17.0	13.7–20.3	51	31.9	28.6–35.1
27	17.6	14.3–20.9	52	32.6	29.1–35.9
28	18.1	14.9–21.6	53	33.0	29.7–36.4
29	18.9	15.6–22.1	54	33.6	30.3–37.0
30	19.4	16.1–22.7	55	34.1	30.9–37.6
31	20.0	16.6–23.3	56	34.9	31.6–38.1
32	20.6	17.1–23.9	57	35.4	32.1–38.7
33	21.1	17.9–24.6	58	36.0	32.7–39.3
34	21.7	18.4–25.1	59	36.6	33.3–39.9

35	22.3	19.0–25.7	60	37.1	33.9–40.6
36	22.9	19.6–26.3	61	37.9	34.6–41.1
37	23.6	20.1–26.9	62	38.4	35.1–41.7
38	24.1	20.6–27.4	63	39.0	35.7–42.3
39	24.7	21.4–28.0	64	39.6	36.3–42.9
40	25.3	22.0–28.6	65	40.1	36.9–43.5

*From Jeanty P, Cantraine F, Cousaert E, et al: The binocular distance: A new way to estimate fetal age. J Ultrasound Med 1984; 3:241–243. Used by permission.

TABLE 5–9.
Outer Orbital Diameter (Binocular Distance) Measurement Table*

Predicted Outer Orbital Diameter, mm	Biparietal Diameter, mm	Mean Gestational Age, wk	Predicted Outer Orbital Diameter, mm	Biparietal Diameter, mm	Mean Gestational Age, wk
13	19	11.6	41	57	23.8
14	20	11.6	41	58	24.3
15	21	12.1	42	59	24.3
16	22	12.6	43	60	24.7
17	23	12.6	43	61	25.2
17	24	13.1	44	62	25.2
18	25	13.6	44	63	25.7
19	26	13.6	45	64	26.2
20	27	14.1	45	65	26.2
21	28	14.6	46	66	26.7
21	29	14.6	46	67	27.2
22	30	15.0	47	68	27.6
23	31	15.5	47	69	28.1
24	32	15.5	48	70	28.6
25	33	16.0	48	71	29.1
25	34	16.5	49	73	29.6
26	35	16.5	50	74	30.0
27	36	17.0	50	75	30.6
27	37	17.5	51	76	31.0
28	38	17.9	51	77	31.5
30	40	18.4	52	78	32.0
31	42	18.9	52	79	32.5
32	43	19.4	53	80	33.0
32	44	19.4	54	82	33.5
33	45	19.9	54	83	34.0
34	46	20.4	54	84	34.4
34	47	20.4	55	85	35.0
35	48	20.9	55	86	35.4
36	49	21.3	56	88	35.9
36	50	21.3	56	89	36.4
37	51	21.8	57	90	36.9
38	52	22.3	57	91	37.3
38	53	22.3	58	92	37.8
39	54	22.8	58	93	38.3
40	55	23.3	58	94	38.8
40	56	23.3	59	96	39.3
			59	97	39.8

*From Mayden KL, Tortora M, Berkowitz RL, et al: Orbital diameters: A new parameter for prenatal diagnosis and dating. Am J Obstet Gynecol 1982; 144:289–297. Used by permission.

THE CEREBELLAR DIMENSIONS

The cerebellum has been evaluated in two articles,[168, 169] one in number form from 15 to 39 weeks[168] and one as a graph from 14 to 32 weeks.[169] With real-time ultrasound, both used the standard transaxial image of the head, obtaining the cavum septi pellucidi and thalamus as midline structures and then rotating the transducer slightly posterior and inferior to image the posterior fossa (Fig 5–14). Both articles measured the transaxial cerebellar diameter with Smith et al.[169] also measuring the anteroposterior diameter. McLeary et al.[168] compared the cerebellum to the biparietal diameter while Smith et al.[169] compared the cerebellum only to the menstrual age. Both showed a continued growth of the cerebellum through the second and third trimester, with slowing near term. McLeary et al.[168] claimed to have no difficulty in imaging the cerebellum regardless of fetal age, while Smith et al.[169] found the cerebellum more difficult to image and measure after 30 weeks, because its borders became less distinct.

The usefulness of the cerebellar measurements is in its comparison to the biparietal diameter. Since both the biparietal diameter and cerebellum are imaged using the same scanning technique, the cerebellum becomes a potentially useful measurement to confirm the biparietal diameter and to determine if there is abnormality in the posterior fossa. While not shown in these articles, failure to demonstrate all or part of the cerebellum could be a sign of cerebellar hypoplasia or of decreased cerebellar growth.

A table comparing the transverse dimension of the cerebellum to the biparietal diameter is recommended[168] (Table 5–10). It is thought that these data are probably valid, since the graph by Smith et al.[169] correlated closely from 15 to 30 weeks, deviating only by less than a millimeter at 15 weeks to no more than 3 mm at 30 weeks. More work is needed to confirm the work by McLeary et al.,[168] however, since, after 30 weeks, there is no confirmation of their results.

SUBARACHNOID CISTERNS

The fetal subarachnoid cisterns have been extensively studied throughout the second and third trimesters.[170] Visualization of the cisterns is variable. Some are more successfully identified in the second trimester, some in the third trimester, and some throughout both.[170] Knowledge of these cisterns is important so that their identification as normal fluid-filled spaces avoids the incorrect diagnosis of abnormality. In addition, if these cisterns are prominent and dilated ventricles are present, the diagnosis of communicating hydrocephalus can be suggested.[170]

Of particular importance is the large cistern of the posterior fossa, termed the cisterna magna. It is located caudad to the cerebellum, between the cerebellum and the base of the occipital bone. Images of this region are obtained in the same manner as that used to visualize the cerebellum. After obtaining the standard biparietal diameter image with the cavum septi pellucidi and thalamus as midline structures, the transducer is angled posteriorly and inferiorly (Fig 5–15,A).

Two articles evaluated the normal cisterna magna,[171, 172] one in number form

52 Second and Third Trimester Obstetrical Measurements

from 15 weeks to 36 weeks[172] and the other in graph form from 14 to 32 weeks.[171] It was noted that this cistern could be identified in greater than 90% of fetuses from 15 to 28 weeks.[172] After 29 and 33 weeks, respectively, the ability to image this region declined sharply to 58% and 33%.[172] Nevertheless, when imaged, the depth of the cisterna magna from the posterior aspect of the cerebellum to the occipital bone measured 5 mm in average diameter with a range of ±3 mm[172] (Fig 15–15,B). No cisterna magna measured more than 10 mm in size.[172] Although the graph by Smith et al.[171] tended to confirm these observations, it shows a 2 SD maximum of 15 mm in size at 30 weeks. It is not certain whether this was an actual measurement or, more probably, a calculated theoretical number.

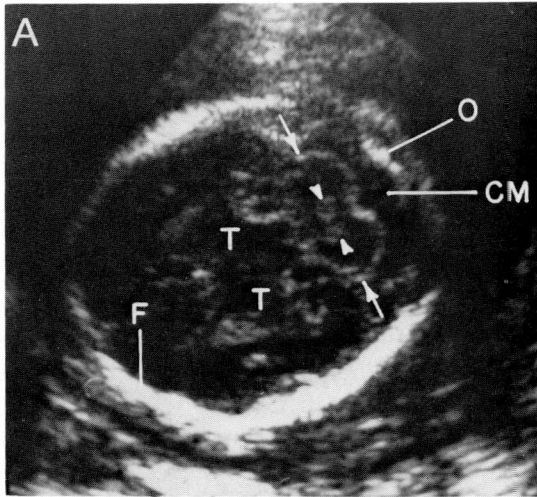

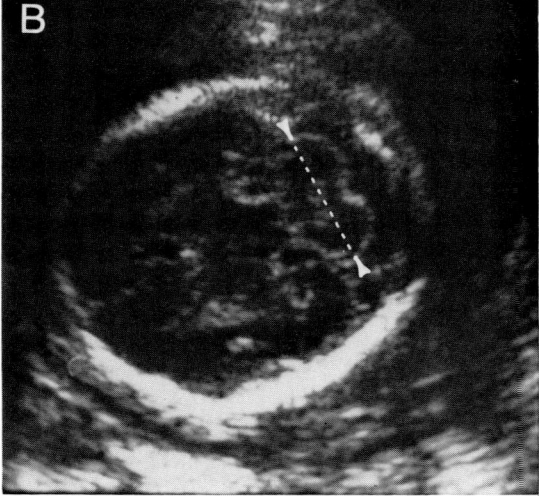

FIG 5–14.
Transaxial image of the fetal head at 30 weeks, rotated slightly posterior and inferior to image the cerebellum *(arrows).* **A,** cerebellum is located immediately posterior to the thalami *(T).* The hyperechoic midline cerebellar structure is the vermis *(arrowheads).* **B,** same image as **A** showing the transverse dimension of the cerebellum *(arrowheads* and *dotted line).* F indicates frontal bone; O, occipital bone; CM, cisterna magna.

TABLE 5–10.
Fetal Cerebellar Transverse Diameter Measurement Table*

Cerebellar Transverse Diameter, mm	Biparietal Diameter, mm	
	Predicted Mean Value	Range of 16%–84%, 1SD
15	34.7	31.5–38.0
16	37.2	34.0–40.6
17	39.8	36.4–43.2
18	42.2	38.8–45.7
19	44.6	41.1–48.1
20	46.9	43.4–50.5
21	49.2	45.6–52.8
22	51.4	47.8–55.0
23	53.5	49.9–57.2
24	55.6	51.9–59.3
25	57.6	53.9–61.3
26	59.5	55.8–63.3
27	61.5	57.7–65.2
28	63.3	59.5–67.1
29	65.1	61.3–68.8
30	66.8	63.0–70.6
31	68.4	64.7–72.2
32	70.0	66.3–73.8
33	71.6	67.8–75.3
34	73.0	69.3–76.8
35	74.4	70.7–78.2
36	75.8	72.1–79.5
37	77.1	73.4–80.8
38	78.3	74.4–82.0
39	79.5	75.9–83.1
40	80.6	77.0–84.2
41	81.7	78.1–85.2
42	82.6	79.1–86.2
43	83.6	80.1–87.1
44	84.4	81.0–87.9
45	85.3	81.9–88.6
46	86.0	82.7–89.3
47	86.7	83.5–89.9
48	87.3	84.2–90.5
49	87.9	84.8–91.0

(Continued.)

TABLE 5–10 (cont.).

Cerebellar Transverse Diameter, mm	Biparietal Diameter, mm	
	Predicted Mean Value	Range of 16%–84%, 1SD
50	88.4	85.4–91.4
51	88.8	85.9–91.8
52	89.2	86.4–92.1
53	89.6	86.8–92.3
54	89.8	87.2–92.5

*From McLeary RD, Kuhns LR, Barr M, Jr: Ultrasonography of the fetal cerebellum. *Radiology* 1984; 151:439–442. Used by permission.

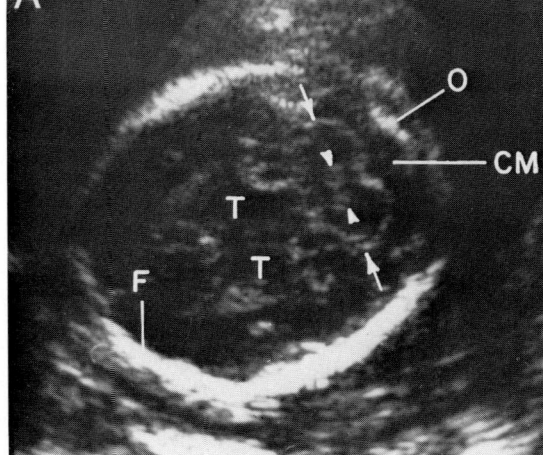

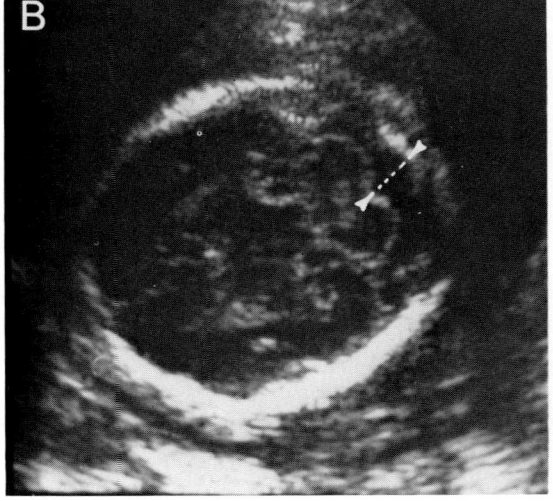

FIG 5–15.
Transaxial image of the fetal head at 30 weeks, rotated slightly posterior and inferior to image the cerebellum *(arrows)* and the cisterna magna *(CM)*. **A,** cisterna magna is located immediately posterior to the cerebellum, between it and the occipital bone *(O)*. **B,** same image as A showing the depth of the cisterna magna *(arrowheads* and *dotted line)*. F indicates frontal bone; *T,* thalami; *arrowheads,* vermis of cerebellum.

The value of both imaging and measuring the cisterna magna is important, since it can be used to detect and confirm posterior fossa abnormalities. Cerebellar hypoplasia, communicating hydrocephalus, and Dandy Walker cysts could enlarge this space.[172, 173] Conversely, if the cisterna magna cannot be imaged or is less than 2 mm, especially prior to 28 weeks, this would suggest a spina abnormality with secondary Arnold-Chiari type II malformation.[172] It must be emphasized, though, that a prominent cisterna magna without any other findings might also be a normal variant.[172]

REFERENCES

Biparietal Diameter
1. Durkan JP, Russo GL: Ultrasonic fetal cephalometry: Accuracy, limitations, and applications. *Obstet Gynecol* 1966; 27:399–403.
2. Willocks J, Donald I, Duggan TC, et al: Fetal cephalometry by ultrasound. *J Obstet Gynaecol Br Commonwealth* 1964; 71:11–20.
3. Kohorn EI: An evaluation of ultrasonic fetal cephalometry. *Am J Obstet Gynecol* 1967; 97:553–559.
4. Taylor ES, Holmes JH, Thompson HE, et al: Ultrasound diagnostic techniques in obstetrics and gynecology. *Am J Obstet Gynecol* 1964; 90:655–671.
5. Campbell S: Ultrasonic fetal cephalometry during the second trimester of pregnancy. *J Obstet Gynecol Br Commonwealth* 1970; 77:1057–1063.
6. Sabbagha RE: Assessment of differences in sonar biparietal diameter values regarding fetal age and weight. *J Clin Ultrasound* 1973; 1:68–74.
7. Hohler CW, Inglis J, Collins H, et al: Ultrasound biparietal diameter: Defining relationships in normal pregnancy. *NY State J Med* 1976; 76:373–376.
8. Hern WA: Correlation of fetal age and measurements between 10 and 26 weeks of gestation. *Obstet Gynecol* 1984; 63:26–32.
9. Lunt RM, Chard L: Reproducibility of measurement of fetal biparietal diameter by ultrasonic cephalometry. *J Obstet Gynaecol Br Commonwealth* 1974; 81:682–685.
10. Davison JM, Lind T, Farr V, et al: The limitations of ultrasonic fetal cephalometry. *J Obstet Gynaecol Br Commonwealth* 1981; 80:769–775.
11. Docker MF, Settatree RS: Comparison between linear array real time ultrasonic scanning and conventional compound scanning in the measurement of the fetal biparietal diameter. *Br J Obstet Gynaecol* 1977; 84:924–929.
12. Levi S, Smets P: Intra-uterine fetal growth studied by ultrasonic biparietal measurements: The percentiles of biparietal distribution. *Acta Obstet Gynecol Scand* 1973; 52:193–198.
13. Cooperberg PL, Chow T, Kite V, et al: Biparietal diameter: A comparison of real time and conventional B-scan techniques. *J Clin Ultrasound* 1976; 4:421–423.
14. Fescina RH, Ucieda FJ: Reliability of fetal anthropometry by ultrasound. *J Perinatal Med* 1980; 8:93–98.
15. Watmough D, Crippin D, Mallard JR: A critical assessment of ultrasonic fetal cephalometry. *Br J Radiol* 1974; 47:24–33.
16. Johnson ML, Dunne MG, Mack LA, et al: Evaluation of fetal intracranial anatomy by static and real-time ultrasound. *J Clin Ultrasound* 1980; 8:311–318.
17. Shepard M, Filly RA: A standardized plane for biparietal diameter measurement. *J Ultrasound Med* 1982; 1:145–150.
18. Hadlock FP, Deter RL, Harrist RB, et al: Fetal biparietal diameter: Rational choice of plane of section for sonographic measurement. *AJR* 1982; 138:871–874.
19. Hughey M, Sabbagha RE: Cephalometry by real-time imaging: A critical evaluation. *Am J Obstet Gynecol* 1978; 131:825–830.

20. Drumm JE: The prediction of delivery date by ultrasonic measurement of fetal crown-rump length. *Br J Obstet Gynecol* 1977; 84:1–5.
21. Campbell S, Warsof SL, Little D, et al: Routine ultrasound screening for the prediction of gestational age. *Obstet Gynecol* 1985; 65:613–620.
22. Smazal SF, Weisman LE, Hoppler KD, et al: Comparative analysis of ultrasonographic methods of gestational age assessment. *J Ultrasound Med* 1983; 2:147–150.
23. Kopta MM, May RR, Crane JP: A comparison of the reliability of the estimated date of confinement predicted by crown-rump length and biparietal diameter. *Am J Obstet Gynecol* 1983; 145:562–565.
24. Campbell S: The prediction of fetal maturity by ultrasonic measurement of the biparietal diameter. *J Obstet Gynecol Br Commonwealth* 1969; 76:603–609.
25. Sabbagha RE, Turner H, Rockett H, et al: Sonar BPD and fetal age: Definition of the relationship. *Obstet Gynecol* 1974; 43:7–14.
26. Campbell S, Newman GB: Growth of the fetal biparietal diameter during normal pregnancy. *J Obstet Gynaeol Br Commonwealth* 1971; 78:518–519.
27. Sabbagha RE, Hughey M: Standardization of sonar cephalometry and gestational age. *Obstet Gynecol* 1978; 52:402–406.
28. Wiener SN, Flynn MJ, Kennedy AW, et al: A composite curve of ultrasonic biparietal diameters for estimating gestational age. *Radiology* 1977; 122:781–786.
29. Kurtz AB, Wapner RJ, Kurtz RJ, et al: Analysis of biparietal diameter as an accurate indicator of gestational age. *J Clin Ultrasound* 1980; 8:319–326.
30. Levi S, Erbsman F: Antenatal fetal growth from the nineteenth week: Ultrasonic study of 12 head and chest dimensions. *Am J Obstet Gynecol* 1975; 121:262–268.
31. Weinraub Z, Schneider D, Langer R, et al: Ultrasonographic measurement of fetal growth parameters for estimation of gestational age and fetal weight. *Isr J Med Sci* 1979; 15:829–832.
32. Hellman LF, Kobayashi M, Fillisti L, et al: Growth and development of the human fetus prior to the twentieth week of gestation. *Am J Obstet Gynecol* 1969; 103:784–800.
33. Hoffbauer H: The importance of ultrasonic diagnosis in early pregnancy. *Electromedia* 1970; 3:227–230.
34. Piiroinen O: Studies in diagnostic ultrasound. *Acta Obstet Gynecol Scand [Suppl]* 1975; 55:1–60.
35. Hoffbauer H, Pachaly J, Arabin B, et al: Control of fetal development with multiple ultrasonic body measures. *Contrib Gynecol Obstet* 1979; 6:147–156.
36. Hadlock FP, Deter RL, Harrist RB, et al: Fetal biparietal diameter: A critical re-evaluation of the relation to menstrual age by means of real-time ultrasound. *J Ultrasound Med* 1982; 1:97–104.
37. Wladimiroff JW, Bloemsma CA, Wallenburg HCS: Ultrasonic assessment of fetal head and body sizes in relation to normal and retarded fetal growth. *Am J Obstet Gynecol* 1978; 131:857–860.
38. Wladimiroff JW, Bloemsma CA, Wallenburg HCS: Ultrasonic diagnosis of the large-for-dates infant. *Obstet Gynecol* 1978; 52:285–288.
39. Varma TR: Prediction of delivery date by ultrasound cephalometry. *J Obstet Gynaecol Br Commonwealth* 1973; 80:316–319.
40. Brown RE: *Ultrasonography: Basic Principles and Clinical Applications.* St Louis, Warren H Green Inc, 1975, p 116.
41. Winsberg F: Personal communications, in *Ultrasonography in Obstetrics and Gynecology.* Baltimore, Williams & Wilkins, 1979, p 165.
42. Lee BO, Major FJ, Weingold AB: Ultrasonic determination of fetal maturity at repeat cesarean section. *Obstet Gynecol* 1971; 38:294–297.
43. Hibbard LT, Anderson GV: Clinical applications of ultrasonic fetal cephalometry. *Obstet Gynecol* 1967; 29(6):842–847.

44. Hansmann M: A critical evaluation of the performance of ultrasonic diagnosis in present-day obstetrics. *Gynakologe* 1974; 7:26–35.
45. Aantaa K, Forss M: Determination of biparietal diameter by the ultrasonic b-scan technique. *Acta Obstet Gynecol Scand* 1974; 53:121–124.
46. Hassani SN: *Ultrasound in Gynecology and Obstetrics*. New York, Springer-Verlag, 1979, pp 91–92.
47. Hobbins JC; *Yale Nomogram*. Iselin, NJ, Seimens Corporation, Electro Medical Division, 1979.
48. Flamme P: Ultrasonic fetal cephalometry: Percentiles curve. *Br Med J* 1972; 3:384–385.
49. Yiu-Chiu V, Chiu L: Ultrasonographic evaluation of normal fetal anatomy and congenital malformations. *J Comput Tomogr* 1981; 5:367–381; 508–509.
50. Persson PH, Grennert L, Gennser G, et al: Normal range curves for the intrauterine growth of the biparietal diameter. *Acta Obstet Gynecol Scand* 1978; 78:15–20.
51. Fescina RH, Ucieda FJ, Cordano MC, et al: Ultrasonic patterns of intrauterine fetal growth in a Latin American country. *Early Hum Dev* 1982; 6:239–248.
52. Garrett W, Robinson D: Assessment of fetal size and growth rate by ultrasonic echoscopy. *Obstet Gynecol* 1979; 38:525–534.
53. Eriksen PS, Secher NJ, Weis-Bentzon M: Normal growth of the fetal biparietal diameter and the abdominal diameter in a longitudinal study. *Acta Obstet Gynecol Scand* 1985; 64:65–70.
54. Jeanty P, Cousaert E, Hobbins JC, et al: A longitudinal study of fetal head biometry. *Am J Perinat* 1984; 1:118–128.
55. Chervenak FA, Jeanty P, Cantraine F, et al: The diagnosis of fetal microcephaly. *Am J Obstet Gynecol* 1984; 149:512–517.
56. Osefo NJ, Chukudebelu WO: Sonar cephalometry and fetal age relationship in the Nigerian woman. *East Afr Med J* 1983; Feb:pp 98–102.
57. Oman SD, Wax Y: Estimating fetal age by ultrasound measurements: An example of multivariate calibration. *Biometrics* 1984; 40:947–960.
58. Sanders M: Personal communications, 1979. Sabaggha RE, Barton FA, Barton, BA: Sonar biparietal diameter: I. Analysis of percentile growth differences in two normal populations using same methodology. *Am J Obstet Gynecol* 1976; 126:479–484.
59. Yagel S, Adoni A, Oman S, et al: A statistical examination of the accuracy of combining femoral length and biparietal diameter as an index of fetal gestational age. *Br J Obstet Gynaecol* 1986; 93:109–115.
60. Persson PH, Weldner BM: Normal range growth curves for fetal biparietal diameter, occipito frontal diameter, mean abdominal diameters and femur length. *Acta Obstet Gynecol Scand* 1986; 65:759–761.
61. Kossoff G, Garrett WJ, Radovanovich G: Grey scale echography in obstetrics and gynaecology. *Australas Radiol* 1974; 18:63–111.
62. Deter RL, Harrist RB, Hadlock FP, et al: Longitudinal studies of fetal growth with the use of dynamic image ultrasonography. *Am J Obstet Gynecol* 1982; 143:545–554.
63. Thompson HE, Holmes JH, Gottesfeld KR, et al: Fetal development as determined by ultrasonic pulse echo techniques. *Am J Obstet Gynecol* 1965; 92:44–52.
64. Campbell S, Dewhurts CJ: Diagnosis of the small-for-dates fetus by serial ultrasonic cephalometry. *Lancet* 1971; 2:1002–1006.
65. Willocks J, Dunsmore IR: Assessment of gestational age and prediction of dysmaturity by ultrasonic fetal cephalometry. *J Obstet Gynaecol Br Commonwealth* 1971; 78:804–808.
66. Bartolucci L: Biparietal diameter of the skull and fetal weight in the second trimester: An allometric relationship. *Am J Obstet Gynecol* 1975; 122:439–445.

67. Willocks J: The study of fetal growth by serial cephalometry and estriol measurements. *J Reprod Med* 1971; 6:84–88.
68. Queenan JT, Kubarych SF, Cook LN, et al: Diagnostic ultrasound for detection of intrauterine growth retardation. *Am J Obstet Gynecol* 1976; 124:865–873.
69. Chapman MG, Sheat JH, Furness ET, et al: Routine ultrasound screening in early pregnancy. *Med J Aust* 1979; 2:62–63.
70. Issel EP, Prenzlau P, Bayer H, et al: The measurement of fetal growth during pregnancy by ultrasound (b-scan). *J Perinatal Med* 1975; 3:269–275.
71. Aantaa K, Forss M: Growth of the fetal biparietal diameter in different types of pregnancies. *Radiology* 1980; 137:167–169.
72. Ogata ES, Sabbagha R, Metzger BE, et al: Serial ultrasonography to assess evolving fetal macrosomia: Studies in 23 pregnancy diabetic women. *JAMA* 1980; 243:2405–2408.
73. Ojala A, Ylostalo P, Jouppila P, et al: Fetal cephalometry by ultrasound in normal and complicated pregnancy. *Ann Chir Gynaecol Fenniae* 1970; 59:71–75.
74. Murata Y, Martin CB: Growth of the biparietal diameter of the fetal head in diabetic pregnancy. *Am J Obstet Gynecol* 1973; 115:252–256.
75. Pap G, Pap L: Ultrasonic estimation of gestational age and fetal weight. *Paediatr Acad Sci Hung* 1979; 20:119–135.
76. Pap G, Szoke J, Pap L: Intrauterine growth retardation: Ultrasonic diagnosis. *Acta Paediatr Hung* 1983; 24:7–15.
77. Parker AJ, Davies P, Mayho AM, et al: The ultrasound estimation of sex-related variations of intrauterine growth. *Am J Obstet Gynecol* 1984; 149:665–669.
78. Walton SM: Ethnic considerations in ultrasonic scanning of fetal biparietal diameters. *Aust NZ J Obstet Gynaecol* 1981; 21:82–83.
79. Wittman BK, Robinson HP, Aitchison T, et al: The value of diagnostic ultrasound as a screening test for intrauterine growth retardation: Comparison of nine parameters. *Am J Obstet Gynecol* 1979; 134:30–35.
80. Jordaan HVF: Biological variation in the biparietal diameter and its bearing on clinical ultrasonography. *Am J Obstet Gynecol* 1978; 131:53–58.
81. Pedersen JF: Ultrasound evidence of sexual difference in fetal size in first trimester. *Br Med J* 1980; 281:1253.
82. Parker AJ: Assessment of gestational age of the Asian fetus by the sonar measurement of crown-rump length and biparietal diameter. *Br J Obstet Gynaecol* 1982; 89:836–838.
83. Dubowitz LMS, Goldberg C: Assessment of gestation by ultrasound in various stages of pregnancy in infants differing in size and ethnic origin. *Br J Obstet Gynaecol* 1981; 88:255–259.
84. Meire HB, Farrant P: Ultrasound demonstration of an unusual fetal growth pattern in Indians. *Br J Obstet Gynaecol* 1981; 88:260–263.
85. Okupe RF, Coker OO, Gbajumo SA: Assessment of fetal biparietal diameter during normal pregnancy by ultrasound in Nigerian women. *Br J Obstet Gynaecol* 1984; 91:629–632.
86. Munoz WP, Moore PJ, MacKinnon A, et al: Biparietal diameter and menstrual age in the black population attending Edendale Hospital. *J Clin Ultrasound* 1986; 14:681–688.
87. Sabbagha RE: *Ultrasound in High-Risk Obstetrics.* Philadelphia, Lea & Febiger, 1979, p 38.

Unusual Head Shape
88. Hadlock FP, Deter RL, Harrist RB, et al: Fetal biparietal diameter: Rational choice of plane of section for sonographic measurement. *AJR* 1982; 138:871–874.
89. Kossoff G, Garrett WJ, Radovanovich G: Grey scale echography in obstetrics and gynaecology. *Australas Radiol* 1974; 18:63–111.

90. Hoffbauer H, Pachaly J, Arabin B, et al: Control of fetal development with multiple ultrasonic body measures. *Contrib Gynecol Obstet* 1979; 6:147–156.
91. Levi S, Erbsman F: Antenatal fetal growth from the nineteenth week: Ultrasonic study of 12 head and chest dimension. *Am J Obstet Gynecol* 1975; 121:262–268.
92. Fescina RH, Ucieda FJ, Cordano MC, et al: Ultrasonic patterns of intrauterine fetal growth in a Latin American country. *Early Hum Dev* 1982; 6:239–248.
93. Garrett W, Robinson D: Assessment of fetal size and growth rate by ultrasonic echoscopy. *Obstet Gynecol* 1979; 38:525–534.
94. Jeanty P, Cousaert E, Hobbins JC, et al: A longitudinal study of fetal head biometry. *Am J Perinat* 1984; 1:118–128.
95. Chervenak FA, Jeanty P, Cantraine F, et al: The diagnosis of fetal microcephaly. *Am J Obstet Gynecol* 1984; 149:512–517.
96. Persson PH, Weldner BM: Normal range growth curves for fetal biparietal diameter, occipito frontal diameter, mean abdominal diameters and femur length. *Acta Obstet Gynecol Scand* 1986; 65:759–761.
97. Hansmann M: A critical evaluation of the performance of ultrasonic diagnosis in present-day obstetrics. *Gynakologe* 1974; 7:26–35.
98. Deter RL, Harrist RB, Hadlock FP, et al: The use of ultrasound in the assessment of normal fetal growth: A review. *J Clin Ultrasound* 1981; 9:481–493.
99. *Dorland's Illustrated Medical Dictionary*, ed 24. Philadelphia, WB Saunders Co, 1957, pp 217, 444.
100. Hastings Ince JG: On the value of cephalometry in the estimation of foetal weight: Based on measurements of 1010 infants. *J Obstet Gynaecol Br Emp* 1939; 46:1003–1009.
101. Jordaan HVF: The differential enlargement of the neurocranium in the full-term fetus. *S Afr Med J* 1976; 50:1978–1981.
102. Haas LL: Roentgenological skull measurements and their diagnostic applications. *AJR* 1952; 67:197–209.
103. Hadlock FP, Deter RL, Carpenter RJ, et al: Estimating fetal age: Effect of head shape on BPD. *AJR* 1981; 137:83–85.
104. Shields JR, Medearis AL, Bear MB: Fetal head and abdominal circumferences: Effect of profile shape on the accuracy of ellipse equations. *J Clin Ultrasound* 1987; 15:241–244.
105. Kasby CB, Poll V: The breech head and its ultrasound significance. *Br J Obstet Gynaecol* 1982; 89:106–110.
106. Wolfson RN, Zador IE, Halvorsen P, et al: Biparietal diameter in premature rupture of membranes: Errors in estimating gestational age. *J Clin Ultrasound* 1983; 11:371–374.
107. Doubilet PM, Greenes RA: Improved prediction of gestational age from fetal head measurements. *AJR* 1984; 142:797–800.

Head Circumference

108. Hadlock FP, Deter RL, Carpenter RJ, et al: Estimating fetal age: Effect of head shape on BPD. *AJR* 1981; 137:83–85.
109. Usher R, McLean F: Intrauterine growth of live-born Caucasian infants at sea level: Standards obtained from measurements in 7 dimensions of infants born between 25 and 44 weeks of gestation. *Pediatrics* 1969; 74:901–910.
110. Lubchenco LO, Hansmann C, Boyd E: Intrauterine growth in length and head circumference as estimated from live births at gestational ages from 26 to 42 weeks. *Pediatrics* 1966; 37:403–408.
111. Babson SG, Benda GI: Growth graphs for the clinical assessment of infants of varying gestational age. *Pediatrics* 1976; 89:814–820.
112. Gairdner D: Ultrasonic fetal cephalometry. *Br Med J* 1972; 3:585.
113. Hadlock FP, Kent WR, Loyd JL, et al: An evaluation of two methods for measur-

ing fetal heads and body circumferences. J Ultrasound Med 1982; 1:359–360.
114. Shields JR, Medearis AL, Bear MB: Fetal head and abdominal circumferences: Ellipse calculations versus planimetry. J Clin Ultrasound 1987; 15:237–239.
115. DeVore GR, Platt LD: Choosing the correct equation for computing the head circumference from two diameters: The effect of head shape. Am J Obstet Gynecol 1984; 148:221.
116. Birnholz JC: On calculating the perimeter of an ellipse. J Clin Ultrasound 1984; 12:55–56.
117. Shields JR, Medearis AL, Bear MB: Fetal head and abdominal circumferences: Effect of profile shape on the accuracy of ellipse equations. J Clin Ultrasound 1987; 15:241–244.
118. Hoffbauer H, Pachaly J, Arabin B, et al: Control of fetal development with multiple ultrasonic body measures. Contrib Gynecol Obstet 1979; 6:147–156.
119. Deter RL, Harrist RB, Hadlok FP, et al: Longitudinal studies of fetal growth with the use of dynamic image ultrasonography. Am J Obstet Gynecol 1982; 143:545–554.
120. Deter RL, Harrist RB, Hadlock FP, et al: The use of ultrasound in the assessment of normal fetal growth: A review. J Clin Ultrasound 1981; 9:481–493.
121. Levi S, Erbsman F: Antenatal fetal growth from the nineteenth week: Ultrasonic study of 12 head and chest dimensions. Am J Obstet Gynecol 1975; 121:262–268.
122. Weinraub Z, Shneider D, Langer R, et al: Ultrasonographic measurement of fetal growth parameters for estimation of gestational age and fetal weight. Isr J Med Sci 1979; 15:829–832.
123. Fescina RH, Ucieda FJ, Cordano MC, et al: Ultrasonic patterns of intrauterine fetal growth in a Latin American country. Early Hum Dev 1982; 6:239–248.
124. Jeanty P, Cousaert E, Hobbins JC, et al: A longitudinal study of fetal head biometry. Am J Perinat 1984; 1:118–128.
125. Chervenak FA, Jeanty P, Cantraine F, et al: The diagnosis of fetal microcephaly. Am J Obstet Gynecol 1984; 149:512–517.
126. Parker AJ, Davies P, Mayho AM, et al: The ultrasound estimation of sex-related variations of intrauterine growth. Am J Obstet Gynecol 1984; 149:665–669.
127. Campbell S, Thoms A: Personal communications. Fetal head circumference against gestational age, in Metrewelli Practical Clinical Ultrasound, Chicago, 1978, p 114.
128. Athey PA, Hadlock FP, in Harshberger SE (ed): Ultrasound in Obstetrics and Gynecology. St Louis, CV Mosby, 1981, p 269.
129. Hadlock FP, Deter RL, Harrist RB, et al: Fetal head circumference: Relation to menstrual age. AJR 1982; 138:649–653.
130. Deter RL, Harrist RB, Hadlock FP, et al: Fetal head and abdominal circumferences: II. A critical reevaluation of the relationship to menstrual age. J Clin Ultrasound 1982; 10:365–372.
131. Fescina RH, Martell M: Intrauterine and extrauterine growth of cranial perimeter in term and preterm infants. Am J Obstet Gynecol 1983; 147:928–932.
132. Ott WJ: The use of ultrasonic fetal head circumference for predicting expected date of confinement. J Clin Ultrasound 1984; 12:411–415.
133. van Egmond-Linden A, Wladimiroff JW, Niermeijer MF, et al: Fetal hydrocephaly: Diagnosis, prognosis and management. Ultrasound Med Biol 1986; 12:939–944.
134. Deter RL, Harrist, RB, Hadlock FP, Carpenter RJ; Fetal head and abdominal circumferences: I. Evaluation of measurement errors. J Clin Ultrasound 1982; 10:357–363.
135. Crane JP, Kopta MM: Prediction of intrauterine growth retardation via ultrasonically measured head/abdominal circumference ratios. Obstet Gynecol 1979; 54:597–601.

136. Law RG, MacRae KD: Head circumference as an index of fetal age. *J Ultrasound Med* 1982; 1:281–288.

Head Area

137. Kossoff G, Garrett WJ, Radovanovich G: Grey scale echography in obstetrics and gynaecology. *Australas Radiol* 1974; 18:63–111.
138. Levi S, Erbsman F: Antenatal fetal growth from the nineteenth week: Ultrasonic study of 12 head and chest dimensions. *Am J Obstet Gynecol* 1975; 121:262–268.
139. Weinraub Z, Schneider D, Langer R, et al: Ultrasonographic measurement of fetal growth parameters for estimation of gestational age and fetal weight. *Isr J Med Sci* 1979; 15:829–832.
140. Fescina RH, Ucieda FJ, Cordan MC, et al: Ultrasonic patterns of intrauterine fetal growth in a Latin American country. *Early Hum Dev* 1982; 6:239–248.
141. Garrett W, Robinson D: Assessment of fetal size and growth rate by ultrasonic echoscopy. *Obstet Gynecol* 1979; 38:525–534.
142. Wladimiroff JW, Bloemsma CA, Wallenburg HCS: Ultrasonic assessment of fetal growth. *Acta Obstet Gynecol Scand* 1977; 56:37–42.
143. Varma TR, Taylor H, Bridges C: Ultrasound assessment of fetal growth. *Br J Obstet Gynecol* 1979; 86:623–632.
144. Rossavik IK, Deter RL, Hadlock FP: Mathematical modeling of fetal growth: III. Evaluation of head growth using the head profile area. *J Clin Ultrasound* 1987; 15:23–30.

Head Volume

145. Marinez DA, Barton JL: Estimation of fetal body and fetal head volumes: Description of technique and nomograms for 18 to 41 weeks of gestation. *Am J Obstet Gynecol* 1980; 137:78–84.
146. Rossavik IK, Deter RL: Mathematical modeling of fetal growth: I. Basic principles. *J Clin Ultrasound* 1984; 12:529–533.
147. Rossavik IK, Deter RL: Mathematical modeling of fetal growth: II. Head cube (A), abdominal cube (B) and their ratio (A/B). *J Clin Ultrasound* 1984; 12:535–545.
148. DuBose TJ: Fetal biometry: Vertical calvarial diameter and calvarial volume. *J Diagn Med Sonogr* 1985; 1:205–217.
149. O'Keeffe DF, Garite TJ, Elliott JP, et al: The accuracy of estimated gestational age based on ultrasound measurement of biparietal diameter in preterm premature rupture of membranes. *Am J Obstet Gynecol* 1985; 151:309–312.

Ventricular Size

150. Hanson J, Levander B, Liliequist B: Size of the intracerebral ventricles as measured with computer tomography, encephalography and echoventriculography. *Acta Radiol [Suppl] (Stockh)* 1975; 346:98–106.
151. Skolnick ML, Rosenbaum AE, Matzuk T, et al: Detection of dilated cerebral ventricles in infants: A correlative study between ultrasound and computed tomography. *Radiology* 1979; 131:447–451.
152. Johnson ML, Dunne MG, Mack LA, et al: Evaluation of fetal intracranial anatomy by static and real-time ultrasound. *J Clin Ultrasound* 1980; 8:311–318.
153. vanEgmond-Linden A, Wladimiroff JW, Niermeijer MF, et al: Fetal hydrocephaly: Diagnosis, prognosis and management. *Ultrasound Med Biol* 1986; 12:939–944.
154. Jeanty P, Dramaix-Wilmet M, Delbeke D, et al: Ultrasonic evaluation of fetal ventricular growth. *Neuroradiology* 1981; 21:127–131.
155. Hadlock FP, Deter RL, Park SK: Real-time sonography: Ventricular and vascular anatomy of the fetal brain in utero. *Am J Neuroradiol* 1980; 1:507–511.
156. McGahan JP, Phillips HE: Ultrasonic evaluation of the size of the trigone and the fetal ventricle. *J Ultrasound Med* 1983; 2:315–319.
157. Denkhaus H, Winsberg F: Ultrasonic measurement of the fetal ventricular system. *Radiology* 1979; 131:781–787.

158. Jorgensen C, Ingemarsson I, Svalenius E, et al: Ultrasound measurement of the fetal cerebral ventricles: A prospective, consecutive study. *J Clin Ultrasound* 1986; 14:185–190.
159. Pretorius DH, Drose JA, Manco-Johnson ML: Fetal lateral ventricular ratio determination during the second trimester. *J Ultrasound Med* 1986; 5:121–124.
160. Johnson ML, Mack LA, Rumack CM, et al: B-mode echoencephalography in the normal and high risk infant. *AJR* 1979; 133:375–381.
161. Chinn DH, Callen PW, Filly RA: The lateral cerebral ventricle in early second trimester. *Radiology* 1983; 148:529–531.

Ocular Dimensions

162. Benacerraf BR, Frigoletto FD Jr, Bieber FR: The fetal face: Ultrasound examination. *Radiology* 1984; 153:495–497.
163. Birnholz JC: Ultrasonic fetal ophthalmology. *Early Hum Dev* 1985; 12:199–209.
164. Jeanty P, Dramaix-Wilmet M, Van Gansbeke N, et al: Fetal ocular biometry by ultrasound. *Radiology* 1982; 143:513–516.

Orbital Dimensions

165. Jeanty P, Dramaix-Wilmet M, Van Gansbeke N, et al: Fetal ocular biometry by ultrasound. *Radiology* 1982; 143:513–516.
166. Jeanty P, Cantraine F, Cousaert E, et al: The binocular distance: A new way to estimate fetal age. *J Ultrasound Med* 1984; 3:241–243.
167. Mayden KL, Tortora M, Berkowitz RL, et al: Orbital diameters: A new parameter for prenatal diagnosis and dating. *Am J Obstet Gynecol* 1982; 144:289–297.

Cerebellar Dimensions

168. McLeary RD, Kuhns LR, Barr M Jr: Ultrasonography of the fetal cerebellum. *Radiology* 1984; 151:439–442.
169. Smith PA, Johansson D, Tzannatos C, et al: Prenatal measurement of the fetal cerebellum and cisterna cerebellomedullaris by ultrasound. *Prenat Diagn* 1986; 6:133–141.

Subarachnoid Cisterns

170. Pilu G, DePalma L, Romero R, et al: The fetal subarachnoid cisterns: An ultrasound study with report of a case of congenital communicating hydrocephalus. *J Ultrasound Med* 1986; 5:365–372.
171. Smith PA, Johansson D, Tzannatos C, et al: Prenatal measurement of the fetal cerebellum and cisterna cerebellomedullaris by ultrasound. *Prenat Diagn* 1986; 6:133–141.
172. Mahony BS, Callen PA, Filly RA, et al: The fetal cisterna magna. *Radiology* 1984; 153:773–776.
173. Comstock CH, Boal DB: Enlarged fetal cisterna magna: Appearance and significance. *Obstet Gynecol* 1985; 66(suppl):25S–28S.

Chapter 6

Fetal Body Measurements

THORACIC DIAMETER

Seven articles have measured the thoracic diameter, comparing it to gestational age,[1-7] three throughout the second and third trimesters[1, 4, 5] and the others from 21 weeks or beyond to term. Measurements have been obtained from static scanners in five,[1-4, 7] three giving actual numbers,[1, 2, 7] with one in graph[4] and one in equation[3] form. The other two[5, 6] used real-time scanners, both in graph form. All showed an increase in thoracic diameter with increasing gestational age.

Six of the articles obtained thoracic measurements in the transaxial projection at the region of cardiac motion or just above the diaphragm,[2-7] three with SD.[2, 4, 5] In the last article,[1] the thoracic diameter was obtained from a long axis view of the fetus. Since the exact internal anatomical landmarks and the points of measurement were not mentioned, this article will not be considered further. The AP dimension was measured in four articles,[2-4, 7] with four measuring the transaxial diameter.[2, 5-7] Only 3 specifically stated that the thoracic measurements were taken outer to outer edge.[2, 5, 6]

The results of these measurements are diverse. The AP dimensions varied among the articles by 6 mm at 24 weeks to 12 mm at term, while the transaxial diameters varied by as much as 20 mm throughout gestation. Because of these discrepancies, it is thought that the thoracic diameter measurements are not accurate enough to be routinely used. The abdominal measurements, on the other hand, have been much more extensively evaluated, have at least the same or smaller standard deviations, and are therefore recommended instead.

THORACIC CIRCUMFERENCE

Five articles have compared thoracic circumference to gestation age,[1-3, 7, 8] 1 from 12 to 40 weeks,[1] 3 from 20 weeks to post-term,[2, 7, 8] and 1 from 32 weeks to term.[3] Three[1, 2, 7] presented their data in number form, with the other two using equations[3] on graphs[8] instead. Two[2, 8] also gave standard deviations. All except one[8] were evaluated with static scanners, all giving numbers that increased with increasing gestational age. Four[2, 3, 7, 8] measured the circumference in transaxial projection at the region of cardiac motion from the outer limits of the thoracic cage. The last article[1] measured the fetus in long axis. This article failed to state at what level the measurements were obtained and whether the outer margins were used.

When the numbers were compared, it was found that Weinraub et al.,[3] Hansmann,[7] and Nimrod et al.[8] had numbers uniformly below the other two by 5–7 mm at every gestational age. The Levi and Erbsman[2] and Hoffbauer[1] articles were fairly close, from 22 to 32 weeks, but after that time diverged, until at term the Hoffbauer[1] measurements were 2.5 mm larger.

When all of these articles were then compared to the newborn measurements of Usher and McLean,[9] none was close. It is therefore thought that the thoracic circumference does not have enough data or close enough grouping to be used in clinical practice. The abdominal measurements have been more widely evaluated, appear to have at least the same, if not smaller, standard deviations and are recommended instead.

THORACIC AREA

Six articles have measured the thoracic area, comparing it to gestational age.[10–15] One was in number form,[11] one as an equation,[12] 2 in number and graph form,[13, 14] and the other 2 in graph form alone.[10, 15] An additional article by Wladimiroff et al.[16] published a graph of the thoracic area which appears identical to a graph in another of his articles[13] and will not be discussed further.

All data were obtained on static scanners. The measurements started from either the mid–second trimester[11, 13] or the early third trimester[10, 12, 14, 15] and continued until term, all showing increase in thoracic area with increasing gestational age. Five of these articles stated the exact anatomical position used to obtain the measurements,[11–15] two at the level of the heart[11, 12, 15] and two below the cardiac pulsations.[13, 14] This latter position, below the cardiac pulsations, while termed thoracic, is more likely to be in the upper abdomen. These two articles[13, 14] will therefore be analyzed in both the thoracic area and abdominal area sections. All used a planimeter or map reader to obtain area measurements. While only one stated that the outer margins of the thoracic cage were measured,[11] even that article failed to state exactly where the measurements were obtained and actually referred to the thoracic area as a "trunk" measurement.

The thoracic area numbers were quite discrepant and no definite pattern could be established. Surprisingly, even the numbers from the two articles by Wladimiroff[13, 14] were divergent. Because no definite trend could be established, it is thought that the thoracic area measurement should not be used routinely.

ABDOMINAL DIAMETER

Eight articles have measured the diameter of the fetal abdomen,[17–24] five in number form,[17, 19, 21, 22, 24] one as a graph,[23] and one in equation form.[18] All showed an increase in the abdominal diameter with increasing gestational age.

Hoffbauer et al.[17] evaluated the transverse abdominal diameter throughout the second and third trimesters in both the "small and large" dimensions (presumably AP and transverse). Neither the part of the abdomen nor the abdominal boundaries used to take these measurements were described. Weinraub et al.[18] measured the AP diameter of the abdomen but failed to mention the exact anatomical position used and whether the measurements were taken outer to outer diameter. Garrett and Robinson[20] evaluated the fetal abdominal diameter from 23 to 36 weeks, measuring the transaxial abdominal diameter at the area above the kidney and below the heart, which is in the region of the liver, presumably outer to outer diameter. Because of these inconsistencies, these three articles will not be considered further.

Of the remaining five articles,[19, 21-24] Fescina et al.[19] evaluated the AP and transverse diameters, Grandjean et al.[23] the transverse diameter, and Eriksen et al.,[21] Persson and Weldner,[22] and Tamura et al.[24] averaged the two diameters perpendicular to each other, all at the level of the umbilical vein from early second trimester to term. While the umbilical vein is a reproducible landmark, it is only valid if imaged within the liver, not extending to the anterior abdominal wall and equidistant from the right and left sides of the abdomen (Fig 6–1,A). In that position it is termed the umbilical portion of the left portal vein. All measurements should then be taken outer to outer margins since there is not a reproducible inner margin. If the body is round, only one measurement needs to be taken (Fig 6–1,B). If the body is ovoid, however, two measurements perpendicular to each other (preferable transverse and AP) are averaged (Fig 6–2).

Four of these five articles were precise in their anatomical position and in their outer to outer measurements,[21-24] while the fifth was vague in its description of the umbilical vein position and the margins used.[19] When their numbers were compared, the Grandjean et al.[23] numbers tapered off after 35 weeks, and Fescina et al.[19] did not give a standard deviation with the mean. These latter two articles[19, 23] therefore will also not be considered further.

The remaining three articles by Eriksen et al.,[21] Persson and Weldner,[22] and Tamura et al.[24] had closely grouped mean numbers, and all gave a standard deviation range. They all compared their measurements to the gestational age; two were longitudinal studies, one examining their patients every 2 to 4 weeks[21] or triweekly.[22] The third study was a cross-sectional analysis.[24] In addition, all showed a close one-to-one relationship (in millimeters) to the biparietal diameter until approximately 30 weeks, the biparietal measurements taken from either their own article[21] or compared to the table of Kurtz et al.[25] In the last trimester, all revealed an increase in body size to 15 mm or more greater than the biparietal diameter by term.

The major differences among these three articles[21, 22, 24] was that Tamura et al.[24] compared their measurements only to gestational age, while Eriksen et al.[21] and Persson and Weldner[22] compared the mean abdominal measurements to both biparietal diameter and gestational age. This latter approach has more clinical usefulness. Therefore, Eriksen et al.[21] and Persson and Weldner[22] are the two preferable studies, and either would suffice for appropriate mean abdominal diameter measurements. The only difference in the two articles[21, 22] is that the Eriksen et al.[21] article was performed using approximately twice the number of measurements. Because of their larger numbers, the standard deviation of this article would be expected to be smaller. It is not. While this find-

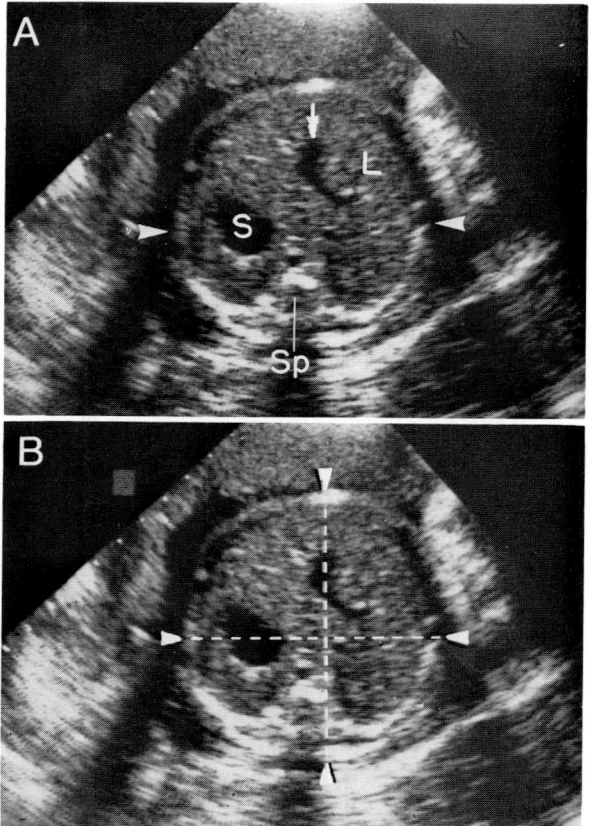

FIG 6–1.
Transaxial scan of the upper fetal abdomen in a 30-week fetus. **A,** round abdomen with the umbilical portion of the left portal vein *(arrow)* positioned within the liver *(L)*, not extending to the anterior abdominal wall and equidistant from the lateral abdominal walls *(arrowheads)*. S indicates stomach; *Sp,* spine. **B,** same image as **A** showing the outer diameter measurements, denoted by arrowheads and dotted lines. The two lines are perpendicular to each other, one anteroposterior (AP) and the other transverse. Since the body is round, only one of the two is needed for an adequate abdominal diameter measurement.

ing is puzzling, the table by Eriksen et al.[21] is nevertheless recommended (Table 6–1).

ABDOMINAL CIRCUMFERENCE

Abdominal circumference measurements, initially used in the evaluation of the newborn,[26] now have been used extensively in utero. In two articles comparing the accuracies of prenatal and postnatal ultrasound abdominal circumferences,[27, 28] the measurements were found to correlate closely with errors of no greater than 6%. This percentage is misleading, however, since in one article[27] the prenatal measurements were always 6% greater, while in the other[28] the fetal measurements were both higher and lower. These inaccuracies contrast sharply with the higher correlation of prenatal and postnatal head circumference measurements. At least part of this inaccuracy is technical, since: (1) the neonatal abdominal circumference measurement is taken only during expiration, whereas the respiration phase of the fetus could not be determined;[28] (2) in obtaining the neonatal measurements, there can be slight tightening or relaxing of the measurement tape, resulting in neonatal measurement discrepancies of 5 to 10 mm;[28] and (3) the newborn measurements are taken in the mid-abdomen at the level of the umbilicus,[27] while fetal abdominal measurements are obtained higher at the level of the fetal liver.[27, 29]

Despite these discrepancies, there have been 15 *in utero* analyses of abdominal circumference in 16 articles.[28-43] Of these, while Campbell and Wilkin[41] initially presented their data in graph form, their numbers were published by

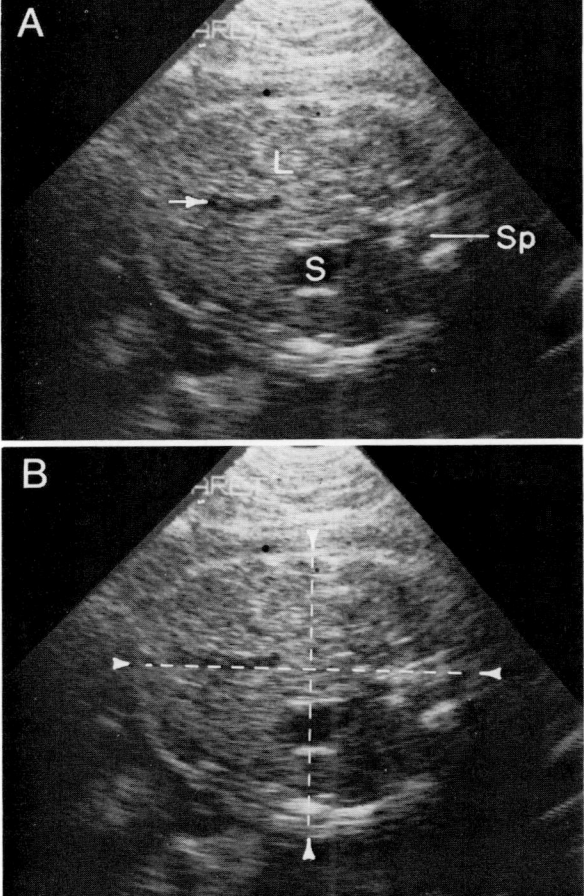

FIG 6–2.
Transaxial scan of the upper abdomen in a 32-week fetus with oligohydramnios. **A,** ovoid abdomen with the umbilical portion of the left portal vein *(arrow)* positioned within the liver *(L)* equidistant from the lateral abdominal walls. S indicates stomach; *Sp,* spine. **B,** same image as **A** showing the outer diameter measurements perpendicular to one another *(arrowheads* and *dotted lines).* Since the body is ovoid, both measurements should be taken and averaged to obtain the abdominal diameter.

TABLE 6–1.
Abdominal Diameter Measurement Table*

Gestational Age, wk	Predicted Mean Biparietal Diameter, mm	Average Abdominal Diameter, mm	
		Predicted Mean	Range From 5th to 95th Percentile
13	25.6	22.7	18.2–27.2
14	28.5	26.4	21.7–31.1
15	31.5	30.1	25.3–34.9
16	34.6	33.7	28.6–38.8
17	37.7	37.3	32.0–42.7
18	40.9	40.9	35.4–46.5
19	44.1	44.5	38.7–50.3
20	47.4	48.0	41.9–54.0
21	50.6	51.4	45.2–57.7
22	53.9	54.9	48.3–61.5
23	57.1	58.3	51.4–65.2
24	60.4	61.7	54.5–68.9
25	63.5	65.0	57.5–72.6
26	66.6	68.4	60.5–76.2
27	70.0	71.7	63.4–79.9
28	72.6	74.9	66.3–83.6
29	75.4	78.2	69.1–87.2
30	78.1	81.4	71.9–90.9
31	80.7	84.6	74.6–94.5
32	83.1	87.7	77.2–98.2
33	85.4	90.8	79.8–101.8
34	87.5	93.9	82.4–105.5
35	89.4	97.0	84.8–109.2
36	91.1	100.1	87.3–112.9
37	92.6	103.1	89.5–116.5
38	93.8	106.1	91.9–120.3
39	94.8	109.0	94.1–124.0
40	95.5	112.0	96.2–127.8

*From Eriksen PS, Sechor NJ, Weis-Bentzon M: Normal growth of fetal biparietal diameter and the abdominal diameter in a longitudinal study: An evaluation of the two parameters in predicting fetal weight. *Acta Obstet Gynecol Scand* 1985; 64:65–70. Used by permission.

Bree and Mariona.[42] Only the Campbell and Wilkin analysis[41] will be considered further, since it could not be determined if the numbers published by Bree and Mariona[42] were obtained from the original authors or extrapolated from their graph. In addition, Athey and Hadlock[36] will not be considered further, since their data were the preliminary results later finalized by Hadlock et al.[29] Last, Ogata et al.[33] will be discussed at the end of this section, when diabetic effects on abdominal circumference will be evaluated.

The remaining 13 articles[28-32, 34, 35, 37-41, 43] analyzed abdominal circumference in both the second and third trimester and found it to increase as the gestational age increased. Seven were given in numbers,[28-30, 32, 37, 40, 41] five in graph form,[34, 35, 38, 39, 43] and one as an equation.[31] Five used static scans,[28, 30, 31, 41, 43] seven used real-time,[29, 32, 34, 37-40] and 1[35] did not state the type of scanner. All the articles except those of Hoffbauer et al.[30] and Meire and Farrant[35] stated that the measurements were obtained at the area of the liver, in particular at either the umbilical portion of the left portal vein or fetal stomach, and that the outer margins of the abdomen were measured with a digitizer (Fig 6-3).

The accuracy in obtaining each measurement has been analyzed. The intraobserver error is not significant, an error of only 0.7% (range, 0% to 1.7%) when one photograph is used, with the measurement error increasing to 1.9% (range, 0.4% to 5.9%) from two photographs.[27, 29] The interobserver error is similarly small, 2.4%, with a range of 0.8% to 4% at 1 SD, thought to be primarily caused by the use of different measuring devices.[27]

Two questions need to be answered about the abdominal circumference measurements: are static and real-time scanners equally accurate in obtaining an abdominal circumference, and can the circumference be measured as accurately using an equation as it can with map reader or digitizer? For the question of real-time vs. static scan accuracy, two articles compared these two methods and found no statistical differences.[44, 45] For the question of equation vs. digitizer, the answer is not as straightforward. The equation for abdominal circumference is the formula for a circumference of a circle[46] (Table 6-2). This equation should be accurate, since in transaxial view the abdomen is either circular or mildly ellipsoidal. In a study of 122 fetal abdomens between 15 and 42 weeks, the abdomens (as expected) were found to be round or mildly ovoid.[47] When the smaller abdominal diameter was divided by the larger abdominal diameter, the range varied from 70.4 to 100, with a median of 89.1 and a 2 SD range of 82.1–96.1.[47]

Three articles performing both computations found a small error of no greater than 6%.[40, 46, 48] One article presented all the numbers from 18 weeks to term, showing that the digitized numbers were always larger, 1.6% larger at 18 weeks increasing to 6% at term.[40] They calculated this discrepancy to be highly significant at $P<.0001$. Another article did not show numbers or state in which direction the error occurred but found the error of 6% not be of great significance, at $P<.05$.[46] The third determined that equations slightly and consistently underestimated the abdominal circumference, a finding of no statistical significance.[48] Since all of the articles had a small error of no greater than 6%, it is statistically puzzling why one article deemed these discrepancies significant and the other two did not. It would not seem, however, that a maximum error of 6% near term should cause large measurement inconsistencies. In addition, while the

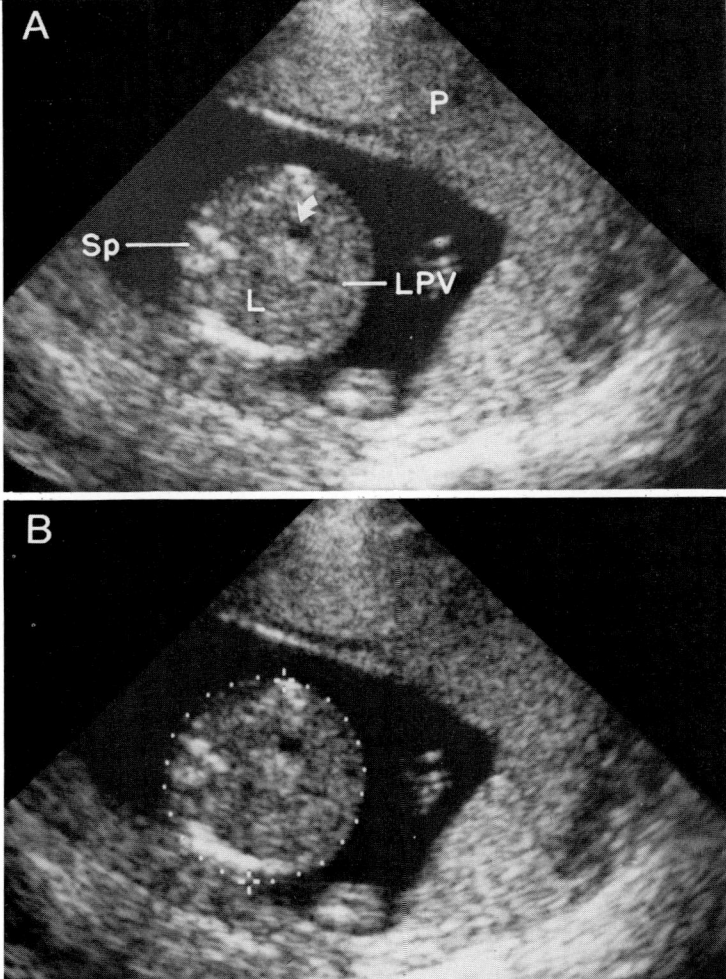

FIG 6–3.
Transaxial image of the upper fetal abdomen in a 22-week fetus. **A,** rounded body with the umbilical portion of the left portal vein *(LPV)* well positioned and midline within the liver *(L)*. Sp indicates spine; P, placenta; *curved arrow,* stomach. **B,** same image as **A** showing *dotted line* created by a digitizer around the outer margins of the abdomen to obtain a circumference measurement.

TABLE 6–2.
Circumference Computations

1. Planimetry
2. Equation for a circle
$$\left(\frac{D_1 + D_2}{2}\right) \pi = (D_1 + D_2) \times 1.57$$

numbers are different for digitized vs. equation-produced abdominal circumference measurements, they still overlapped in the one article in which they were thought significant at less than 1 SD, 25% to 75%.[40] Near term, the increased error might be due to a more crowded and therefore more ellipsoid body. Perhaps a correction factor in the circle circumference equation is needed to compensate for this small error.

When these 13 articles were compared, Hadlock et al.,[29] Deter et al.,[37] Fescina et al.,[32] and the equation-produced numbers of Tamura et al.[40] were found to be very close in their mean numbers. Tamura and Sabbagha,[28] Deter et al.,[38,39] Meire and Farrant,[35] and the digitized values of Tamura et al.[40] had uniformly larger numbers by approximately 3% to 4%, approaching 6% near term. Hoffbauer et al.,[30] Hobbins et al.,[43] Weinraub et al.,[31] and Parker et al.[34] had uniformly smaller numbers by approximately 5% to 8%. Campbell and Wilkin[41] were fairly close from 26 weeks until 32 weeks and then showed marked decrease with a variation of −2.9% at term.

It is thought that the Hadlock, Deter, Tamura, and Fescina articles[29,32,37,40] are most accurate, since they are in the middle of the mean numbers of all other articles. All four gave a range of standard deviations, Tamura et al.[40] from the 10th to 90th percentile and the other three at least at 2 SD.[29,32,37] Of these four articles, Hadlock et al.[29] showed mean abdominal circumferences with the gestational age varying in weeks, increasing from ±1.9 weeks at 12 gestational weeks to ±2.5 weeks by 42 gestational weeks, while the others used mean gestational age with the abdominal circumference varying in centimeters. This latter approach has no practicality in everyday obstetrical ultrasound measurements. Therefore, Hadlock et al.[29] is chosen (Table 6–3) because of its real-world applicability. The discrepancies between an equation-produced circumference and a digitized-produced circumference, while appearing to be small, cannot be resolved at the present time.

The abdominal circumference has been shown to vary with fetal gender, ethnic background and maternal diabetes mellitus in three articles, all in graph form.[33-35] Parker et al.[34] examined 96 pregnant European women and claimed that male fetuses were statistically larger than female fetuses after 28 weeks, increasing to term. However, the only numbers given in this article were at 36 gestational weeks and revealed a difference of only 10 mm with overlap at 1 SD. Meire and Farrant[35] compared Indian to European women and found 30% of the Indian fetuses to be 2 SD below their counterparts throughout pregnancy. No numbers were given. Ogata et al.[33] evaluated the growth of the abdominal circumference from 18 to 40 weeks in 23 diabetics, classes A through C. In 13, there was normal abdominal circumference growth throughout gestation. In the other 10 (43%), "accelerated somatic growth" was noted after 28 to 32 weeks. While the biparietal diameters stayed the same in size, this increase in abdominal circumference was reflected at birth by increased subcutaneous tissues as measured by skinfold thickness and increase in the fetal weight. Clearly, more work is needed in these areas to define the true incidence and severity of these changes.

ABDOMINAL AREA

Eight articles have measured the abdominal area with comparison to gestational age.[49-56] Two have previously been described under "thoracic area."[50,54] Since these articles stated that the thoracic area was measured below the cardiac pulsations, they were most likely measured at the region of the liver.[50,54] An

TABLE 6-3.
Abdominal Circumference Measurement Table*

Abdominal Circumference, mm	Gestational Age, wk	
	Predicted Mean Values†	95% Confidence Limits‡
100	15.6	13.7–17.5
105	16.1	14.2–18.0
110	16.5	14.6–18.4
115	16.9	15.0–18.8
120	17.3	15.4–19.2
125	17.8	15.9–19.7
130	18.2	16.2–20.2
135	18.6	16.6–20.6
140	19.1	17.1–21.1
145	19.5	17.5–21.5
150	20.0	18.0–22.0
155	20.4	18.4–22.4
160	20.8	18.8–22.8
165	21.3	19.3–23.3
170	21.7	19.7–23.7
175	22.2	20.2–24.2
180	22.6	20.6–24.6
185	23.1	21.1–25.1
190	23.6	21.6–25.6
195	24.0	21.8–26.2
200	24.5	22.3–26.7
205	24.9	22.7–27.1
210	25.4	23.2–27.6
215	25.9	23.7–28.1
220	26.3	24.1–28.5
225	26.8	24.6–29.0
230	27.3	25.1–29.5
235	27.7	25.5–29.9
240	28.2	26.0–30.4
245	28.7	26.5–30.9
250	29.2	27.0–31.4
255	29.7	27.5–31.9
260	30.1	27.1–33.1
265	30.6	27.6–33.6
270	31.1	28.1–34.1

TABLE 6–3 (cont.).

Abdominal Circumference, mm	Gestational Age, wk	
	Predicted Mean Values†	95% Confidence Limits‡
275	31.6	28.6–34.6
280	32.1	29.1–35.1
285	32.6	29.6–35.6
290	33.1	30.1–36.1
295	33.6	30.6–36.6
300	34.1	31.1–37.1
305	34.6	31.6–37.6
310	35.1	32.1–38.1
315	35.6	32.6–38.6
320	36.1	33.6–38.6
325	36.6	34.1–39.1
330	37.1	34.6–39.6
335	37.6	35.1–40.1
340	38.1	35.6–40.6
345	38.7	36.2–41.2
350	39.2	36.7–41.7
355	39.7	37.2–42.2
360	40.2	37.7–42.7
365	40.8	38.3–43.3

*From Hadlock FP, Deter RL, Harrist RB, et al: Fetal abdominal circumference as a predictor of menstrual age. *AJR* 1982; 139:367–370. Used by permission.
†Data from Table 3 of original article.
‡Data from Table 4 of original article.

additional article by Wladimiroff et al.[57] has a graph which appears identical to a graph in his other work[50] and will not be discussed further. The eight articles evaluated the fetal abdomen at the area of the umbilical vein within the liver starting at 24 to 29 weeks until term. One article was in number form,[51] two in number and graph form,[50, 54] four in graph form,[52, 53, 55, 56] and one as an equation.[49] All except Weinraub et al.[49] and Wladimiroff et al.,[50] who squared the abdominal diameter, used a planimeter to obtain their mean area measurements. They all gave SD except Weinraub et al.[49]

When these articles were compared, all showed an increase in abdominal area as gestational age progressed to term. The mean values of the two articles by Wladimiroff[50, 54] were in the middle with four uniformly higher,[51, 53, 55, 56] one uniformly lower,[52] and one starting low and becoming higher by 35 weeks.[49] No definite pattern could be established.

Three articles compared abdominal circumference to abdominal area.[50, 58, 59] In a comparison to fetal weight, the abdominal circumference correlated slightly better than the abdominal area.[58, 59] Between 32 and 38 weeks, abdominal circumference was a better predictor of growth rate than abdominal area, with an equal number of false positives.[50, 58] In addition, the intraobserver errors were smaller in calculating abdominal circumference from either the same or different images.[58]

Abdominal area measurements are therefore not of greater accuracy and may be even less accurate than abdominal circumference measurements. Since the abdominal circumference is an easier measurement to obtain and has been more extensively evaluated, area measurements are not recommended.

BODY VOLUME

Three articles have been published comparing body volumes to gestational age.[60–62] One article,[60] in graph form, performed static scans from 18 to 41 weeks and calculated the fetal volume by using the volume for a prolated ellipse, equal to 0.523 multiplied by the length of the fetus (the exact landmarks for obtaining the length are not stated), the transverse and AP diameters (measured in transaxial view from the upper abdomen at the umbilical vein). At 18 weeks, the fetal body volume was 40 cc, increasing steadily to greater than 800 cc by 40 weeks. In the same article, the fetal body volume was compared to the fetal head volume and was found after 29 weeks to increase more than the head volume. The interobserver and intraobserver errors were estimated for the body volume measurements and found to be 6.4 and 6.3 cc, respectively.

In the other two articles,[61, 62] the fetal body volume was computed from two diameters taken in transaxial view at the level of the liver. In graph form, the body volume increased from approximately 10 cc at 12 weeks to approximately 50 cc at 18 weeks to greater than 1,400 cc at term.

Despite the theoretical probability that a body volume is a better method for evaluating overall body size, these formulas (particularly extrapolating a volume from transaxial measurements alone) have not proved accurate. Fetal body volumes are therefore not recommended.

TOTAL FETAL VOLUMES

Two articles have attempted to calculate fetal volume.[63, 64] One combined close interval static scans of the fetus, to compute a total fetal volume.[64] In comparing their in utero results to hydrostatic weight of aborted fetus or birth weight, they found that their formula consistently underestimated the true volume by 10%. The other article[64] used ellipsoid calculations of the head and body.

There were large differences in the volumes between the two articles. While this is an interesting concept, these two methods are so discrepant in technique and results that total fetal volumes are not recommended.

TOTAL FETAL LENGTH

Articles have been published evaluating live premature infants from approximately 24 gestational weeks until term,[65–68] two in number form[65, 66] with the other two in graph form. All measurements were obtained with infants fully extended and measured from the crown (top of the head) to the heel. All articles gave a mean newborn length with a variation around the mean of 2 SD, revealing an overall size increase from approximately 355 mm at 26 weeks to 500 mm by term. This neonatal growth was found to be linear in one article.[67] In the other three, it was biphasic, with a more rapid initial growth until approximately 36 weeks, followed by a decrease until term.[65, 66, 68] Male infants were found to be equal to female in length in one article,[66] with males slightly larger in another two.[65, 68]

There have been seven ultrasound articles evaluating the length of the fetus,[69–75] by either measuring the length of the fetal head and body,[69–72] or by measuring its femoral length.[73–75] The fetus was analyzed throughout the entire second and third trimesters from 12 to 15 weeks until 40 weeks in two articles,[69, 70] while the other five articles evaluated the fetus from 20 or more weeks to term. Three presented the data as numbers,[69, 72, 75] two graphs only,[70, 71] and two in graph and equation form.[73, 74] Only three[70, 73, 75] also had an SD.

Although four[69–72] imaged the fetus with static scans, none specifically mentioned the points from where the measurements were obtained. Presumably, three of these[69, 71, 72] evaluated the full length of the fetus from the top of the head to the bottom of the rump, while the last article[70] only measured the length of the trunk. Nevertheless, when their numbers were compared, particularly the three evaluating the full length of the fetus,[69, 71, 72] two[71, 72] had numbers similar to the full length of the premature infants. This is quite surprising, since the ultrasound measurements could not have incorporated the length of the fetal extremities.

The other three articles[73–75] measured the fetal femur with real-time scanners, all within 72 hours of delivery, one in number form[75] and the other two as graphs.[73, 74] All found a close linear relationship to the neonatal crown-heel length, from approximately 20 weeks until term. While these articles could not be compared with the ones in the preceding paragraph, there may be a value in determining fetal length for the prediction of birth weight or of growth retardation.[75] Further work is needed to verify this data. The Vintzileos et al.[75] table is nevertheless recommended to predict fetal crown-heel length by using the femoral length measurement (Fig 6–4), since it is in number form and over a wider range than the other articles (Table 6–4).

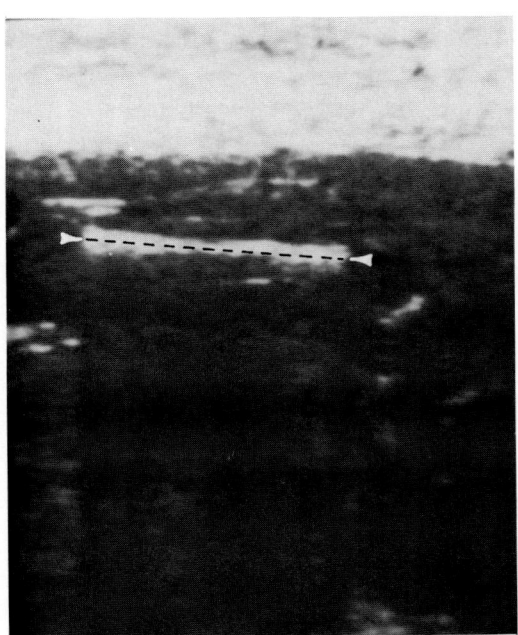

FIG 6–4.
Long-axis image of fetal femur at 30 weeks. The femoral shaft is ossified and the measurement is taken along its longest length, excluding the nonossified proximal and distal epiphyseal cartilages. Measurement denoted by *arrowheads* and *dotted line*.

TABLE 6-4.
Fetal Length Measurement Table—Use of Femur Length to Predict Fetal Crown-Heel Length*

Femur Length, mm	Predicted Fetal Crown-Heel Length, mm		Femur Length, mm	Predicted Fetal Crown-Heel Length, mm	
	Predicted Mean	Range From 5th to 95th Percentile		Predicted Mean	Range From 5th to 95th Percentile
30	239	226–251	61	422	419–425
31	245	233–256	62	428	424–431
32	251	239–262	63	434	430–437
33	257	245–268	64	439	436–443
34	262	252–273	65	445	442–449
35	268	258–279	66	451	447–455
36	274	264–284	67	457	453–461
37	280	270–290	68	463	458–468
38	286	277–295	69	469	464–474
39	292	283–306	70	475	470–480
40	298	289–306	71	481	475–486
41	304	295–312	72	487	481–493
42	310	302–318	73	493	486–499
43	316	308–323	74	498	492–505
44	321	314–329	75	504	497–511
45	327	321–334	76	510	503–518
46	333	327–340	77	516	508–524
47	339	333–345	78	522	514–530
48	345	339–351	79	528	520–536
49	351	346–356	80	534	525–543
50	357	352–362	81	540	531–549
51	363	358–368	82	546	536–555
52	369	364–373	83	552	542–561
53	375	370–379	84	557	547–568
54	380	377–384	85	563	553–574
55	386	383–390	86	569	558–580
56	392	389–396	87	575	564–587
57	398	395–401	88	581	569–593
58	404	401–407	89	587	575–599
59	410	407–413	90	593	580–606
60	416	413–419			

*From Vintzileos AM, Campbell WA, Neckles S, et al: The ultrasound femur as a predictor of fetal length. *Obstet Gynecol* 1984; 64:779–782. Used by permission.

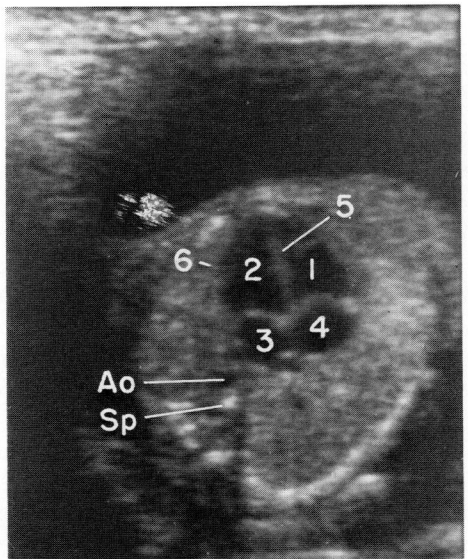

FIG 6–5.
Transaxial image of lower fetal chest in a 25-week fetus showing a four-chamber view of the heart in systole. The left side of the fetus is on the reader's *left*. *1* indicates right ventricle, closest to anterior chest wall; *2,* left ventricle; *3,* left atrium, closest to descending thoracic aorta; *4,* right atrium; *5,* interventricular septum; *6,* left ventricular wall; *Ao,* descending thoracic aorta; *Sp,* spine.

FETAL BODY ORGAN MEASUREMENTS

Heart

Since the late 1970s, high-resolution real-time equipment, frequently with M-mode capabilities, has permitted accurate evaluation of the fetal heart. The planes of section involved in imaging the normal heart and its internal structures have been extensively studied.[76–86] Throughout the second and third trimester, preferably after 16 weeks, the success in visualizing cardiac structures varied with fetal position, fetal heart size (directly related to fetal size), and examiner experience.[83] Visualization of the great vessels, the atrial and ventricular size and function, the AV valves, and the presence and continuity of ventricular and atrial septa was greater than 90%.[78, 82] Only the semilunar valves, aortic arch, ascending and descending aorta, and venae cavae were visualized less frequently, 55% to 87% of the time.[78, 82, 86]

Articles have described as few as two and as many as eight planes of section to evaluate adequately the fetal heart. While detailed descriptions of these sections are beyond the scope of this book, two articles offer comparisons of ultrasound images to diagrams and/or autopsy pictures.[83, 84] Of all the views, the easiest and most routine is the four-chamber image, which offers almost all significant intracardiac information and only fails in its inability to image the great vessels and their values. The procedure for the four-chamber view is as follows: The large size of the fetal liver and the unexpanded lungs causes the fetal heart to lie almost perpendicular to the fetal trunk, a different axis than in children and adults. In transaxial plane, through the lower chest, the four-chamber view visualizes both ventricles, the interventricular septum, both atria, the foramen ovale, the mitral and tricupsid valves, and the descending thoracic aorta (Figs 6–5 and 6–6). The fetal heart is on the left side with the right ventricle positioned anteriorly and closest to the chest wall. If transaxial and obliqued longitudinal views can also be obtained higher in the chest at the cardiac base, continuity of the aortic root to the left ventricle, pulmonary artery to the right ventricle, and the aortic and pulmonic valves can be shown.[84] These views eliminate all major cardiac anomalies except transposition of the great vessels.

Because of the rapid movement of the fetal heart, approximately 120 to 180 beats per minute[87] with frequent additional movements of the fetus, rapid-scanning real-time ultrasound (with scan rates of at least 20 to 30 frames per second) is essential for proper orientation. Since the cardiac structures are relatively small, a high-resolution transducer (at least 3.5 MHz, if not 5.0 MHz) should be used. There has been discussion in the literature as to whether real-time or M-mode should be used to obtain the cardiac measurements. Real-time requires less skill and time for proper orientation and can measure a structure at any angle. Freeze-framing capabilities, however, usually degrade the image. M-mode, on the other hand, scans and records faster but has to be perpendicular to the object imaged. It frequently requires increased time to obtain a measurement.

Real-time imaging is initially required to obtain the proper orientation before M-mode recording is obtained. If the fetus shifts position, real-time may have to be used again to reorient for M-mode. Once oriented correctly, M-mode is superior for arrhythmias, particularly the tachyarrythmias,[86–89] and for the evaluation of valvular motion. It is also slightly better for evaluating the exact phase

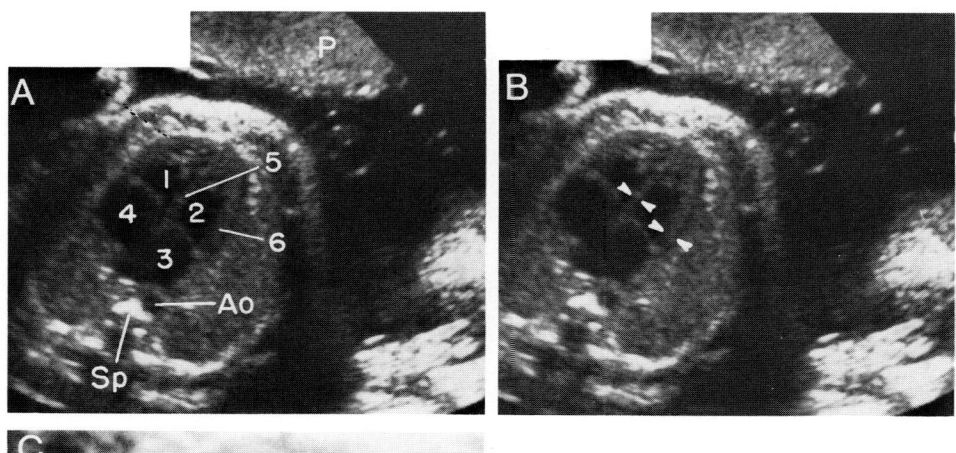

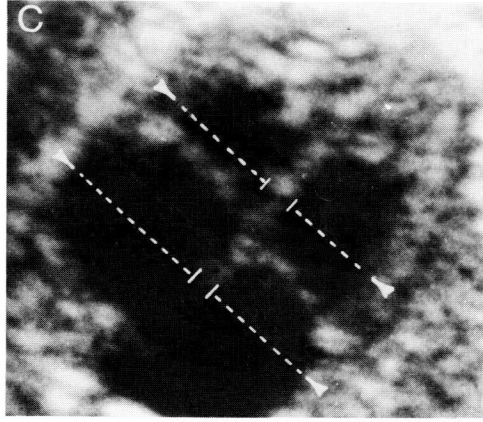

FIG 6–6.
Transaxial scan of lower fetal chest in a 20-week fetus. **A,** a four-chamber view of the heart in diastole is shown. (Note the atria are much larger than in Fig 6–5.) The left side of the fetus is on the reader's *right*. 1 indicates right ventricle, closest to anterior chest wall; 2, left ventricle; 3, left atrium; 4, right atrium; 5, interventricular septum; 6, left ventricular wall; *Ao,* descending thoracic aorta; *Sp,* spine; *P,* placenta. **B,** same image as **A** showing the thickness of the interventricular septum and left ventricular wall *(arrowheads),* measured close to the AV valves. **C,** magnified same image as **A** showing measurements of the inner dimensions of the atria and ventricles, just above and below the AV valves *(arrowheads, perpendicular and dotted lines).*

of the cardiac cycle, systole or diastole. For structural abnormalities, both real-time and M-mode have their advantages, but real-time is favored because of increased ease of scanning. Almost all structural cardiac abnormalities detected by ultrasound in utero have been large. They have been visually obvious, at least 3 to 4 mm in size, and therefore measurements were not necessary. Nevertheless, structural cardiac abnormalities could be so subtle that only abnormal measurements might suggest their diagnosis.

A number of articles have been published describing different normal cardiac parameters.[90-109] Unfortunately, many of these failed to measure the same structures or to use the same phase of the cardiac cycle or same anatomic plane. Levi and Erbsman,[90] using static scans from the mid-second trimester until term, evaluated the outer cardiac AP and transverse diameters, circumference, and area. Suzuke et al.[91] analyzed the heart volume with static scans from 30 weeks to term using the formula approximating the equation for a sphere:

$$4/3 \pi \times AP \text{ dimension}/2 \times (\text{transverse dimension}/2)^2$$

They found their volumes to increase throughout gestation and to correlate well with the biparietal diameter, gestational age, and fetal weight, particularly if the fetus weighed more than 2,500 gm. Although outer cardiac margins were used, the exact anatomical place where these measurements were taken was not stated. Jeanty et al.[92] also measured the outer dimensions of the heart with real-time from 12 to 40 weeks. Their measurements for transverse and longitudinal diameters and for volume were very different from those of Levi and Erbsman,[90] and deviate near term from those of Suzuke et al.[91] DeVore and Platt,[93] taking into account the phase of the cardiac cycle with M-mode, found that cardiac measurements by Jeanty et al.[92] were "random" and inaccurate in over 40% of cases because the phase of the cardiac cycle was not taken into account. DeVore and Platt[93] thought that measurement should only be made in end-diastole or end-systole.

Filkins et al.[94] evaluated the cardiothoracic ratio from 16 to 36 weeks and found that the ratio of the transverse cardiac to transverse thoracic diameters had a constant mean value of 0.50 (range, 0.45 to 0.55) and the ratio of the AP dimensions of the heart to the thorax had a mean value of 0.52 (range, 0.45 to 0.58). These ratios are compelling because of their simplicity. However, the article failed to take in account the phase of the cardiac cycle, an omission that might introduce significant error.[93] In addition, the exact points of measurement were not specified. Using both real-time and M-mode, DeVore et al.,[95] measured the biventricular outer diameter in end-diastole from the four-chamber transaxial view and compared it to the thoracic circumference at the same level. The exact outer borders of the heart and chest were well defined. A graph was created with a mean and 2 SD and was helpful in defining 4 cases of cardiothoracic disproportion. In addition, the head, abdomen, and femur were measured, and graphs were created comparing these parameters to the heart and chest. While the comparison of the heart to chest is undoubtedly valid and of clinical value, numbers were not given, and therefore no table can be recommended. Wladimiroff and McGhie[96] calculated the left ventricular cardiac output and blood flow in the descending aorta by using a combination of real-time and Doppler. Exact points of measurement of the heart were not described and an assumption had

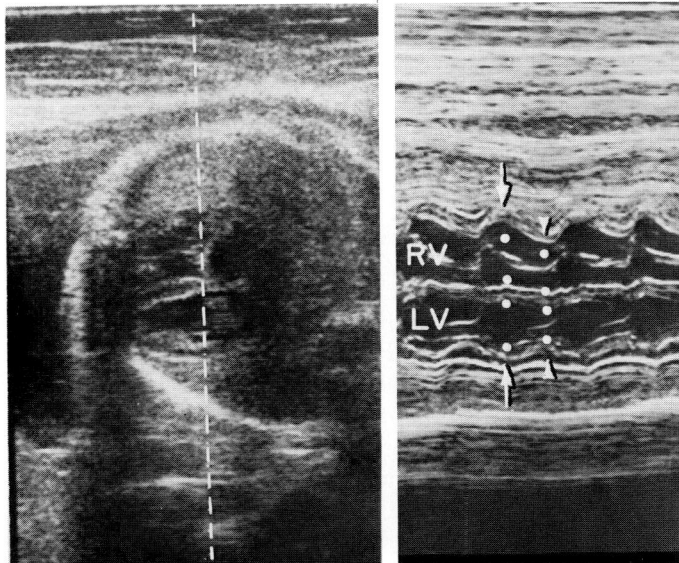

FIG 6–7.
Comparison of inner dimensions of the right and left ventricles. Split image showing a perpendicular four-chamber view of the fetal heart on the left and M-mode tracing on the right. **Left,** *dotted line* oriented through the ventricles just below the AV valves. **Right,** *dots* denote right ventricular *(RV)* and left ventricular *(LV)* inner diameters in both end diastole *(arrows)* and end-systole *(arrowheads)*. Note that they remain approximately 1:1 in both systole and diastole.

to be made of an exact and constant diameter of the descending aorta so that true blood flow could be calculated. These articles will therefore not be considered further.

Ten articles have analyzed the same ventricular cardiac dimension: the left ventricular diameter, the right ventricular diameter, and their ratio.[97–105, 109] Seven of these articles used M-mode after real-time obtained the correct cardiac orientation,[97–103, 105] while the other three used real-time ultrasound exclusively.[97, 104, 109] Six articles evaluated the fetal heart from the early second trimester until term,[97–99, 103, 104, 109] while the other four examined the fetal heart in the third trimester. Five of these articles[97–99, 101, 109] evaluated the maximum transverse diameter of the left ventricle and right ventricle at the AV valves in end-diastole while the remainder measured the ventricular chambers below the area of the mitral and tricuspid valve evaluating the diameters in both end-diastole and end-systole.

There are several points which can be made from these studies. While the left and right ventricular chambers and wall thicknesses increased with increasing gestational age, the ratio of the right to left ventricles remained relatively constant throughout gestation, between 0.85 and 1.3[97, 98, 100, 103, 105, 109] (see Figs 6–5 to 6–7). This ratio was confirmed in a postmortem study.[106] The close similarity between the ventricular dimensions does not suggest dominance of the right ventricle in utero.[103]

In addition, Allan et al.[99] and Vosters et al.[107] evaluated the interventricular septum and found it to increase in both end-diastole and end-systole from 1.0 mm at 16 weeks to 4.0 mm at term (see Figs 6–5 and 6–6). The interventricular septum and left ventricular wall thicknesses, however, grew equally during pregnancy, so that their ratio remained approximately 1 to 1, confirmed in a fetal postmortem study,[106] where a ratio of 1.14 ± 0.34 was found[106] (Figs 6–6,B, and 6–8). It was suggested that if the ratio increased above 1.5, it was abnormal. The exact place to measure the thickness of both was not stated. Using the adult and pediatric echocardiographic positions, however, it is recommended that the measurements be obtained close to the AV valves (see Fig 6–6,B).

Allan et al.[99] and Shime et al.[109] measured the left atrium, Allan et al.[99] and Shime et al.[109] measured the right atrium, and DeVore et al.[108] and Shime et al.[109] measured the aortic root (Figs 6–6,C, 6–9, and 6–10). All showed increase toward term. The aortic and pulmonary arteries were also measured at the valvular regions[97] (see Fig 6–9). While they were compared to fetal weight instead of to either the biparietal diameter or gestational age, they were nevertheless found to be relatively constant throughout gestation with the diameter of the pulmonary and aortic valves increasing from 6 to 8 mm and 5 to 7 mm respectively. This 1–to-1 ratio of the valves has been found to persist after birth.[97] Last, the right-to-left atrium had a ratio of 1:1[109] (see Figs 6–6 and 6–10).

While no tables cover the entire second and third trimester, a table is given so that the reader will have approximate values that can be expected in utero[109] (Table 6–5). In addition, several ratios appear to be of significant value throughout the second and third trimesters, all approximately 1:1 (Table 6–6): the transverse diameter of the right-to-left ventricle (0.85 to 1.3), the interventricular

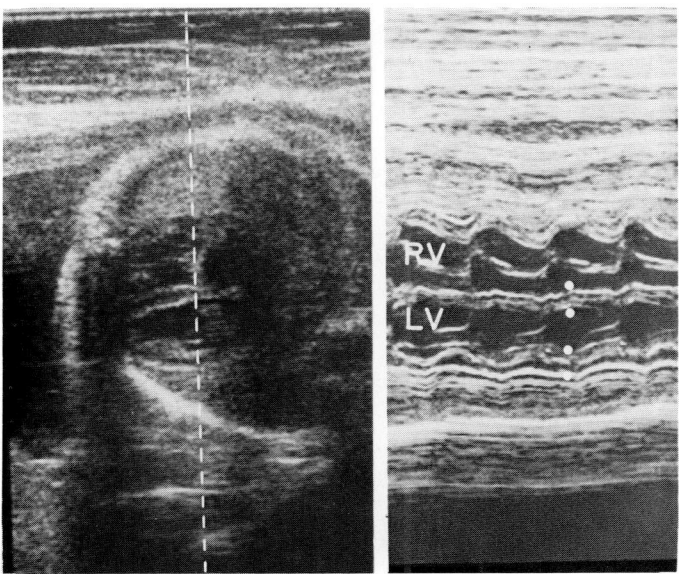

FIG 6–8.
Comparison of interventricular septum to the left ventricular wall thickness. Split image showing a perpendicular four-chamber view of the fetal heart on the left and M-mode tracing on right. **Left,** *dotted line* oriented through the ventricles just below the AV valves. **Right,** *dots* denote the thickness of the interventricular septum and left ventricular wall in diastole. Note that the ratio remains approximately 1:1 in both systole and diastole. *LV* indicates left ventricle; *RV*, right ventricle.

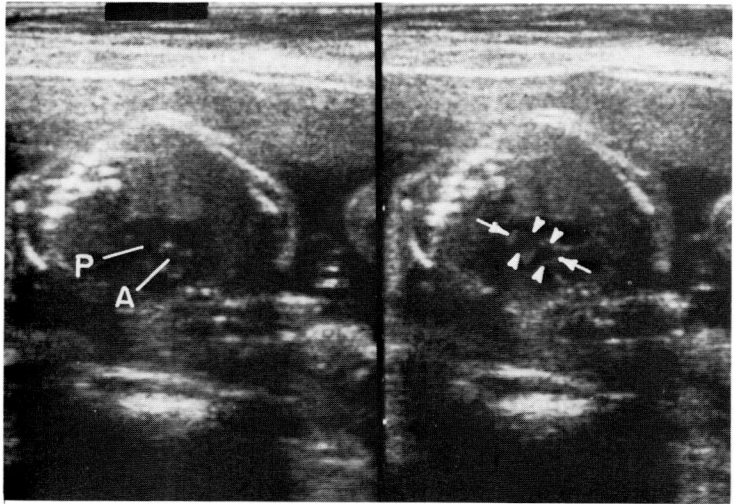

FIG 6–9.
Comparison of the aortic and pulmonary artery diameters. Transaxial images of fetal heart at 30 weeks through the cardiac base. The aorta (A) and pulmonary artery (P) are identified just at or slightly above the aortic and pulmonary valves. Measurements are obtained in any direction of the anechoic rounded structures *(arrows* and *arrowheads)*.

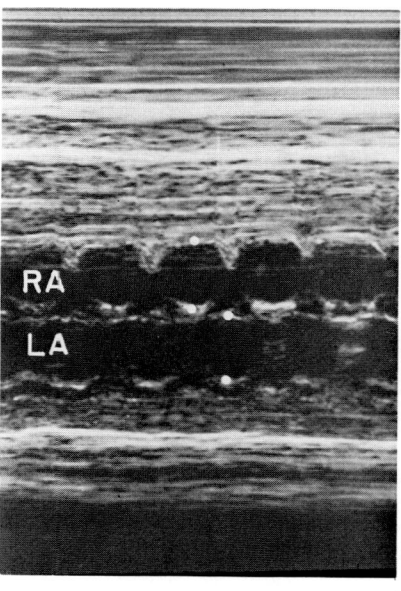

FIG 6–10.
Comparison of the inner dimensions of the right and left atria. M-mode tracing perpendicular through the right atrium *(RA)* and left atrium *(LA)*. *White dots* show the atria in systole. Note the systoles of the atria are at slightly different times.

septum to left ventricular wall thickness (1:1), right-to-left atrium (1:1), and the aortic to pulmonary arteries at the valvular region (1:1). In addition, the interventricular septal thickness should not be greater than 1.0 mm at 16 weeks, increasing to 4.0 mm at term. These ratios and the interventricular septal thickness seem easy to measure, since they appear also to remain constant regardless of the part of the cardiac cycle in which they are measured.

TABLE 6–5.
Fetal Cardiac Measurement Table*

	Linear Increase From 17 to 40 wk, mm		Range From 5th to 95th Percentile
	17 wk	40 wk	
Left ventricle†	4	16	±1.7
Right ventricle†	4	19	±1.8
Left atrium‡	4	16	±1.9
Right atrium‡	6	16	±1.5
Aortic root	2.4	10	±1.3

*From Shime J, Gresser RN, Rakowski H: Quantitative two-dimensional echocardiographic assessment of fetal cardiac growth. Am J Obstet Gynecol 1986; 154:294–300. Used by permission.
†Measurements taken in end-diastole at the tips of the atrioventricular valves just prior to closure in a plane perpendicular to the interventricular septum.
‡Measurements obtained in end-systole just after atrioventricular valve closure using widest visible internal diameter in a plane perpendicular to the interatrial septum.

TABLE 6–6.
Fetal Cardiac Ratios Throughout Second and Third Trimesters

Anatomical Areas	Ratio
Transverse inner diameters of right to left ventricle	0.85:1.3
Transverse inner diameters of right to left atrium	1:1
Thickness of interventricular septum to left ventricular wall	1:1
Inner diameters of aortic to pulmonary arteries (at base of the heart at the valvular region)	1:1

Fetal Liver

The fetal liver has been evaluated in four articles, two in transverse[110, 111] and two in long axis.[112, 113] In the transaxial plane of the fetus, using the left portal vein (actually the umbilical portion of the left portal vein) as a dividing line, the normal left lobe was found to be proportionately larger than in adults. A transverse ratio of the left to right lobes of the liver in utero was found to have a mean value of 1.04 with a range of 0.78 to 1.30.[110] This ratio remained constant throughout gestational life. In adults, this same ratio was performed using computed tomography and was found to be smaller, with a mean value of 0.76. While the size of the liver has been shown to decrease in asymmetric intrauterine growth retardation, as reflected by a decreased abdominal size, the ratio of the left to right lobes did not change in affected fetuses.[111] This implies that both lobes are equally decreased. Therefore while this ratio is of academic interest, it has not been shown to have clinical value.

Two additional articles[112, 113] have measured the fetal liver in long axis from 20 weeks to term. The long axis was detected by first locating the fetal abdominal aorta, and then moving the transducer parallel and to the right to locate the longest length of the liver.[112] The measurement was taken from the right hemidiaphragm to the liver edge (Fig 6–11). The liver length was found to increase from 27 mm to 49 mm, with a range of 2 SD. The rate of growth of the liver was shown to increase throughout gestation and closely paralleled the increase in abdominal circumference.[112] A follow-up study by the same group[113] evaluated 16 isoimmunized fetuses and found liver size and rate of growth to be a valuable indicator of the severity of fetal hydrops. Using the amniotic fluid bilirubin values (also termed Delta OD 450) as their measure of severity, all eight severely affected fetuses had abnormal liver size and growth (more than 5 mm/week). The abdominal circumference and umbilical vein diameter were also measured and found to be less sensitive. While not studied in these articles, the liver length and rate of growth would be expected to be decreased to fetuses with asymmetric growth retardation.

There may be technical factors involved in obtaining consistent measurements. While the caudal edge of the liver seems easy to identify, the dome of the right hemidiaphragm may be difficult to routinely image because of shadowing from ribs or overlying extremities. This could significantly affect the measurements. Nevertheless, this work appears both valid and clinically useful and is therefore recommended[112] (see Fig 6–11; Table 6–7). More work is needed,

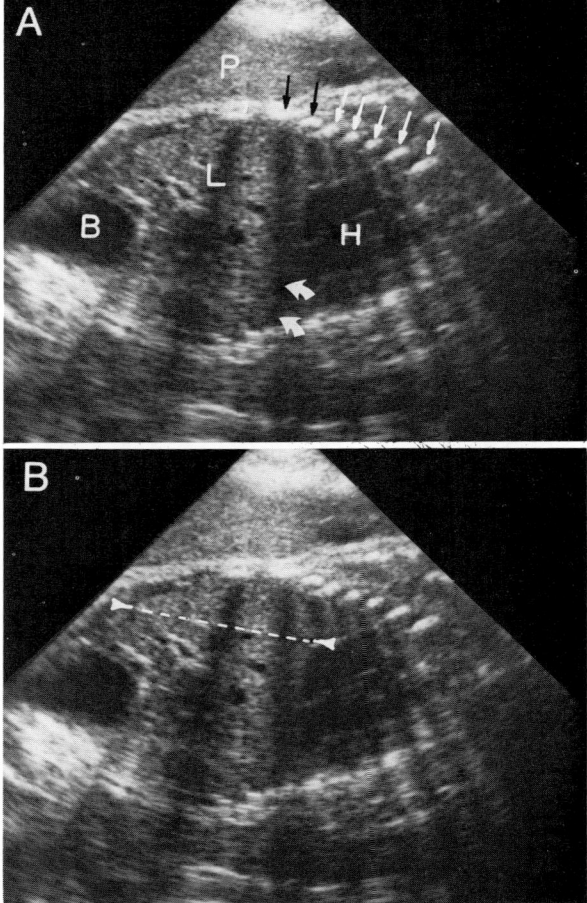

FIG 6–11.
Long axis scan of the body in 25 week fetus. **A,** long axis of the liver *(L)* is identified to the right and parallel to the abdominal aorta. Note that its upper margin is partially obscured by shadowing from the ribs *(arrows)*. H indicates heart; B, fetal bladder; P, placenta. *Curved arrows* denote part of the right hemidiaphragm. **B,** same image as **A** showing measurement of the liver, from top of right hemidiaphragm to caudal tip of liver. Measurement denoted by *arrowheads* and *dotted line.*

particularly near term, at which point only three patients were examined, so that standard deviations can be calculated for each mean measurement.

Fetal Spleen

A recent article[114] stated that the spleen could be routinely imaged as a hyperechoic mass in transverse and coronal views using the stomach, spine, and left hemidiaphragm as landmarks. Measurements were taken in longitudinal, coronal, and transverse dimensions, and the splenic circumferences and volumes were calculated. Mean values in number form, and the 5th to 95th percent ranges were given from 18 weeks to term.

While their table is interesting, it is unlikely that the spleen can be routinely imaged. First, the spleen is not hyperechoic but hypoechoic, and frequently difficult to identify unless surrounded by ascites. Secondly, in transaxial plane,

TABLE 6–7.
Fetal Liver Measurement Table*

Gestational Age, wk	Long-Axis Measurement, mm†	
	True Mean	Range From 5th to 95th Percentile
20	27.3	20.9–33.7
21	28.0	26.5–29.5
22	30.6	23.9–37.3
23	30.9	26.4–35.4
24	32.9	26.2–39.6
25	33.6	28.3–38.9
26	35.7	29.4–42.0
27	36.6	33.3–39.9
28	38.4	34.4–42.4
29	39.1	34.1–44.1
30	38.7	33.7–43.7
31	39.6	33.9–45.3
32	42.7	35.0–50.2
33	42.8	37.2–50.4
34	44.8	37.7–51.9
35	47.8	38.7–56.9
36	49.0	40.6–57.4
37	52.0	45.2–58.8
38	52.9	48.7–57.1
39	55.4	48.7–62.1
40	59.0	—
41	49.3	46.9–51.7

*From Vintzileos AM, Neckles S, Campbell WA, et al: Fetal liver ultrasound measurements during normal pregnancy. *Obstet Gynecol* 1985; 66:477–480. Used by permission.
†Measured in longitudinal plane from top of right hemidiaphragm to tip of right lobe of liver.

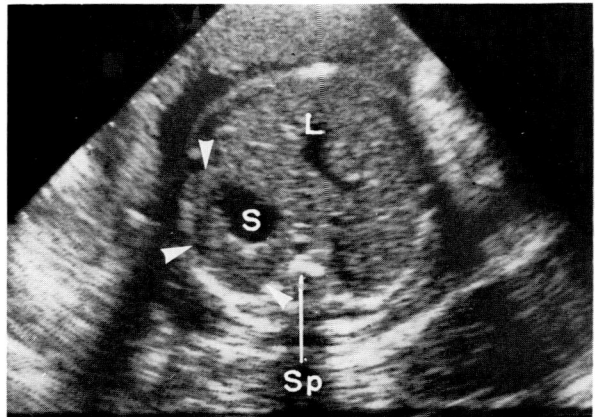

FIG 6–12.
Transaxial scan of the upper abdomen showing the hypoechoic spleen *(arrowheads)* on the left between the distended stomach *(S)*, spine *(Sp)*, and lateral margin of the fetal body. *L* indicates liver.

the stomach, when filled, is the only consistent landmark (Fig 6–12). The long axis of the spleen, obtained by the authors in coronal view, is even more difficult to identify and is totally dependent on fetal position.

The measurements change little from 18 weeks to term. According to the table proposed, an error of 2 to 3 mm in any dimension would cause an error of as much as 20 weeks. Nevertheless, if this work could be duplicated, it would be of value not only in determining normal-sized spleen but also in cases of enlarged spleen. The authors were able to detect splenomegaly in 5 of the most severely affected cases of fetal hydrops. In these cases, however, other abnormalities typical of hydrops, such as ascites, were present, which undoubtedly made splenic visualization easier.

Fetal Adrenal Glands

The fetal adrenal glands were evaluated in three articles.[115–117] While they can be identified as early as 21 gestational weeks, the adrenal glands are not routinely imaged until the third trimester (28 weeks onward). The adrenal glands are ovoid, triangular, or heart-shaped in long axis, with one article[115] claiming to identify both adrenal limbs as oval and disk-shaped in transverse (Fig 6–13). The peripheral cortex is hypoechoic with the central medulla hyperechoic, an echogenicity similar to that of the adjacent kidney (Fig 6–13,C). The adrenals and kidneys should not be confused, however, because their overall shapes and sizes are different.

The adrenal glands are not always easy to image. Because of their position in the high retroperitoneum, frequently only a "peek" at them between the lower ribs is possible (see Fig 6–13). In addition, because of their closeness to the fetal spine, usually only the one closest to the transducer is imaged.

Nevertheless, the adrenal glands have been measured with real-time ultrasound in two articles.[116, 117] Lewis et al.[116] measured the adrenal length from 30 to 39 weeks, presenting their data as numbers. Hata et al.[117] evaluated the length, circumference, and area of the adrenal glands from 22 to 42 weeks, presenting their data in graph form. Both showed an increase in size as the fetus grew to term. In addition, Lewis et al.[116] calculated a ratio of the adrenal-to-renal long axis. In comparison of these two articles,[116, 117] the fetal adrenal glands measured 14 to 16 mm at 30 weeks to 22 to 25 mm at term. The ratio of the long axis of the adrenal to the long axis of the adjacent kidney remained relatively constant, between 0.48 and 0.66 (see Fig 6–13,B). In transaxial view, it was also found that while the adrenal width was very narrow (only several millimeters in thickness), the AP dimension was similar to the kidney (see Fig 6–13,C). When the AP dimension of the adrenal was compared to the AP abdominal diameter at the same level, the ratio was approximately 0.30.[116]

At present, the ranges are too large and not enough cases have been mea-

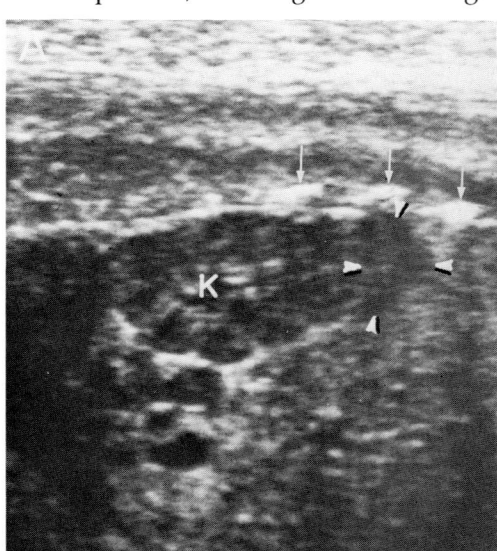
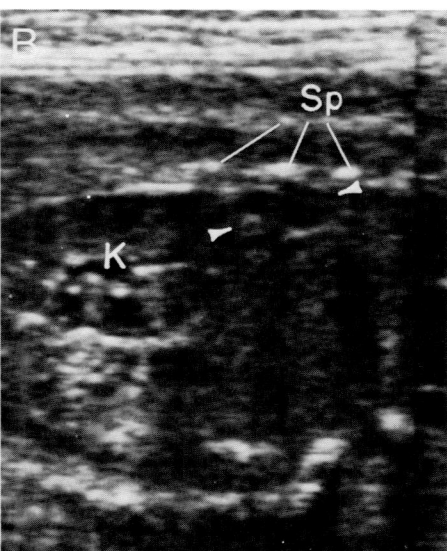
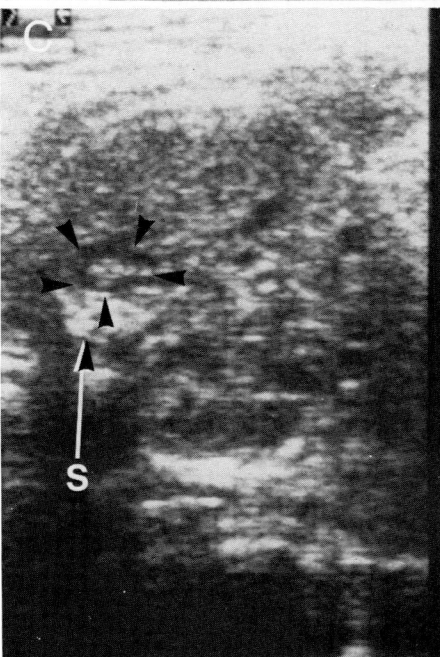

FIG 6–13.
Fetal adrenal glands, imaged in three fetuses greater than 30 weeks. **A,** long-axis scan of the fetal body adjacent to the spine *(arrows)* showing the triangular-shaped adrenal gland *(arrowheads)* in long axis immediately superior to the kidney *(K)*. The adrenal gland is partially obscured by shadowing from the fetal spine. **B,** long-axis scan of the fetal body showing an ovoid shaped adrenal gland *(arrowheads)*, partially obscured by shadowing from the spine *(Sp)*, immediately superior to the kidney *(K)*. Note the adrenal gland is about half the length of the kidney. **C,** transaxial scan of the fetal body showing the thin oval disk-like adrenal gland *(arrowheads)* in the high retroperitoneum adjacent to the fetal spine *(S)*. The other adrenal cannot be imaged because of shadowing from the spine. Note the central hyperechoic medulla and peripheral hypoechoic cortex, similar to the renal echogenicity (see **A**). The transverse shapes of the kidney and adrenal gland are dissimilar, round vs. ovoid, respectively.

sured to recommend a table. In addition, there are no reported cases of abnormal sized adrenal glands detected *in utero*. If small adrenal glands could be imaged, however, this might be an important sign of intrauterine growth retardation. Anderson et al.,[118] evaluating the adrenal weight in stillborn or neonatal autopsy specimens from 22 weeks to term, found that the weight of normal adrenal glands was always higher than comparable adrenal weights in neonates with preeclampsia and antepartum hemorrhage.

Fetal Kidneys

The fetal kidneys have been measured in four articles from the early second trimester until term,[119-122] two in number form,[121, 124] one in graph form,[119] and one with both equations and graphs.[120] Two of these were performed with real-time ultrasound,[120, 122] while the other two were imaged with static scanners.

The fetal kidneys are not routinely seen until 15 weeks.[119] After 17 weeks, they can be imaged in approximately 90% of cases, although they are usually not easily separable from the surrounding tissues (Fig 6-14,A). After 26 weeks, presumably due to increase in hyperechoic perinephric fat, the kidney becomes easily identified[123] (Fig 6-14,B). Quite frequently, except when the fetus is in a back-up position, the kidney closest to the transducer is optimally visualized while the opposite kidney is obscured by the fetal spine.

The kidneys have the same ovoid configuration as that seen in children and adults with an echogenicity similar to the adult kidney. The periphery (cortex) is hypoechoic[119, 121] with a hyperechoic center (renal sinus)[119] (Fig 6-14,C). On occasion the cortex can be further differentiated by identifying the almost totally anechoic medulla. The renal sinus becomes hyperechoic and easily identified by the third trimester, due to deposition of fat.[120, 123]

Three renal measurements have been evaluated, i.e., the length, width, and AP diameter. The renal length is measured in coronal or sagittal plane along the long axis of the kidney, and the AP and transverse diameters obtained in transaxial view (Figs 6-15 and 6-16). This measurement of the AP dimension in transaxial plane is not ideal. To obtain a true AP measurement, it should be measured from the long axis image of the kidney, perpendicular to the renal length (see Fig 6-15,B). Despite this potential shortcoming, all three measurements were analyzed by Jeanty et al.[120] from 20 weeks to term. Two of the three measurements, the renal length and AP dimensions, were evaluated by Lawson et al.[119] and Bertagnoli et al.[122] from 15 weeks and 24 weeks to term, respectively. Grannum et al.[121] measured the kidneys from 16 weeks to term only in transaxial view, calculating three measurements, the AP diameter, transverse diameter and circumference and then comparing them to similar measurements of the fetal abdomen at the same level. Jeanty et al.[120] also calculated the volumes of the fetal kidneys from the prolated ellipse formula.

The data was presented as numbers in only two of the articles[121, 122] with two of the articles[120, 122] including SD. The exact points for measuring the kidney were only specifically stated in one of the articles,[122] but were alluded to in the other three.[119-121] While presumably all the articles measured the kidneys accurately, Bertagnoli et al.[122] stated that the outer to outer margins were used in measuring the renal long axis and the outer to inner margins were used to obtain the AP measurement. How the inner margin could be obtained was not stated.

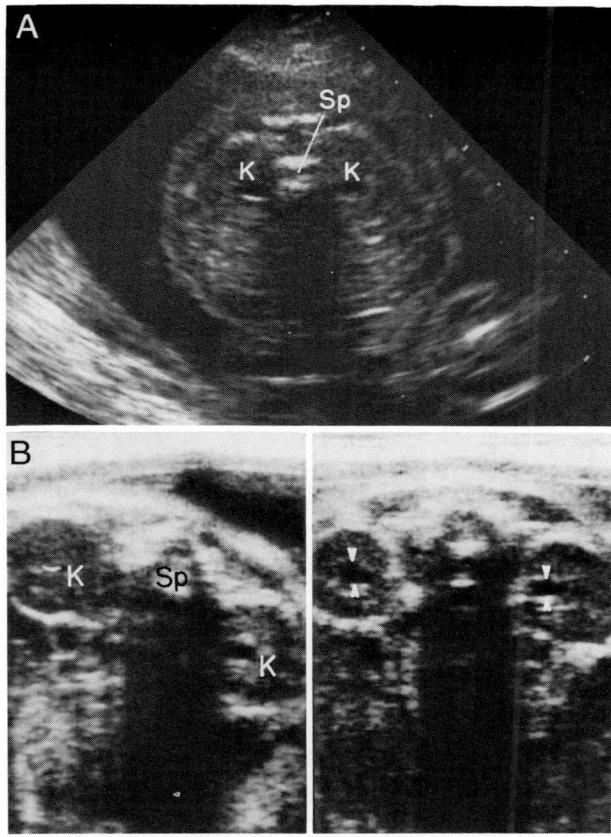

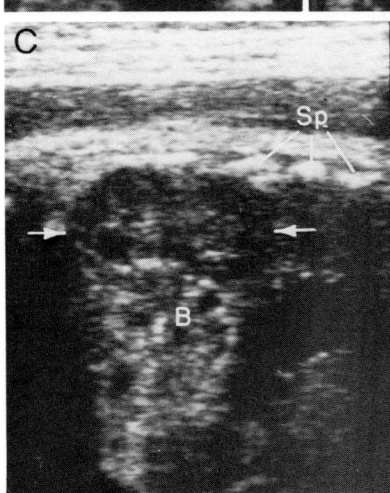

FIG 6–14.
Scans of fetal kidneys. **A,** transaxial image of the fetal body in a 20-week fetus showing the kidneys *(K)* on both sides of the spine *(Sp)*. Note how the kidneys are difficult to separate from the surrounding tissues. **B,** transaxial dual scans of the fetal body in a 35-week fetus. *Left image,* the kidneys *(K)* are easily identified on both sides of the spine *(Sp)* because of the surrounding hyperechoic perinephric fat. *Right image,* an anechoic space in the middle of the hyperechoic central collecting system *(arrowheads),* less than 10 mm in AP diameter, consistent with pyelectasis from normal physiologic reflux. **C,** long-axis scan of the fetal kidney *(arrows)* in a 30-week fetus. Note the hyperechoic central collecting system and hypoechoic peripheral cortex. *B* indicates adjacent bowel.

Grannum et al.,[121] measuring the AP and transverse renal dimensions, did not measure the kidneys in the same straight anteroposterior and transverse axis as used to measure the fetal abdomen. Rather, the renal measurements were taken at an oblique angle.

Despite these differences, the fetal kidney length could be compared from three of the articles.[119, 120, 122] These three showed an increase in the renal length as the fetus increased in gestational age. The variation was very small. At 24 and 40 weeks, the mean length varied from 23 to 25 mm and from 36 to 41 mm, respectively. In the AP dimension, all four articles[119–122] could be compared and discrepancies between articles of only 4 to 5 mm were noted throughout gestation, 11 to 14 mm at 22 weeks to 21 to 25.6 mm at term. In transverse dimension, two articles could be compared,[120, 121] showing only a 3– to 5–mm discrepancy from 22 to 40 weeks, 13 to 16.4 mm, and 23.1 to 28 mm, respectively. The renal volume measurements by Jeanty et al.[120] could not be compared to any other article and did not seem to have any specific advantage in diagnosing fetal renal abnormalities.

The work by Bertagnoli et al. is recommended.[122] Specific numbers of the renal long axis and AP measurements are given with a 2 SD range. While the exact measurement points of the AP measurement are slightly in question and

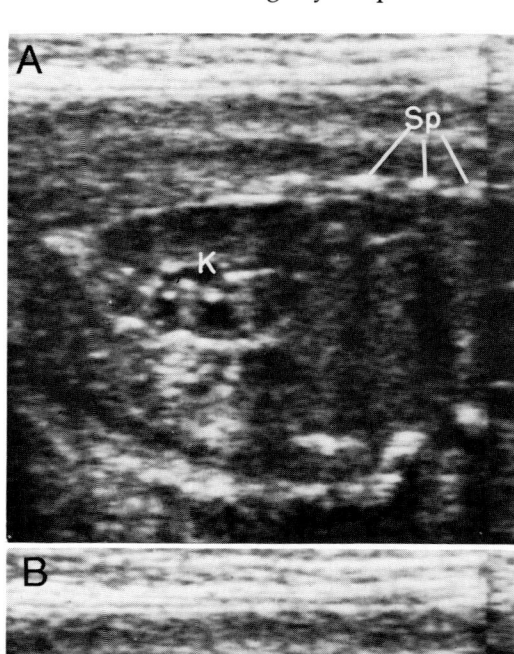

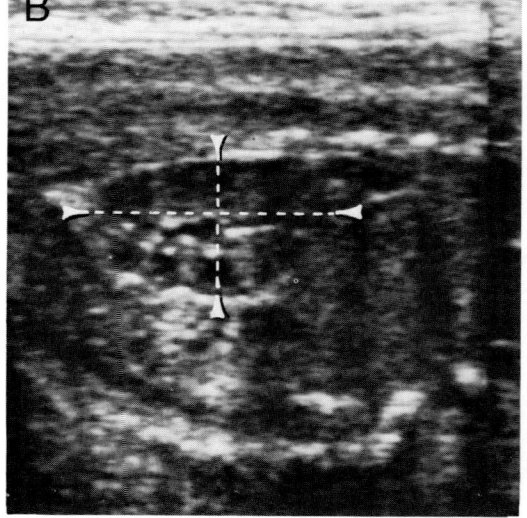

FIG 6–15.
Long-axis scan of the fetal body, adjacent to the spine *(Sp)*, in a 32-week fetus. **A,** long-axis scan of the kidney *(K)* with hyperechoic central collecting system and hypoechoic peripheral cortex. **B,** same image as **A** showing the length and perpendicular AP measurements *(arrowheads* and *dotted line)*.

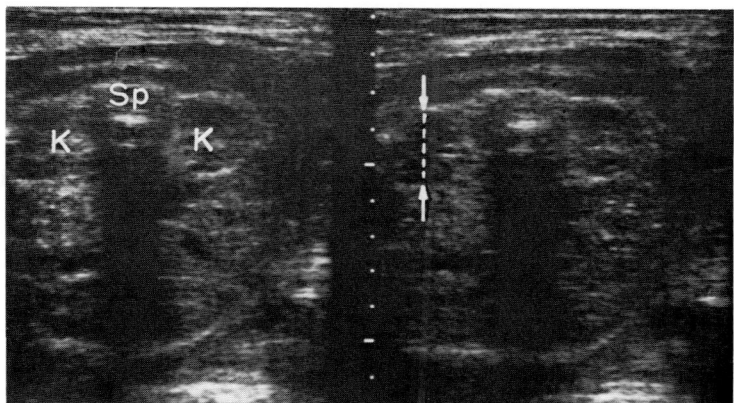

FIG 6–16.
Transaxial dual scans of fetal body. *Left image,* the kidneys *(K)* are imaged on both sides of the spine *(Sp)*. *Right image* (same image as that on the left) shows the AP measurement *(arrowheads* and *dotted line)*. The AP measurement taken from a transaxial scan is not as precise as that taken from a long-axis scan, such as Figure 6–15,B.

a predicted rather than a true mean is used, the study was performed on a large number of patients, both cross-sectionally and longitudinally. Of the two types of studies, the numbers are so close that the longitudinal study was chosen because of the possibility that it might be more accurate (Table 6–8).

The renal to abdomen ratios proposed by Grannum et al.[121] are also of practical value for the evaluation of changes in fetal renal size (Table 6–9). The authors stated that a ratio of the renal to abdominal circumference was constant throughout pregnancy, between 0.27 to 0.30. A similar ratio could be calculated from their data when the AP and transverse dimensions were compared (Fig 6–17). The AP diameter of the kidney divided by the AP diameter of the abdomen gave a ratio of 0.25 to 0.31, while the ratio of the transverse dimension of the kidney to abdomen was 0.27 to 0.31. As a result, any of these ratios could be used with equal accuracy. It must be emphasized, however, that in addition to these measurements, changes in renal echogenicity, particularly anechoic spaces, are also signs of fetal renal disease.

Occasionally an anechoic space can be identified within the renal sinus (see Fig 6–14,B). While Lawson et al.[119] thought that this was a normal finding after 30 weeks and should not be mistaken for hydronephrosis, there is no doubt that this is pyelectasis.[124] This mild pyelectasis, while benign, is undoubtedly due to physiologic reflux in utero. It is a normal finding, present when the fetal urinary bladder is partially or totally distended. On occasion, this can be seen to resolve as the fetus spontaneously voids.

Three articles evaluated this anechoic space from 19 to 20 weeks to term and found that if the measure of the intrarenal collecting system were 9 mm or less an anteroposterior direction, there was no obstruction and all of these cases were normal at birth.[124–126] Some normal fetus even had a separation of the collecting system of 11 mm. If however the pyelectasis were greater than 10 mm and/or associated with dilated ureters, persistance of urinary bladder distension, or oligohydramnios, obstructive uropathy should be seriously considered.[125–128]

TABLE 6–8.
Fetal Kidney Measurement Table*

Gestational Age, wk	Renal Measurements With Range of 5th to 95th Percentile, mm (2 SD)†			
	Length		Anteroposterior Diameter	
	Predicted Mean	2 SD	Predicted Mean	2 SD
22	—	—	11.1	8.7–13.5
23	—	—	11.5	9.1–13.9
24	24.4	22.0–26.8	11.9	9.5–14.3
25	25.0	22.6–27.4	12.4	10.0–14.8
26	25.7	23.3–28.1	13.0	10.6–15.4
27	26.4	24.0–28.8	13.5	11.1–15.9
28	27.2	24.8–29.6	14.2	11.8–16.6
29	28.0	25.6–30.4	14.8	12.4–17.2
30	28.8	26.4–31.2	15.5	13.1–17.9
31	29.6	27.2–32.0	16.3	13.9–18.7
32	30.4	28.0–32.8	17.1	14.7–19.5
33	31.3	28.9–33.7	18.0	15.6–20.4
34	32.2	29.8–34.6	18.9	16.5–21.3
35	33.1	30.8–35 4	19.9	17.5–22.3
36	34.1	31.8–36.4	20.9	18.5–23.3
37	35.1	32.8–37.4	22.0	19.6–24.4
38	36.1	33.8–38.4	23.2	20.8–25.6
39	37.1	34.8–39.4	24.4	22.0–26.8
40	38.2	35.9–40.5	25.7	23.3–28.1
41	39.3	37.0–41.6	—	—
42	40.4	38.1–42.7	—	—

*From Bertagnoli L, Lalatta F, Gallicchio R, et al: Quantitative characterization of the growth of the kidneys. J Clin Ultrasound 1983; 11:349–356. Used by permission.
†Longitudinal study used.

TABLE 6–9.
Renal to Abdominal Ratio—Range Throughout Second and Third Trimester*

	Ratio
Renal-to-abdominal circumferences	0.27:0.30
Renal-to-abdominal anteroposterior diameters	0.25:0.31
Renal-to-abdominal transverse diameters	0.27:0.31

*Adapted from Grannum P, Bracken M, Silverman R, et al: Assessment of fetal kidney size in normal gestation by comparison of ratio of kidney circumference to abdominal circumference. Am J Obstet Gynecol 1980; 136:249–254.

Fetal Urinary Bladder

When distended, the configuration of the fetal urinary bladder is either ovoid or round (Fig 6–18). It has been evaluated in two articles[129, 130] from 32 to 41 weeks with static scanners. The volume of the urinary bladder was calculated by using the equation for a sphere. The hourly urine output was computed and found to increase toward term, 12.2 ml at 32 weeks increasing to 28.2 ml at term.[129] The urinary bladder has been observed to fill and empty in cycles from 50 to 155 minutes.[130] It normally filled at a constant rate, with voiding occurring within seconds but occasionally over 30 minutes.[130] This finding may be important in detecting growth retardation since the same article found that 47% of 62 affected fetuses had decreased urine output.[130]

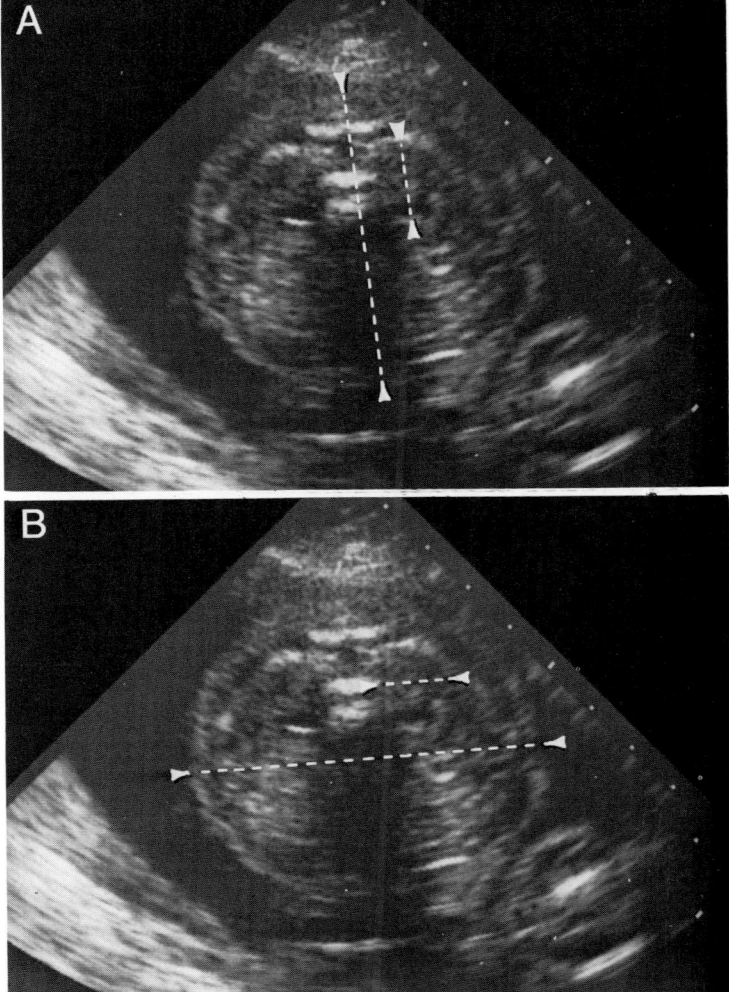

FIG 6–17.
Transaxial scans of the fetal body at the region of the kidneys. **A,** comparison of the AP dimensions of the body and a kidney *(arrowheads* and *dotted lines)*. The kidney is approximately 30% of the body. **B,** comparison of the transverse dimension of the body and a kidney *(arrowheads* and *dotted lines)*. The kidney is approximately 30% of the body.

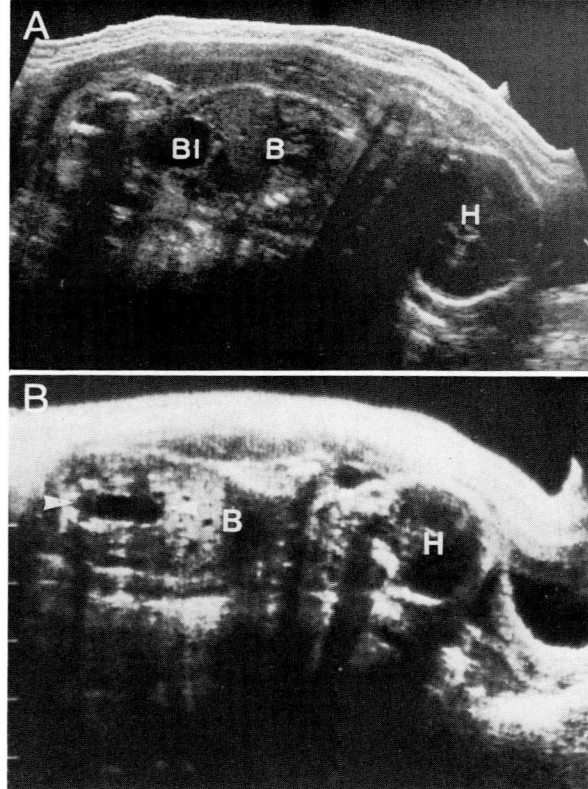

FIG 6–18.
Long-axis scans of two different fetuses in the third trimester, both in cephalic presentation, with different-shaped bladders. **A,** rounded bladder *(Bl).* **B,** ovoid bladder *(arrowheads).* H indicates fetal head; B, fetal body.

In the evaluation of renal anomalies, the urinary bladder plays a pivotal role.[131] When both kidneys are obstructed, the bladder will be either persistently distended or empty, depending upon the level of obstruction. When the kidneys are not functioning, the urinary bladder will not be identified, even over a $1\frac{1}{2}$–hour period, scanned at 10– to 15–minute intervals. On occasion, a rudimentary bladder can be identified filled with a small amount of fluid. Nevertheless, regardless of the type of renal problem, failure of the bladder to change size over time, despite close interval observation, strongly implies bilateral renal abnormalities.

If nonfunctioning kidneys are a consideration, it has been suggested that 20 to 40 mg of Lasix (furosemide), a diuretic that crosses the placental barrier, could be given intravenously to the mother. While some observers have suggested that Lasix may not affect the immature fetal renal tubules, a series by Dubbins et al.[131] reported three cases of suspected bilateral renal agenesis that were proved to have nonfunctioning kidneys with this Lasix challenge test. In all cases of significant bilateral renal dysfunction and obstruction, an additional finding of marked oligohydramnios is almost always present.

Fetal Bowel

The normal fetal bowel has been evaluated in one article.[132] Using real-time ultrasound, 130 fetuses were scanned from 16 weeks to term. The colon was found to be filled with meconium and could be imaged as early as 22 weeks but not consistently identified until 28 weeks (Fig 6–19). From then until term, it appeared as a hypo- to almost completely anechoic tubular structure situated around the perimeter of the abdominal cavity. The diameter of the colon, depicted in a graph, progressively increased in internal diameter as the fetus matured, increasing from an average of 4 to 6 mm at 22 weeks to 10 to 18 mm at term[132] (see Fig 6–19). The colon showed no peristalsis and persisted without change. No colon segment exceeded 18 mm in diameter, even at term.

The small bowel loops in the midabdomen were less frequently identified. None were seen earlier than 28 weeks and even at term could only be identified in 30% of cases. When imaged, no loop exceeded 7 mm in inner diameter or 15 mm in length. Since peristalsis occurred, these loops were only transiently seen.

The authors felt that any persistent loop of small bowel or any prominent small or large bowel loop, larger than 7 mm and 15 mm in internal diameter, respectively, should be considered pathological. This article appears valid and clinically useful. More work is needed, however, before a table can be recommended.

FETAL EXTREMITY MEASUREMENTS

In the late 1960s and early 1970s, measurements of fetal long bones were performed from abdominal radiographs of pregnant women[133–135] with addi-

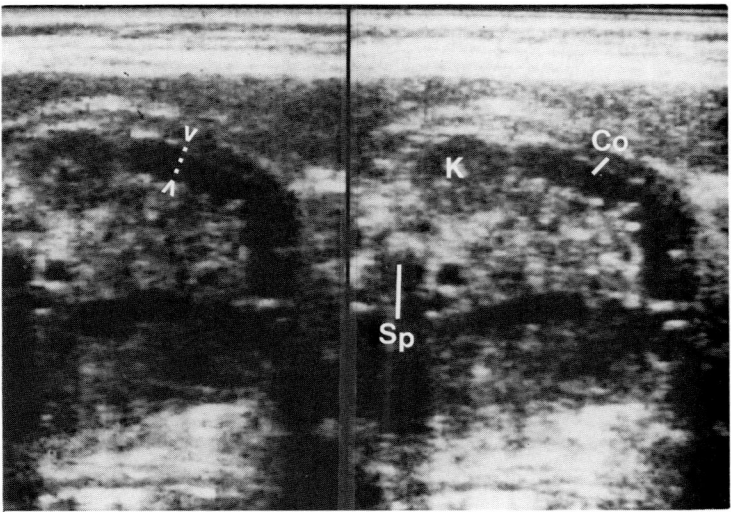

FIG 6–19.
Transaxial dual-image scan of the fetal body through the lower abdomen in a 38-week fetus. *Right image,* the prominent colon *(Co)* is situated at the periphery of the abdomen, filled with hypoechoic meconium. *Sp* indicates spine; *K,* kidney. *Left image,* the inner diameter measurement of the colon *(arrowheads* and *dotted lines).*

tional comparison to radiographs of premature newborn children.[136] While there was difficulty with magnification and orientation, the bones detected on the radiographs correlated well with gestational age.[133, 136] Since 1980, with the advent of high-resolution real-time ultrasound, numerous articles have been published analyzing the length of the fetal long bones. Three of these compared ultrasound to radiographs on aborted fetuses and found good correlation,[137–139] with one demonstrating a correlation coefficient of 0.998.[138] Although there was a high degree of accuracy using radiographs and ultrasound, ultrasound is preferable. There is no ionizing radiation, and real-time ultrasound allows movement of the transducer to ensure that the longest extremity lengths are routinely imaged. The femur, humerus, ulna, radius, radius-ulna complex, tibia, fibula, and tibia-fibula complex have been measured. The femur is the most commonly measured bone, however, since it is the longest tubular bone and the easiest consistently to image.

The technique for obtaining the femoral length is as follows. After the long axis of the fetus is identified, the transducer is turned 90° to produce a cross-sectional image of the fetal trunk. The transducer is moved down the fetus

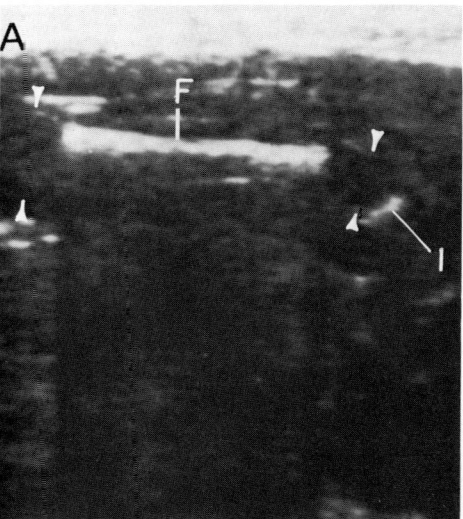

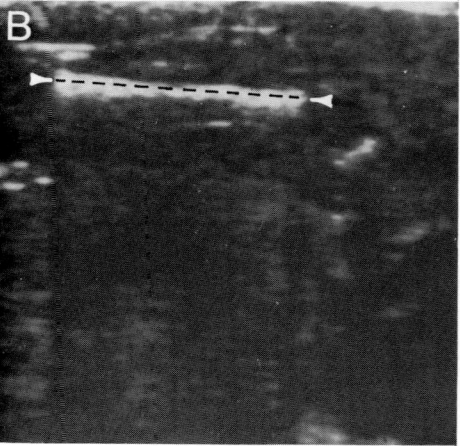

FIG 6–20.
Ultrasound scan of the long axis of a femur (F). **A,** the hyperechoic linear structure is the ossified shaft (diaphysis). The hypoechoic ends of the femur (arrowheads) are rounded structures. On the reader's *left* is the distal epiphyseal cartilage, and on the reader's *right* the proximal epiphyseal cartilage adjacent to the ilium (I). **B,** same image as **A** showing the measurement of the shaft (arrowheads and dotted line).

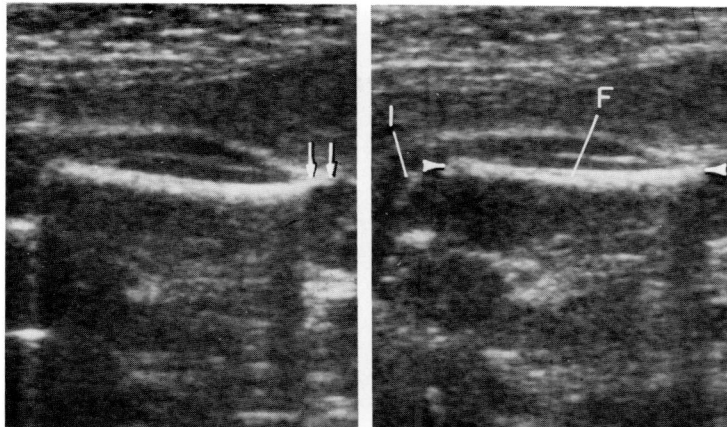

FIG 6–21.
Long-axis dual scans of the femur *(F)*. *Right image,* the hyperechoic diaphysis is denoted by arrowhead. The ilium *(I)* shows the proximal end. *Left image,* a slightly different scan plane again shows the femur shaft. In addition, a hyperechoic nonosseous extension *(arrows)* is imaged distally, falsely elongating the femoral measurement. This is termed the "distal femur point."

toward the rump, maintaining the 90° angle until the lower spine and iliac crest are identified. Since the femur is usually flexed at approximately 30°–45°, the transducer is rotated until a full femoral length is imaged. The hyperechoic linear structure represents the ossified portion of the femoral diaphysis and corresponds to the femoral length measurement from the greater trochanter to the femoral condyles[140] (Fig 6–20). The greater trochanter and the condyles do not ossify in utero but can be imaged as rounded hypoechoic masses at each end of the diaphysis, termed the epiphyseal cartilages (Fig 6–20,A). They should not be included in the femoral length measurement. Ideally the hyperechoic diaphysis and hypoechoic cartilages should all be imaged to assure the examiner that the entire diaphysis is seen and its measurement accurate.[141]

This same article pointed out that occasionally a "distal femur point" is imaged, a nonosseous extension continuing from the distal end of the diaphysis toward the knee[141] (Fig 6–21). In examining a cadaver fetal femur, this distal spur was found to be a specular reflector from the smooth surface of the lateral aspect of the distal epiphyseal cartilage. It is not ossified and should not be included in the femoral length measurement because it would falsely overestimate the femoral length by as much as 3 weeks.[141]

The normal diaphysis of the femur has a straight lateral border and a curved medial border,[142] incorrectly termed mild physiologic bowing,[137] and often observed after 18 weeks (Fig 6–22). A straight measurement of the femur taken from one end of the diaphysis to the other should disregard this area of curvature (Fig 6–22,C). If included, however, the measurement would only increase by a maximum of 2 mm in length[143] (Fig 6–22,D). Lastly, after 30 weeks, a punctate hyperechoic distal femoral epiphysis may be observed.[144] While this is frequently a sign of fetal maturity, it is distinctly separate from the distal end of the diaphysis and should not be included in the femoral length measurement (Fig 6–23).

The other fetal extremities are more difficult to routinely image. The humerus does not have a constant angle of flexion with the fetal trunk. It can usually be identified by imaging the fetal spine in the upper thoracic-lower cervical region,

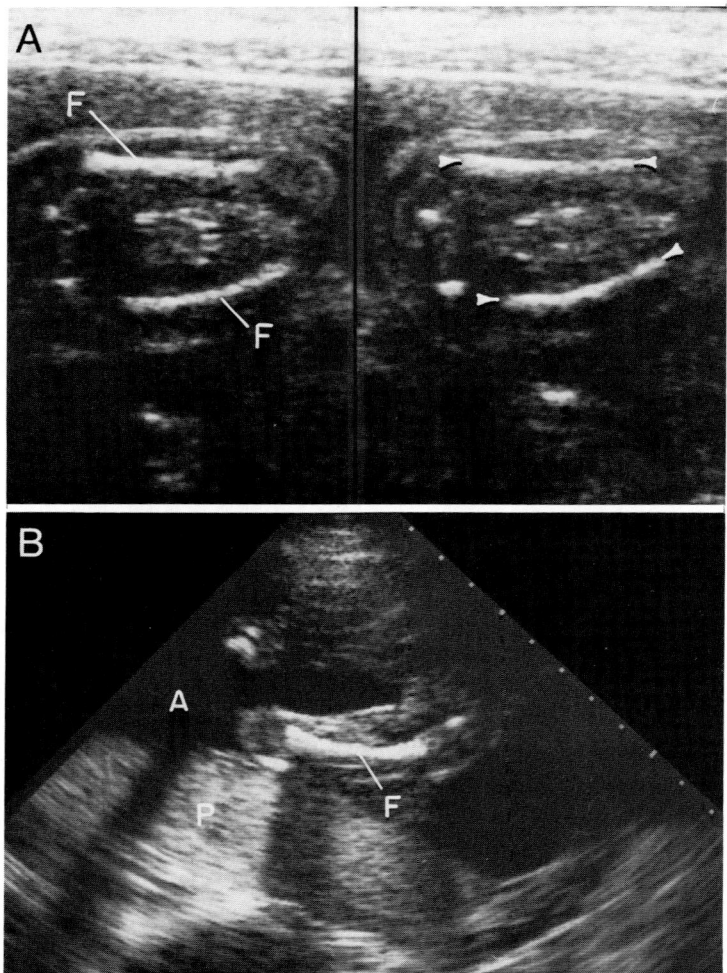

FIG 6–22.
The straight lateral and curved medial borders of the femurs *(F)*. **A,** long-axis dual scans. *Left image,* the fetus is lying on its side so that the upper femur is imaged on its lateral and the lower femur on its medial border. *Right image,* both femurs (regardless of curvature) are measured from one end of the diaphysis to the other *(arrowheads)*. **B,** the medial curved border of the femur of a different fetus. A indicates amniotic fluid; P, placenta. *(Continued.)*

identifying the scapula, and then rotating the transducer until the long axis of the humerus is obtained (Fig 6–24). Just as with the femur, only the humeral shaft (diaphysis) is ossified. The shaft is therefore measured, disregarding the nonossified ends. The forearm (radius and ulna) and distal leg (tibia and fibula) are the most difficult to image due to the paucity of adjacent landmarks and to the often rapid movements of the fetus and extremities (Figs 6–25 and 6–26). While only the diaphyseal shafts are ossified and thus measured, the bones are not the same length. In the leg, the tibia is longer than the fibula and in the forearm the ulna is longer than the radius. To make certain that the correct bone is measured, both should be imaged. The fibula is situated lateral to the tibia

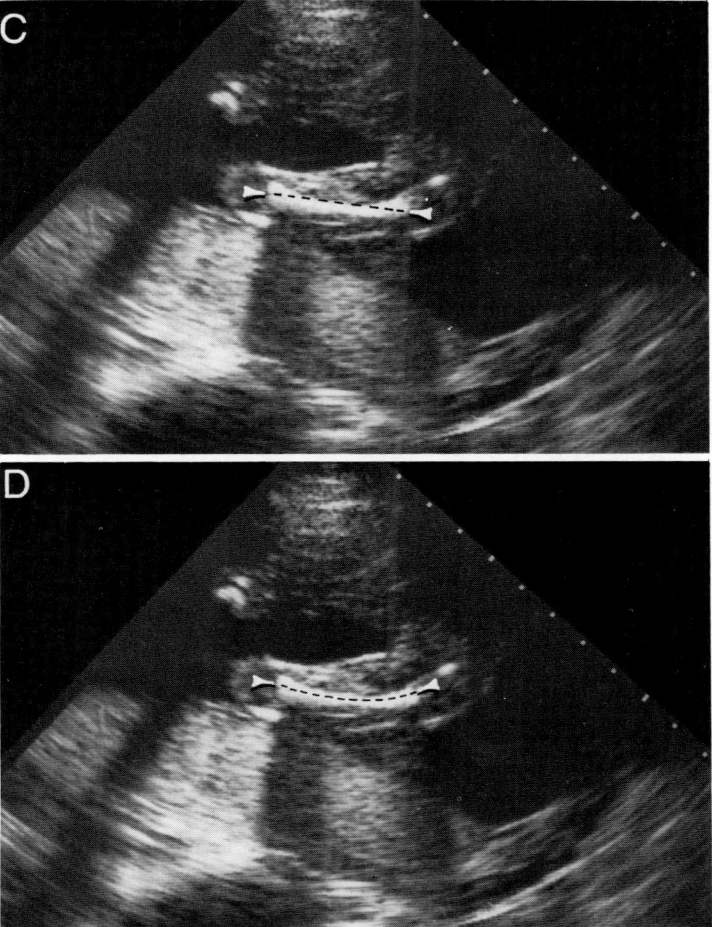

FIG 6–22 (cont.).
C, same image as **B** showing the correct straight measurement, disregarding the curve of the diaphysis *(arrowheads* and *dotted line)*. **D,** same image as **B** showing the incorrect curved measurement along the curved medial border of the diaphysis *(arrowheads* and *dotted lines)*. Even if this mistake is made, it only adds 2 mm to the femur length.

and is a little thinner.[145] The ulna always appears longer than the radius proximally, while distally they meet at the same level.

Unless the fetus is in a face-up or face-down orientation, all the fetal extremities are often not imaged. More commonly, the fetus is in an oblique or lateral lie, so that only the limbs closest to the transducer are identified, while the limbs further away are partially obscured by the fetal body and spine. Nevertheless, at least one femur can be measured in almost every case. Since it is rare to have different-sized femurs in the same fetus, one femur accurately represents the length of both. This femoral length serves two purposes, as a predictor of gestational age and as an indicator of skeletal dysplasias and asymmetric intrauterine growth retardation. Rarely one femur is either fractured or hypoplastic, the latter occurring secondary to maternal diabetes mellitus.

The femoral length has been found to be a good predictor of gestational age. In one article,[138] the growth of the femur was within ±6.7 days of the menstrual age at the 95% confidence level and therefore a reliable predictor of fetal age.[138] In two other articles, when the femoral length was compared to the menstrual history,[146, 147] the femoral length could be used as an adjunctive test in establishing fetal age, since it was found to be ±11.6 days between 18 and 24 weeks, increasing to ±22.7 days by 36 to 42 weeks.[146] More recently, Wolfson et al.[148] compared the biparietal diameter (uncorrected in shape) to the femoral length and found them equal estimators of gestational age. In evaluating 30 growth retarded fetuses, Woo et al.[149] confirmed that the femoral length was as accurate as the biparietal diameter. Surprisingly, Yeh and co-workers[150] thought that the femoral measurement was more precise than the biparietal diameter. While this was confirmed by Tse and Lee[151] using the original data of Yeh et al.,[150] several aspects of the initial work appear inaccurate: their evaluation was limited to a linear regression analysis,[152] unspecified calculations were used, and the correlation coefficient between the biparietal diameter and gestational age was unusually low, at 0.35. In two works by another group, the femoral length was also interpreted as being more accurate than the biparietal diameter.[153, 154] This, too, is unimpressive, since the femur length accuracy up to 31 gestational weeks was poor at ±2.75 weeks.[153] When combined with the biparietal diameter, accuracies of only ±2.5 weeks up to 32 weeks and ±2.75 weeks up to 34 weeks were obtained.[153] Therefore, in summary, the femoral length has approximately the same accuracy as the biparietal diameter and can be used as an alternative measurement, especially when the head is an unusual shape or is difficult to image because of an unusual position.

The reproducibility of femoral length measurements has also been investigated. Three consecutive measurements of the femur, regardless of its length, have been found to have an error of only 0.8 mm, with a range of 0.1 to 1.5 mm.[138] Several factors may produce measurement errors. False shortening of the femur may result from tangential sections so that the full femoral length is not imaged.[138] Overestimation of the femoral length has been proposed by excessive use of power or gain during scanning, which falsely thickened and lengthened the bone,[138] or by incorporating proximal or distal ossification centers

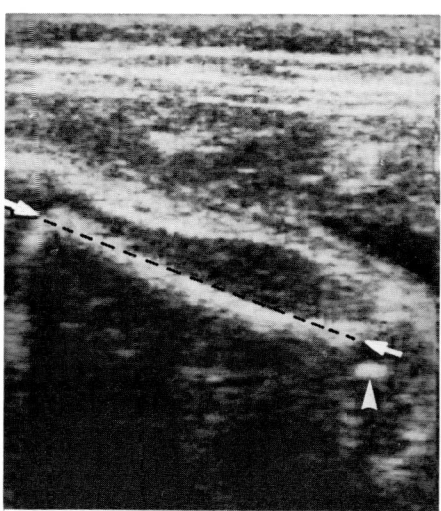

FIG 6–23.
Long axis of a femur at 37 weeks. The measurement of the hyperechoic diaphysis (arrowheads and dotted line) is performed from one end to the other, disregarding the separate hyperechoic distal femoral epiphysis (arrowhead).

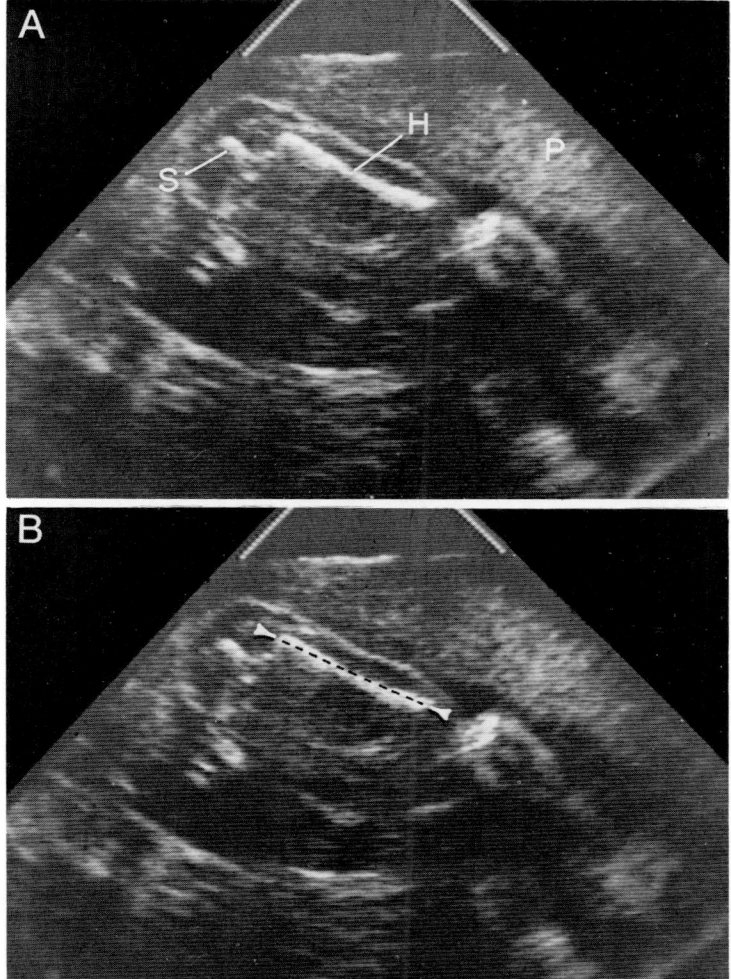

FIG 6–24.
Ultrasound scan of the long axis of the humerus (H). **A,** the hyperechoic linear structure is the ossified diaphysis of the humerus. The hypoechoic ends have not ossified. S indicates scapula, denoting proximal end of humerus; P, placenta. **B,** same image as **A** showing the measurement of the shaft (*arrowheads* and *dotted line*).

into the femoral length measurement.[137] Measuring the "distal femur point" may also falsely lengthen the femur.[141]

The technical factor that has been most investigated because of its potential effect on femoral length has been the type of transducer used to obtain the measurement. Four articles have been published evaluating the accuracy of femoral measurements using mechanical sector scanners vs. linear and phased array (sector or linear) scanners.[155–158] All articles state that the vertical (parallel to the ultrasound beam) measurement errors were small, within 6%, while horizontal (perpendicular to the beam) measurements were more discrepant. Two of the articles[155, 156] stated that in the horizontal plane the mechanical sector scanners were in error within the focal zone by up to 8 mm and outside the focal zone by as much as 26 mm, or 47%! Increased inaccuracies could also occur at the lateral margins of the image. All of these errors made the femur falsely larger. The other two articles,[157, 158] however, found no significant measurement errors, even when the femur was horizontally positioned. The reasons for the marked contradictions among these studies cannot be ascertained but may be due to incorrect equipment calibration,[155] a problem that gets worse with some mechanical sector scanners as the transducer ages. At the present time, while there is no doubt that linear and phased-array scanners are accurate, mechanical sector scanners can be used. Errors using a mechanical sector scanner should

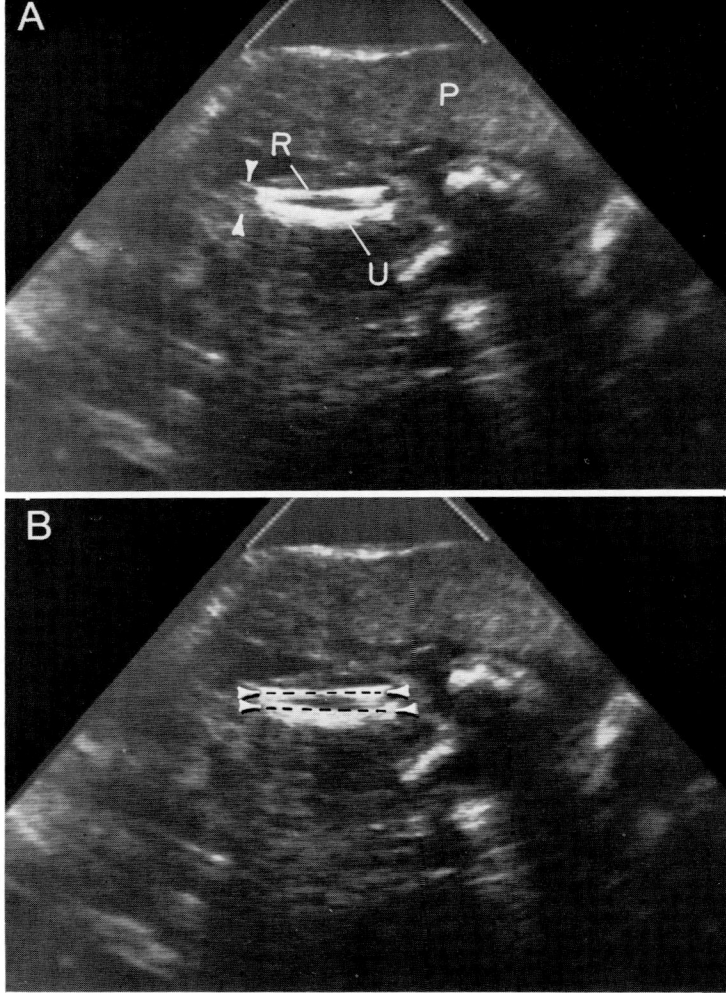

FIG 6–25.
Ultrasound scan of the long axis of the forearm, imaging both the radius (R) and ulna (U). **A,** the radius and ulna are of different lengths, the ulna longer. Both hyperechoic diaphyseal shafts meet at the wrist where the nonossified hypoechoic carpal bones *(arrowheads)* are located. P indicates placenta. **B,** same image as **A** showing the measurements of the shafts of the radius and ulna *(arrowheads* and *dotted lines)*.

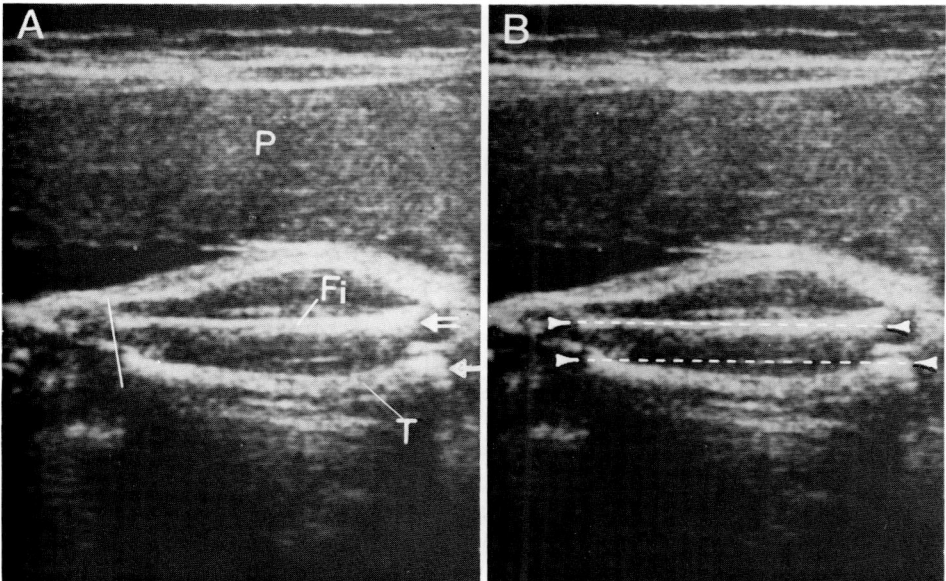

FIG 6–26.
Ultrasound scan of the long bones of the distal leg, the fibula *(Fi)* and tibia *(T)*. **A,** fibula and tibia are of different lengths, the tibia longer and thicker. Both hyperechoic diaphyseal shafts meet at the ankle *(straight line)*, with the proximal end of the tibia *(arrow)* longer than the fibula *(double arrow)*. P indicates placenta. **B,** same image as **A** showing the measurements of the shafts of the tibia and fibula, disregarding their curves *(arrowheads* and *dotted lines)*.

be minimized by imaging the femur within the focal zone and in the middle of the image.

As an indicator of abnormality, any true femoral length shortening is strongly suggestive of either a skeletal dysplasia[159–162] or intrauterine growth retardation.[163] Skeletal dysplasias can be detected by observing the limb's length, growth, mineralization and overall contour. Almost all skeletal dysplasias affect the femurs bilaterally, regardless of what other body parts are also involved. While there is not a great deal known about the in utero development of most skeletal dysplasias, it can be stated that if an abnormality is detected in the femur, the femur is abnormal; a normal examination, however, does not entirely exclude a subtle abnormality or one that may manifest itself later in gestation or after birth.[162,164] For example, heterozygous achondroplasia has been documented by an abnormal femoral length at 27 weeks in cases that had been normal at 16 to 23 gestational weeks.[161, 162, 164] Skeletal dysplasias have also been detected by observing deformity of the long bones in achondrogenesis,[162] fractures of the long bones in osteogenesis imperfecta,[160, 162] and in demineralization of the axial skeleton in such entities as hypophosphatasia.[162] If these abnormalities had not been detected, however, the skeletal dysplasia could not have been ruled out.

In symmetric growth retardation, all the fetal parameters including the femoral length lag behind the correct gestational age.[163] In asymmetric growth retardation, while the fetal body will be affected first, the head and femur measurements will also be affected in severe cases. A recent article comparing pregnant women with sickle cell trait (Hb AS) to a matched group with sickle cell anemia (Hb AA) found that fetuses with the sickle cell trait had the same size biparietal diameter but somewhat smaller femoral lengths.[165] While the birth weights of the sickle cell trait babies were lower, they could not be growth retarded, since their head sizes were normal. If substantiated, this finding could have clinical value.

The femoral length has been evaluated in 21 articles, 14 in number form,[137, 140, 145, 147, 153, 154, 166–173] and 7 in graph form.[138, 139, 150, 152, 161, 174, 175] Three articles by Jeanty et al.[140, 168, 169] were given in table form in reference 169, so the other two references will not be considered further. While Hohler and Quetel[175] compared their own work to that of O'Brien and Queenan[171] in reference 152, their numbers are slightly different, and both reference 152 and 175 will be considered further.

Of the remaining 19 articles,[137–139, 145, 147, 150, 152–154, 161, 166, 167, 169–175] only 15 evaluated the femoral length from the early to mid-second trimester, prior to 20 weeks, to term.[139, 145, 147, 150, 152–154, 166, 167, 169–174] The remaining articles analyzed the femur only through portions of the second and third trimesters. Fifteen articles used linear-array real-time scanners, three[137, 138, 173] were performed with a mechanical sector scanner, and the last[153] did not state what type of scanner was used. When all these articles were compared, there was fairly close grouping of the femoral length throughout gestation, with all articles showing an increase in femur length as the gestation progressed to term. At 16 weeks, for example, 17 articles[137–139, 145, 147, 150, 152–154, 166, 167, 169–174] gave femoral lengths that measured between 18 and 24 mm except one,[150] which was 4 mm larger. At term, all 19 articles gave femoral measurements with a close range, between 75 and 80 mm, except three,[153, 154, 173] which were as much as 5 mm smaller. Of interest, considering the controversy about the use of mechanical sector scanners, was the finding that the articles using the sector scanners[137, 138, 173] did not significantly differ from the other articles except in the work by Haines et al.,[173] which found a decreased femoral length after 36 weeks. Even this observation does not confirm the controversy of femoral length measurements, since a mechanical sector scanner error is expected to produce a longer, not a shorter, femur.

Two additional aspects of femur length should also be considered; i.e., the amount of variation around each mean measurement point and the overall shape of the growth curve, linear or curvilinear. In general, the articles that showed an increased variability in the femur measurements toward term also showed a more curvilinear growth, comparable to that of the biparietal diameter.[145, 147, 152–154, 166, 171, 173] The articles that demonstrated linear growth did not show increased variation.[138, 139, 167, 169, 170, 174, 175] There were only four exceptions. Two articles[159, 175] demonstrated curvilinear growth without increased variation toward term, with the two others showing linear growth with increased variation.[137, 161] The reasons for differences between types of curves cannot be determined. While the tables for both types of curves appear to be acceptable, a curvilinear growth seems to be more physiologic.

Since, as previously discussed, there are two reasons to obtain a femoral length—i.e., to establish a fetal age especially when the head cannot be adequately imaged and to evaluate head to skeleton disproportions—two tables are recommended[145, 170] (Tables 6–10 and 6–11). The results of both are close, both giving their results in number form with a 2 SD range in weeks. The article by Merz et al.,[145] however, seems preferable, since the growth of the femur is curvilinear, the true rather than the predicted mean is used, and the femur

TABLE 6–10.
Fetal Long Bone Measurement Table*

Gestational Age, wk	True Mean and Range From 5th to 95th Percentile, mm (2 SD)					
	Biparietal Diameter		Femur		Humerus	
	Mean	2 SD	Mean	2 SD	Mean	2 SD
13	23	20–26	11	9–13	10	8–12
14	27	24–30	13	11–15	12	10–14
15	30	29–31	15	13–17	14	12–16
16	33	31–35	19	16–22	17	15–19
17	37	34–40	22	19–25	20	16–24
18	42	37–47	25	22–28	23	20–26
19	44	40–48	28	25–31	26	23–29
20	47	43–51	31	28–34	29	26–32
21	50	45–55	35	31–39	32	28–36
22	55	50–60	36	33–39	33	30–36
23	58	53–63	40	36–44	37	34–40
24	61	56–66	42	39–45	38	34–42
25	64	59–69	46	43–49	42	38–46
26	68	63–73	48	44–52	43	40–46
27	70	67–73	49	46–52	45	43–47
28	73	68–78	53	48–58	47	43–51
29	76	71–81	53	48–58	48	44–52
30	77	71–83	56	53–59	50	45–55
31	82	75–89	60	54–66	53	49–57
32	85	79–91	61	55–68	54	50–58
33	86	82–90	64	59–69	56	51–61
34	89	84–94	66	60–72	58	53–63
35	89	82–96	67	61–73	59	53–65
36	91	84–98	70	63–77	60	54–66
37	93	84–102	72	68–76	61	57–65
38	95	89–101	74	68–80	64	61–67
39	95	89–101	76	68–84	65	59–71
40	99	92–107	77	73–81	66	62–70
41	97	91–103	77	73–81	66	62–70
42	100	95–105	78	71–83	68	61–75

*From Merz E, Kim-Kern M, Pehl S: Ultrasonic mensuration of fetal limb bones in the second and third trimesters. J Clin Ultrasound 1987; 15:175–183. Used by permission.

TABLE 6–11.
Femur and Humerus Measurement Table*

Bone Length, mm	Femur		Humerus	
	Predicted Mean Value	Range From 5th to 95th Percentile	Predicted Mean Value	Range From 5th to 95th Percentile
10	12.6	10.4–14.9	12.6	9.9–15.3
11	12.9	10.7–15.1	12.9	10.1–15.6
12	13.3	11.1–15.6	13.1	10.4–15.9
13	13.6	11.4–15.9	13.6	10.9–16.1
14	13.9	11.7–16.1	13.9	11.1–16.6
15	14.1	12.0–16.4	14.1	11.4–16.9
16	14.6	12.4–16.9	14.6	11.9–17.3
17	14.9	12.7–17.1	14.9	12.1–17.6
18	15.1	13.0–17.4	15.1	12.6–18.0
19	15.6	13.4–17.9	15.6	12.9–18.3
20	15.9	13.7–18.1	15.9	13.1–18.7
21	16.3	14.1–18.6	16.3	13.6–19.1
22	16.6	14.4–18.9	16.7	13.9–19.4
23	16.9	14.7–19.1	17.1	14.3–19.9
24	17.3	15.1–19.6	17.4	14.7–20.1
25	17.6	15.4–19.9	17.9	15.1–20.6
26	18.0	15.9–20.1	18.1	15.6–21.0
27	18.3	16.1–20.6	18.6	15.9–21.4
28	18.7	16.6–20.9	19.0	16.3–21.9
29	19.0	16.9–21.1	19.4	16.7–22.1

30	19.4	17.1–21.6	19.9	17.1–22.6
31	19.9	17.6–22.0	20.3	17.6–23.0
32	20.1	17.9–22.3	20.7	18.0–23.6
33	20.6	18.3–22.7	21.1	18.4–23.9
34	20.9	18.7–23.1	21.6	18.9–24.3
35	21.1	19.0–23.4	22.0	19.3–24.9
36	21.6	19.4–23.9	22.6	19.7–25.1
37	22.0	19.9–24.1	22.9	20.1–25.7
38	22.4	20.1–24.6	23.4	20.6–26.1
39	22.7	20.6–24.9	23.9	21.1–26.6
40	23.1	20.9–25.3	24.3	21.6–27.1
41	23.6	21.3–25.7	24.9	22.0–27.6
42	23.9	21.7–26.1	25.3	22.6–28.0
43	24.3	22.1–26.6	25.7	23.0–28.6
44	24.7	22.6–26.9	26.1	23.6–29.0
45	25.0	22.9–27.1	26.7	24.0–29.6
46	25.4	23.1–27.6	27.1	24.6–30.0
47	25.9	23.6–28.0	27.7	25.0–30.6
48	26.1	24.0–28.4	28.1	25.6–31.0
49	26.6	24.4–28.9	28.9	26.0–31.6
50	27.0	24.9–29.1	29.3	26.6–32.0
51	27.4	25.1–29.6	29.9	27.1–32.6
52	27.9	25.6–30.0	30.3	27.6–33.1
53	28.1	26.0–30.4	30.9	28.1–33.6
54	28.6	26.4–30.9	31.4	28.7–34.1

(Continued.)

TABLE 6–11 (cont.).
Femur and Humerus Measurement Table*

Bone Length, mm	Gestational Age, wk			
	Femur		Humerus	
	Predicted Mean Value	Range From 5th to 95th Percentile	Predicted Mean Value	Range From 5th to 95th Percentile
55	29.1	26.9–31.3	32.0	29.1–34.7
56	29.6	27.2–31.7	32.6	29.9–35.3
57	29.9	27.7–32.1	33.1	30.3–35.9
58	30.3	28.1–32.6	33.6	30.9–36.4
59	30.7	28.6–32.9	34.1	31.4–36.9
60	31.1	28.9–33.3	34.9	32.0–37.6
61	31.6	29.4–33.9	35.3	32.6–38.1
62	32.0	29.9–34.1	35.9	33.1–38.7
63	32.4	30.1–34.6	36.6	33.9–39.3
64	32.9	30.7–35.1	37.1	34.4–39.9
65	33.4	31.1–35.6	37.7	35.0–40.6
66	33.7	31.6–35.9	38.3	35.6–41.1
67	34.1	32.0–36.4	38.9	36.1–41.7
68	34.6	32.4–36.9	39.6	36.9–42.3
69	35.0	32.6–37.1	40.1	37.4–42.9
70	35.6	33.3–37.7	—	—
71	35.9	33.7–38.1	—	—
72	36.4	34.1–38.6	—	—
73	36.9	34.6–39.0	—	—
74	37.3	35.1–39.6	—	—

75	37.7	—
76	38.1	—
77	38.6	—
78	39.1	—
79	39.6	—
80	40.0	—
		35.6–39.9
		36.0–40.4
		36.4–40.9
		36.9–41.3
		37.3–41.7
		37.9–42.1

*From Jeanty P, Rodesch F, Delbeke D, et al: Estimation of gestational age from measurements of fetal long bones. J Ultrasound Med 1984; 3:75–79. Used by permission.

length is compared directly to the biparietal diameter. Nevertheless, both are valid studies giving different orientations. Merz et al.[145] compared the mean gestational age to the mean and SD range of both the biparietal diameter and femur. This table allows direct comparison of head to body and better predictions of any disproportions. Jeanty et al.[170] compared the mean femur length to the mean and range of the gestational age. Their table (see Table 6-11) is better for establishing gestational age based on the femur measurement.

Similar work analyzing the growth of the humerus has been reported in five articles.[137, 145, 168, 170, 174] All showed an increase in the size of the humerus as the fetus grows to term. Three gave their results in numbers,[145, 168, 170] with the other two in graph form.[137, 174] The same two tables are recommended, one showing curvilinear growth[145] and one linear growth[170] (see Tables 6-10 and 6-11). Both compare the humerus to the mean and a 2 SD range, Merz et al.,[145] using a true mean and comparing the humeral length directly to the biparietal diameter. The numbers between the articles are only slightly discrepant, up to 3 mm different at term. The reasons for this difference cannot be ascertained but at term this represents an error of no more than 5%, probably not significant.

The ulna, radius, tibia, and fibula have been evaluated in five articles.[137, 139, 145, 169, 170] As with the femur and humerus, these bones also increase in size as the fetus grows. The same two articles[145, 170] are again recommended and for the same reasons (Tables 6-12 to 6-15). Jeanty et al.[170] evaluated the ulna and tibia and Merz et al.[145] measured all four bones. There are discrepancies between the two articles in ulna and tibia measurements, increasing to 4 mm at term. This error is approximately 6% and is of questionable significance. Further work will be needed to establish which table, if either, is more accurate.

A recent article has evaluated the overall length of the fetal foot, comparing it to the gestational age.[176] The foot was measured in either plantar or longitudinal view from the heel to the great toe throughout the second and third trimester. There was close correlation when compared to both a previous pathologic series, reported in the article, and to the gestational age. The data was presented as a graph and in number form. While these data are of interest, it has not been established if this measurement is any more reliable than the other established bony measurements, especially the femoral length. In addition, while not discussed by the authors, this measurement should be technically difficult to obtain because of constant fetal movements.

Ossification centers can also be measured (see Fig 6-23). Not only their detection but also their size is helpful in establishing gestation age.[177, 178] In one article,[177] when the distal femoral epiphyseal ossification center measured ≥6 mm (they did not say how the measurements were taken, presumably longest dimension), the fetus was mature with an amniotic fluid lecithin/sphingomyelin ratio of ≥2.0. At term, this same article found the ossifications centers to be the following sizes: calcaneal, 13 to 16 mm; talar, 9 to 12 mm; distal femoral, 6 to 9 mm; and proximal tibial, 4 to 6 mm.[177] These two articles also showed that when both the distal femoral and proximal tibial epiphyses were present and measured 5 and 3 mm in longest axes, respectively, the fetus should be at least 34 to 35 weeks of age.[177, 178] While not confirmed, these numbers could therefore have clinical significance, especially as a parameter to establish fetal age in the third trimester.

TABLE 6–12.
Fetal Long Bone (Radius and Ulna) Measurement Table*

Gestational Age, wk	True Mean and Range From 5th to 95th Percentile, mm (2 SD)					
	Biparietal Diameter		Radius		Ulna	
	Mean	2 SD	Mean	2 SD	Mean	2 SD
13	23	20–26	6	4–8	8	5–11
14	27	24–30	8	6–10	10	8–12
15	30	29–31	11	10–12	12	11–13
16	33	31–35	14	11–17	16	13–19
17	37	34–40	15	12–18	17	14–20
18	42	37–47	19	17–21	22	19–25
19	44	40–48	21	18–24	24	21–27
20	47	43–51	24	22–26	27	24–30
21	50	45–55	27	23–31	30	26–34
22	55	50–60	28	23–33	31	27–35
23	58	53–63	31	27–35	35	33–37
24	61	56–66	33	29–37	36	32–40
25	64	59–69	35	32–38	39	35–43
26	68	63–73	36	32–40	40	37–43
27	70	67–73	37	34–40	41	39–43
28	73	68–78	39	35–43	44	39–49
29	76	71–81	40	35–45	45	41–49
30	77	71–83	41	35–47	47	44–50
31	82	75–89	42	39–45	49	45–53
32	85	79–91	44	38–50	50	44–56
33	86	82–90	45	40–50	52	49–55
34	89	84–94	47	42–53	54	49–59
35	89	82–96	48	42–54	54	50–58
36	91	84–98	49	44–54	55	52–58
37	93	84–102	51	48–54	56	52–60
38	95	89–101	51	46–56	58	52–64
39	95	89–101	53	48–58	60	54–66
40	99	92–107	53	50–56	60	55–65
41	97	91–103	56	52–60	63	58–68
42	100	95–105	57	52–62	65	60–70

*From Merz E, Kim-Kern M, Pehl S: Ultrasonic mensuration of fetal limb bones in the second and third trimesters. *J Clin Ultrasound* 1987; 15:175–183. Used by permission.

TABLE 6–13.
Ulna Measurement Table*

Ulna Length, mm	Gestational Age, wk		Ulna Length, mm	Gestational Age, wk	
	Predicted Mean Values	Range From 5th to 95th Percentile		Predicted Mean Values	Range From 5th to 95th Percentile
10	13.1	10.6–16.1	41	26.7	23.6–29.7
11	13.6	10.6–16.4	42	27.1	24.1–30.3
12	13.9	10.9–16.9	43	27.7	24.7–30.9
13	14.4	11.1–17.3	44	28.3	25.1–31.3
14	14.6	11.6–17.7	45	28.9	25.9–31.9
15	15.0	11.9–18.0	46	29.4	26.3–32.4
16	15.4	12.3–18.4	47	29.9	26.9–33.0
17	15.7	12.7–18.9	48	30.6	27.4–33.6
18	16.1	13.1–19.1	49	31.1	28.0–34.1
19	16.6	13.6–19.6	50	31.6	28.6–34.7
20	16.9	13.9–20.0	51	32.1	29.1–35.3
21	17.3	14.3–20.6	52	32.9	29.7–35.9
22	17.7	14.7–20.9	53	33.4	30.3–36.4
23	18.1	15.1–21.1	54	34.0	30.9–37.0
24	18.6	15.6–21.6	55	34.6	31.6–37.7
25	19.0	16.0–22.0	56	35.1	32.1–38.3
26	19.4	16.4–22.6	57	35.9	32.9–38.9
27	19.9	16.9–22.9	58	36.4	33.4–39.6
28	20.3	17.3–23.4	59	37.1	34.0–40.1
29	20.9	17.7–23.9	60	37.7	34.6–40.9
30	21.1	18.1–24.3	61	38.3	35.3–41.4
31	21.7	18.6–24.9	62	39.0	35.9–42.0
32	22.1	19.1–25.1	63	39.6	36.6–42.7
33	22.7	19.6–25.7	64	40.3	37.1–43.3
34	23.1	20.1–26.1			
35	23.6	20.6–26.7			
36	24.1	21.1–27.1			
37	24.6	21.4–27.7			
38	25.1	22.1–28.1			
39	25.6	22.6–28.7			
40	26.1	23.1–29.1			

*From Jeanty P, Rodesch F, Delbeke D, et al: Estimation of gestational age from measurements of fetal long bones. J Ultrasound Med 1984; 3:75–79. Used by permission.

TABLE 6–14.
Fetal Long Bone (Tibia and Fibula) Measurement Table*

Gestational Age, wk	True Mean and Range From 5th to 95th Percentile, mm (2 SD)					
	Biparietal Diameter		Tibia		Fibula	
	Mean	2 SD	Mean	2 SD	Mean	2 SD
13	23	20–26	9	7–11	8	6–10
14	27	24–30	10	8–12	9	6–12
15	30	29–31	13	11–15	12	10–14
16	33	31–35	16	13–19	15	12–18
17	37	34–40	18	15–21	17	15–19
18	42	37–47	22	19–25	21	18–24
19	44	40–48	25	22–28	23	20–26
20	47	43–51	27	25–29	26	24–28
21	50	45–55	30	26–34	29	25–33
22	55	50–60	32	29–35	31	28–34
23	58	53–63	36	34–38	34	32–36
24	61	56–66	37	34–40	36	33–39
25	64	59–69	40	37–43	39	35–43
26	68	63–73	42	39–45	40	37–43
27	70	67–73	44	41–47	42	39–45
28	73	68–78	45	41–49	44	41–47
29	76	71–81	46	43–49	45	42–48
30	77	71–83	48	43–53	47	44–50
31	82	75–89	51	48–54	49	44–54
32	85	79–91	52	48–56	51	47–55
33	86	82–90	54	49–59	53	50–56
34	89	84–94	57	52–62	55	51–59
35	89	82–96	58	54–66	56	52–60
36	91	84–98	60	54–66	56	51–61
37	93	84–102	61	57–65	60	56–64
38	95	89–101	62	59–65	60	56–64
39	95	89–101	64	57–71	61	55–67
40	99	92–107	65	62–68	62	61–63
41	97	91–103	66	62–70	63	58–68
42	100	95–105	68	63–73	67	60–74

*From Merz E, Kim-Kern M, Pehl S: Ultrasonic mensuration of fetal limb bones in the second and third trimesters. J Clin Ultrasound 1987; 15:175–183. Used by permission.

TABLE 6–15.
Tibia Measurement Table*

Tibia Length, mm	Gestational Age, wk		Tibia Length, mm	Gestational Age, wk	
	Predicted Mean Values	Range From 5th to 95th Percentile		Predicted Mean Values	Range From 5th to 95th Percentile
10	13.4	10.6–16.3			
11	13.7	10.9–16.6	41	25.7	22.9–28.6
12	14.1	11.1–17.0	42	26.1	23.3–29.1
13	14.4	11.6–17.3	43	26.6	23.7–29.6
14	14.9	11.9–17.7	44	27.1	24.1–30.3
15	15.1	12.1–18.0	45	27.6	24.6–30.6
16	15.6	12.6–18.4	46	28.0	25.1–30.9
17	15.9	13.0–18.9	47	28.4	25.6–31.4
18	16.1	13.3–19.1	48	29.0	26.1–31.6
19	16.6	13.7–19.6	49	29.4	26.6–32.3
20	17.0	14.1–19.9	50	29.9	27.0–32.9
21	17.4	14.6–20.3	51	30.4	27.6–33.3
22	17.9	14.9–20.7	52	30.9	28.0–33.9
23	18.1	15.1–21.1	53	31.4	28.6–34.3
24	18.6	15.6–21.4	54	31.9	29.0–34.9
25	18.9	16.0–21.9	55	32.4	29.6–35.3
26	19.3	16.4–22.1	56	32.9	30.0–35.9
27	19.7	16.9–22.6	57	33.4	30.6–36.3
28	20.1	17.1–23.0	58	33.9	31.0–36.9
29	20.6	17.6–23.6	59	34.4	31.6–37.3
30	21.0	18.1–23.9	60	34.9	32.0–37.9
31	21.4	18.6–24.3	61	35.4	32.6–38.3
32	21.9	18.9–24.7	62	35.9	33.0–39.4
33	22.1	19.3–25.1	63	36.6	33.6–39.4
34	22.6	19.7–25.6	64	37.0	34.1–39.9
35	23.1	20.1–26.0	65	37.6	34.6–40.5
36	23.6	20.6–26.4	66	38.0	35.1–41.0
37	23.9	21.0–26.9	67	38.6	35.7–41.6
38	24.4	21.6–27.3	68	39.1	36.1–42.0
39	24.9	21.9–27.7	69	39.7	36.9–42.6
40	25.3	22.4–28.1			

*From Jeanty P, Rodesch F, Delbeke D, et al: Estimation of gestational age from measurements of fetal long bones. J Ultrasound Med 1984; 3:75–79. Used by permission.

OTHER OSSEOUS STRUCTURES

Clavicle

A recent article has been published measuring the length of the fetal clavicle.[179] A table in number form with a mean predicted value and a 2 SD range was given from 15 to 40 weeks. The clavicle was measured from the ossified ends, disregarding any curve in the bone, and found to correlate linearly with gestational age. While this is an interesting measurement, the authors failed to discuss the degree of difficulty and technical expertise needed to make this measurement. In addition, while they suggested its potential usefulness in detecting both congenital anomalies and shoulder dystocia during delivery, no abnormal cases were analyzed.

SOFT TISSUE MEASUREMENTS: ARMS, LEG, NECK

Fetal subcutaneous fat has been observed radiographically and correlated with weight from 32 weeks to term.[180] The mean numbers for the buttocks and upper dorsal "shoulder hump" at 36 weeks and at term were 3 to 5 mm and 3 to 4 mm, respectively. It was also noted that this fat thickness decreased in cases of fetal starvation.

Fetal subcutaneous tissues have also been evaluated by fetoscopy, attempting to predict fetal weight.[181] The scalp thickness at the vertex of the head and the ratio of the thigh soft tissue thickness on the extensor surface to the cross-sectional diameter of the femur have been measured. It was found that the fetal scalp soft tissues correlated well to fetal weight. When the subcutaneous tissues were less than 3.4 mm, the fetus weighed less than 2,500 gm. When more than 3.4 mm, the soft tissue thickness of the scalp was predictive of a fetus greater than 2,500 gm.[180] When the ratio of the soft tissues of the thigh to the femoral diameter were analyzed, there was also a high degree of correlation to weight. If the ratio were greater than 4.2, all fetuses weighed more than 3,000 gm.

Seven ultrasound articles have attempted to evaluate the soft tissues, five of the extremities,[182-186] and two of the back of the neck.[187, 188] For the thigh measurements, one article[182] measured the transaxial diameter with static scans, and, while not stating exactly where the measurements were taken, found that the soft tissue diameter of the entire thigh increased in a linear fashion from 24 to 38 weeks.[182] Vintzileos et al.[183] measured the transverse thigh and calf circumferences from 20 weeks to term. Both articles presented their data in number form with 2 SD ranges. The measurements were taken at somewhat arbitrary places, mid-thigh and below the knee, and both incorporated the bone, muscle, and subcutaneous tissue in their measurements. Jeanty et al.[184] measured the midlevel of the arm and thigh and determined the transverse and AP thicknesses. In addition, the subcutaneous thickness and the humeral and femoral length and thickness were also measured. Limb volumes were computed in equation and graph form and found to correlate with gestational age. Of interest in their article was the finding that a subcutaneous tissue thickness in the arm of greater than 6 mm and in the thigh of greater than 10 mm, in the absence of edema, was suspicious for macrosomia. Last, two articles from the same group[185, 186] analyzed the transverse thigh circumference from 12 weeks to term, using a "transition plane" in the femur at the junction of the upper and middle third of the thigh to take their measurements. The data were presented in number form, with a mean and 2 SD. They found a close correlation to gestational age, 13 mm at 22 weeks, increasing to 31 mm at term.[185] They also found that their numbers were larger than those of Vintzileos et al.[183] and Jeanty et al.,[184] as much as 9 mm at 23 weeks to 30 mm at term, which they attributed to different methodologies. The reason for these differences, however, cannot be ascertained from the articles. Because of these marked differences, no measurement is recommended at present.

Two articles by Benacerraf et al.[187, 183] measured the skin or soft tissue thickness at the back of the neck behind the occiput in second trimester pregnancies. They found the normal range to be 1 to 5 mm, with only one false positive result in more than 1,700 normal fetuses. In ten cases of Down's syndrome, diagnosed by abnormal karyotype from the amniotic fluid, skin thickening greater than 5 mm was present in four. The exact place to take the measurement and the difficulties in imaging this area were not discussed.

The subcutaneous tissues have a wide range of normal. However, they can be considered to be increased if greater than 6 mm in the arm, 10 mm in the thigh, and 5 mm in the back of the neck. These are very large numbers, usually not exceeded in the majority of abnormal fetuses even when severely affected. In addition, it would be helpful to have a lower limit of skin thickness to aid in the diagnosis of growth retardation. At present, these are not available. No numbers are therefore recommended.

REFERENCES

Thoracic Diameter and Circumference
1. Hoffbauer H, Pachaly J, Arabin B, et al: Control of fetal development with multiple ultrasonic body measures. *Contrib Gynecol Obstet* 1979; 6:147–156.
2. Levi S, Erbsman F: Antenatal fetal growth from the nineteenth week: Ultrasonic study of 12 head and chest dimensions. *Am J Obstet Gynecol* 1975; 121:262–268.
3. Weinraub Z, Schneider D, Langer R, et al: Ultrasonographic measurement of fetal growth parameters for estimation of gestational age and fetal weight. *Isr J Med Sci* 1979; 15:829–832.
4. Issel EP, Prenzlau P, Bayer H, et al: The measurement of fetal growth during pregnancy by ultrasound (b-scan). *J Perinat Med* 1975; 3:269–275.
5. Pap G, Pap L: Ultrasonic estimation of gestational age and fetal weight. *Paediatr Acad Sci Hung* 1979; 20:119–135.
6. Pap G, Szoke J, Pap L: Intrauterine growth retardation: Ultrasonic diagnosis. *Acta Paediatr Hung* 1983; 24:7–15.
7. Hansmann M: A critical evaluation of the performance of ultrasonic diagnosis in present-day obstetrics. *Gynakologe* 1974; 7:26–35.
8. Nimrod C, Davies D, Iwanicki S, et al: Ultrasound prediction of pulmonary hypoplasia. *Obstet Gynecol* 1986; 68:495–498.
9. Usher R, McLean F: Intrauterine growth of live-born Caucasian infants at sea level: Standards obtained from measurements in 7 dimensions of infants born between 25 and 44 weeks of gestation. *Pediatrics* 1969; 74:901–910.

Thoracic Area
10. Kossoff G, Garrett WJ, Radovanovich G: Grey scale echography in obstetrics and

gynaecology. *Austral Radiol* 1974; 18:63–111.
11. Levi S, Erbsman F: Antenatal fetal growth from the nineteenth week: Ultrasonic study of 12 head and chest dimensions. *Am J Obstet Gynecol* 1975; 121:262–268.
12. Weinraub Z, Schneider D, Langer R, et al: Ultrasonographic measurement of fetal growth parameters for estimation of gestational age and fetal weight. *Israel J Med Sci* 1979; 15:829–832.
13. Wladimiroff JW, Bloemsma CA, Wallenburg HCS: Ultrasonic assessment of fetal head and body sizes in relation to normal and retarded fetal growth. *Am J Obstet Gynecol* 1978; 131:857–860.
14. Wladimiroff JW, Bloemsma CA, Wallenburg HCS: Ultrasonic assessment of fetal growth. *Acta Obstet Gynecol Scand* 1977; 56:37–42.
15. Varma TR, Taylor H, Bridges C: Ultrasound assessment of fetal growth. *Br J Obstet Gynaecol* 1979; 86:623–632.
16. Wladimiroff JW, Bloemsma CA, Wallenburg HCS: Ultrasonic diagnosis of the large-for-dates infant. *Obstet Gynecol* 1978; 52:285–288.

Abdominal Diameter
17. Hoffbauer H, Pachaly J, Arabin B, et al: Control of fetal development with multiple ultrasonic body measures. *Contrib Gynecol Obstet* 1979; 6:147–156.
18. Weinraub Z, Schneider D, Langer R, et al: Ultrasonographic measurement of fetal growth parameters for estimation of gestational age and fetal weight. *Isr J Med Sci* 1979; 15:829–832.
19. Fescina RH, Ucieda FJ, Cordano MC, et al: Ultrasonic patterns of intrauterine fetal growth in a Latin American country. *Early Hum Dev* 1982; 6:239–248.
20. Garrett W, Robinson D: Assessment of fetal size and growth rate by ultrasonic echoscopy. *Obstet Gynecol* 1979; 38:525–534.
21. Eriksen PS, Secher NJ, Weis-Bentzon M: Normal growth of the fetal biparietal diameter and the abdominal diameter in a longitudinal study. *Acta Obstet Gynecol Scand* 1985; 64:65–70.
22. Persson PH, Weldner BM: Normal range growth curves for fetal biparietal diameter, occipito frontal diameter, mean abdominal diameters and femur length. *Acta Obstet Gynecol Scand* 1986; 65:759–761.
23. Grandjean H, Sarramon MF, De Mouzon J, et al: Detection of gestational diabetes by means of ultrasonic diagnosis of excessive fetal growth. *Am J Obstet Gynecol* 1980; 138:790–792.
24. Tamura RK, Sabbagha RE, Pan WH, et al: Ultrasonic fetal abdominal circumference: Comparison of direct versus calculated measurement. *Obstet Gynecol* 1986; 67:833–835.
25. Kurtz AB, Wapner RJ, Kurtz RJ, et al: Analysis of biparietal diameter as an accurate indicator of gestational age. *J Clin Ultrasound* 1980; 8:319–326.

Abdominal Circumference
26. Usher R, McLean F: Intrauterine growth of live-born Caucasian infants at sea level: Standards obtained from measurements in 7 dimensions of infants born between 25 and 44 weeks of gestation. *Pediatrics* 1969; 74:901–910.
27. Deter RL, Harrist RB, Hadlock FP, et al: Fetal head and abdominal circumferences: I. Evaluation of measurement errors. *J Clin Ultrasound* 1982; 10:357–363.
28. Tamura RK, Sabbagha RE: Percentile ranks of sonar fetal abdominal circumference measurements. *Am J Obstet Gynecol* 1980; 138:475–479.
29. Hadlock FP, Deter RL, Harrist RB, et al: Fetal circumference as a predictor of menstrual age. *AJR* 1982; 139:367–370.
30. Hoffbauer H, Pachaly J, Arabin B, et al: Control of fetal development with multiple ultrasonic body measures. *Contrib Gynecol Obstet* 1979; 6:147–156.
31. Weinraub Z, Schneider D, Langer R, et al: Ultrasonographic measurement of fetal growth parameters for estimation of gestational age and fetal weight. *Isr J Med Sci* 1979; 15:829–832.

32. Fescina RH, Ucieda FJ, Cordano MC, et al: Ultrasonic patterns of intrauterine fetal growth in a Latin American country. *Early Hum Dev* 1982; 6:239–248.
33. Ogata ES, Sabbagha R, Metzger BE, et al: Serial ultrasonography to assess evolving fetal macrosomia: Studies in 23 pregnancy diabetic women. *JAMA* 1980; 243:2405–2408.
34. Parker AJ, Davies P, Mayho AM, et al: The ultrasound estimation of sex-related variations of intrauterine growth. *Am J Obstet Gynecol* 1984; 149:665–669.
35. Meire HB, Farrant P: Ultrasound demonstration of an unusual fetal growth pattern in Indians. *Br J Obstet Gynaecol* 1981; 88:260–263.
36. Athey PA, Hadlock FP, in Harshberger SE (ed): *Ultrasound in Obstetrics and Gynecology*. St Louis, CV Mosby, 1981, p 269.
37. Deter RL, Harrist RB, Hadlock FP, et al: Fetal head and abdominal circumferences: II. A critical reevaluation of the relationship to menstrual age. *J Clin Ultrasound* 1982; 10:365–372.
38. Deter RL, Harrist RB, Hadlock FP, et al: Longitudinal studies of fetal growth with the use of dynamic image ultrasonography. *Am J Obstet Gynecol* 1982; 143:545–554.
39. Deter RL, Harrist RB, Hadlock FP, et al: The use of ultrasound in the assessment of normal fetal growth: A review. *J Clin Ultrasound* 1981; 9:481–493.
40. Tamura RK, Sabbagha RE, Pan WH, et al: Ultrasonic fetal abdominal circumference: Comparison of direct versus calculated measurement. *Obstet Gynecol* 1986; 67:833–835.
41. Campbell S, Wilkin D: Ultrasonic measurement of fetal abdomen circumference in the estimation of fetal weight. *Br J Obstet Gynaecol* 1975; 82:689–697.
42. Bree RL, Mariona FG: The role of ultrasound in the evaluation of normal and abnormal fetal growth. *Semin Ultrasound* 1980; 1:264–277.
43. Hobbins JC, Grannum PAT, Berkowitz RL, et al: Ultrasound in the diagnosis of congenital anomalies. *Am J Obstet Gynecol* 1979; 134:331–345.
44. Clement D, Silverman R, Scott D, et al: Comparison of abdominal circumference measurements by real-time and B-scan techniques. *J Clin Ultrasound* 1981; 9:1–3.
45. Weiner CP, Sabbagha RE, Tamur RK, et al: Sonographic abdominal circumference: Dynamic versus static imaging. *Am J Obstet Gynecol* 1981; 139:953–955.
46. Hadlock FP, Kent WR, Loyd JL, et al: An evaluation of two methods for measuring fetal heads and body circumferences. *J Ultrasound Med* 1982; 1:359–360.
47. Shields JR, Medearis AL, Bear MB: Fetal head and abdominal circumferences: Effect of profile shape on the accuracy of ellipse equations. *J Clin Ultrasound* 1987; 15:241–244.
48. Shields JR, Medearis AL, Bear MB: Fetal head and abdominal circumferences: Ellipse calculations versus planimetry. *J Clin Ultrasound* 1987; 15:237–239.

Abdominal Area
49. Weinraub Z, Schneider D, Langer R, et al: Ultrasonographic measurement of fetal growth parameters for estimation of gestational age and fetal weight. *Isr J Med Sci* 1979; 15:829–832.
50. Wladimiroff JW, Bloemsma CA, Wallenburg HCS: Ultrasonic assessment of fetal head and body sizes in relation to normal and retarded fetal growth. *Am J Obstet Gynecol* 1978; 131:857–860.
51. Fescina RH, Ucieda FJ, Cordano MC, et al: Ultrasonic patterns of intrauterine fetal growth in a Latin American country. *Early Hum Dev* 1982; 6:239–248.
52. Garrett W, Robinson D: Assessment of fetal size and growth rate by ultrasonic echoscopy. *Obstet Gynecol* 1979; 38:525–534.
53. Wittman BK, Robinson HP, Aitchison T, et al: The value of diagnostic ultrasound as a screening test for intrauterine growth retardation: Comparison of nine parameters. *Am J Obstet Gynecol* 1979; 134:30–35.

54. Wladimiroff JW, Bloemsma CA, Wallenburg HCS: Ultrasonic assessment of fetal growth. *Acta Obstet Gynecol Scand* 1977; 56:37–42.
55. Varma TR, Taylor H, Bridges C: Ultrasound assessment of fetal growth. *Br J Obstet Gynaecol* 1979; 86:623–632.
56. Rossavik IK, Deter RL, Hadlock FP: Mathematical modeling of fetal growth: IV. Evaluation of trunk growth using the abdominal profile area. *J Clin Ultrasound* 1987; 15:31–35.
57. Wladimiroff JW, Bloemsma CA, Wallenburg HCS: Ultrasonic diagnosis of the large-for-dates infant. *Obstet Gynecol* 1978; 52:285–288.
58. Woo JSK, Liang ST, Wan CW, et al: Abdominal circumference vs abdominal area—which is better? *J Ultrasound Med* 1984; 3:101–105.
59. Selbing A, Wichman K, Ryden G: Screening for detection of intra-uterine growth retardation by means of ultrasound. *Acta Obstet Gynecol Scand* 1984; 63:543–548.

Body Volume
60. Marinez DA, Bartown JL: Estimation of fetal body and fetal head volumes: Description of technique and nomograms for 18 to 41 weeks of gestation. *Am J Obstet Gynecol* 1980; 137:78–84.
61. Rossavik IK, Deter RL: Mathematical modeling of fetal growth: I. Basic principles. *J Clin Ultrasound* 1984; 12:529–533.
62. Rossavik IK, Deter RL: Mathematical modeling of fetal growth: II. Head cube (A), abdominal cube (B) and their ratio (A/B). *J Clin Ultrasound* 1984; 12:535–545.

Total Fetal Volumes
63. Marinez DA, Bartown JL: Estimation of fetal body and fetal head volumes: Description of technique and nomograms for 18 to 41 weeks of gestation. *Am J Obstet Gynecol* 1980; 137:78–84.
64. Deter RL, Harrist RB, Hadlock FP, et al: Longitudinal studies of fetal growth using volume parameters determined with ultrasound. *J Clin Ultrasound* 1984; 12:313–324.

Total Fetal Length
65. Usher R, McLean F: Intrauterine growth of live-born Caucasian infants at sea level: Standards obtained from measurements in 7 dimensions of infants born between 25 and 44 weeks of gestation. *Pediatrics* 1969; 74:901–910.
66. Lubchenco LO, Hansmann C, Boyd E: Intrauterine growth in length and head circumference as estimated from live births at gestational ages from 26 to 42 weeks. *Pediatrics* 1966; 37:403–408.
67. Babson SG, Benda GI: Growth graphs for the clinical assessment of infants of varying gestational age. *Pediatrics* 1976; 89:814–820.
68. Wong KS, Scott KE: Fetal growth at sea level. *Biol Neonate* 1972; 20:175–188.
69. Hoffbauer H, Pachaly J, Arabin B, et al: Control of fetal development with multiple ultrasonic body measures. *Contrib Gynecol Obstet* 1979; 6:147–156.
70. Issel EP, Prenzlau P, Bayer H, et al: The measurement of fetal growth during pregnancy by ultrasound (b-scan). *J Perinat Med* 1975; 3:269–275.
71. Ojala A, Ylostalo P, Jouppila P, et al: Fetal cephalometry by ultrasound in normal and complicated pregnancy. *Ann Chir Gynaecol Fenniae* 1970; 59:71–75.
72. Hansmann M: A critical evaluation of the performance of ultrasonic diagnosis in present-day obstetrics. *Gynakologe* 1974; 7:26–35.
73. Ott WJ: Fetal femur length, neonatal crown-heel length, and screening for intrauterine growth retardation. *Obstet Gynecol* 1985; 65:460–464.
74. Hadlock FP, Deter RL, Roecker E, et al: Relation of fetal femur length to neonatal crown-heel length. *J Ultrasound Med* 1984; 3:1–3.
75. Vintzileos AM, Campbell WA, Neckles S, et al: The ultrasound femur length as a predictor of fetal length. *Obstet Gynecol* 1984; 64:779–782.

Fetal Body Organ Measurements

76. Yamaguchi DT, Lee FYL: Ultrasonic evaluation of the fetal heart: A report of experience and anatomic correlation. *Am J Obstet Gynecol* 1979; 134:422–430.
77. DeVore GR, Donnerstein RL, Kleinman CS, et al: Fetal echocardiography: I. Normal anatomy as determined by real-time-directed M-mode ultrasound. *Am J Obstet Gynecol* 1982; 144:249–259.
78. Shime J, Bertrand M, Hagen-Ansert S, et al: Two-dimensional and M-mode echocardiography in the human fetus. *Am J Obstet Gynecol* 1984; 148:679–685.
79. DeVore GR, Donnerstein RL, Kleinman CS, et al: Fetal echocardiography: II. The diagnosis and significant of a pericardial effusion in the fetus using real-time-directed M-mode ultrasound. *Am J Obstet Gynecol* 1982; 144:693–699.
80. Nimrod C, Nicholson S, Machin G, et al: In utero evaluation of fetal cardiac structure: A preliminary report. *Am J Obstet Gynecol* 1984; 148:516–518.
81. DeVore GR, Siassi B, Platt L: Fetal echocardiography: III. The diagnosis of cardiac arrhythmias using real-time-directed M-mode ultrasound. *Am J Obstet Gynecol* 1983; 146:792–799.
82. Lange LW, Sahn DJ, Allen HD, et al: Qualitative real-time cross-sectional echocardiographic imaging of the human fetus during the second half of pregnancy. *Circulation* 1980; 62:799–806.
83. Allan LD, Tynan MJ, Campbell S, et al: Echocardiographic and anatomical correlates in the fetus. *Br Heart J* 1980; 44:444–451.
84. Axel L: Real-time sonography of fetal cardiac anatomy. *AJR* 1983; 141:283–288.
85. Allan LD, Crawford DC, Anderson RH, et al: Echocardiographic and anatomical correlations in fetal congenital heart disease. *Br Heart J* 1984; 52:542–548.
86. Sandor GGS, Farquarson D, Wittman B, et al: Fetal echocardiography: Results in high-risk patients. *Obstet Gynecol* 1986; 67:358–364.
87. Allan LD, Crawford DC, Anderson RH, et al: Evaluation and treatment of fetal arrhythmias. *Clin Cardiol* 1984; 7:467–473.
88. Kleinman CS, Donnerstein RL, Jaffe CC, et al: Fetal echocardiography: A tool for evaluation of in utero cardiac arrhythmias and monitoring of in utero therapy: Analysis of 71 patients. *Am J Cardiol* 1983; 51:237–243.
89. Kleinman CS, Donnerstein RL, DeVore GR, et al: Fetal echocardiography for evaluation of in utero congestive heart failure: A technique for study of nonimmune fetal hydrops. *N Engl J Med* 1982; 306:568–575.
90. Levi S, Erbsman F: Antenatal fetal growth from the nineteenth week: Ultrasonic study of 12 head and chest dimensions. *Am J Obstet Gynecol* 1975; 121:262–268.
91. Suzuki K, Minei LJ, Schnitzer LE; Ultrasonographic measurement of fetal heart volume for estimation of birthweight. *Obstet Gynecol* 1974; 43:867–871.
92. Jeanty P, Romero R, Cantraine F, et al: Fetal cardiac dimensions: A potential tool for the diagnosis of congenital heart defects. *J Ultrasound Med* 1984; 3:359–364.
93. DeVore GR, Platt LD: The random measurement of the transverse diameter of the fetal heart: A potential source of error. *J Ultrasound Med* 1985; 4:335–341.
94. Filkins KA, Brown TF, Levine OR: Real time ultrasonic evaluation of the fetal heart. *Int J Gynaecol Obstet* 1981; 19:35–39.
95. DeVore GR, Horenstein J, Platt LD: Fetal echocardiography: VI. Assessment of cardiothoracic disproportion—A new technique for the diagnosis of thoracic hypoplasia. *Am J Obstet Gynecol* 1986; 155:1066–1071.
96. Wladimiroff JW, McGhie J: Ultrasonic assessment of cardiovascular geometry and function in the human fetus. *Br J Obstet Gynaecol* 1981; 88:870–875.
97. Sahn DJ, Lange LW, Allen HD, et al: Quantitative real-time cross-sectional echocardiography in the developing human fetus and newborn. *Circulation* 1980; 62:588–597.
98. DeVore GR, Siassi B, Platt LD: Fetal echocardiography: IV. M-mode assessment

of ventricular size and contractility during the second and third trimesters of pregnancy in the normal fetus. *Am J Obstet Gynecol* 1984; 150:981–988.
99. Allan LD, Joseph MC, Boyd EGCA, et al: M-mode echocardiography in the developing human fetus. *Br Heart J* 1982; 47:573–583.
100. Wladimiroff JW, McGhie JS: M-mode ultrasonic assessment of fetal cardiovascular dynamics. *Br J Obstet Gynaecol* 1981; 88:1241–1245.
101. Kleinman CS, Donnerstein RL: Ultrasonic assessment of cardiac function in the intact human fetus. *J Am Coll Cardiol* 1985; 5:845–945.
102. Wladimiroff JW, Vosters R, Stewart PA: Fetal echocardiography: Basic and clinical considerations. *Ultrasound Med Biol* 1984; 10:315–327.
103. St John Sutton MG, Gewitz MH, Shah B, et al: Quantitative assessment of growth and function of the cardiac chambers in the normal human fetus: A prospective longitudinal echocardiographic study. *Circulation* 1984; 69:645–654.
104. Azancot A, Caudell TP, Allen HD, et al: Analysis of ventricular shape by echocardiography in normal fetuses, newborns and infants. *Circulation* 1983; 68:1201–1211.
105. Wladimiroff JW, Vosters R, McGhie JS: Normal cardiac ventricular geometry and function during the last trimester of pregnancy and early neonatal period. *Br J Obstet Gynaecol* 1982; 839–844.
106. Leslie J, Shen S, Thornton JC, et al: The human fetal heart in the second trimester of gestation: A gross morphometric study of normal fetuses. *Am J Obstet Gynecol* 1983; 145:312–316.
107. Vosters R, Wladimiroff JW, Versprille A: M-mode ultrasound recording of perinatal geometry and dynamics of the cardiac interventricular septum. *Eur J Obstet Gynecol Reprod Biol* 1984; 16:299–308.
108. DeVore GR, Siassi B, Platt LD: Fetal echocardiography: V. M-mode measurements of the aortic root and aortic valve in second and third-trimester normal human fetuses. *Am J Obstet Gynecol* 1985; 152:543–550.
109. Shime J, Gresser CD, Rakowski H: Quantitative two-dimensional echocardiographic assessment of fetal cardiac growth. *Am J Obstet Gynecol* 1986; 154:294–300.
110. Gross BH, Harter LP, Filly RA: Disproportionate left hepatic lobe size in the fetus: Ultrasonic demonstration. *J Ultrasound Med* 1982; 1:79–81.
111. Gross BH, Filly RA, Harter LP: Inability of relative fetal hepatic lobar size to diagnose intrauterine growth retardation. *J Ultrasound Med* 1982; 1:299–300.
112. Vintzileos AM, Neckles S, Campbell WA, et al: Fetal liver ultrasound measurements during normal pregnancy. *Obstet Gynecol* 1985; 66:477–480.
113. Vintzileos AM, Campbell WA, Storlazzi E, et al: Fetal liver ultrasound measurements in isoimmunized pregnancies. *Obstet Gynecol* 1986; 68:162–167.
114. Schmidt W, Yarkoni S, Jeanty P, et al: Sonographic measurements of the fetal spleen: Clinical implications. *J Ultrasound Med* 1985; 4:667–672.
115. Rosenberg ER, Bowie JD, Andreotti RF, et al: Sonographic evaluation of fetal adrenal glands. *AJR* 1982; 139:1145–1147.
116. Lewis E, Kurtz AB, Dubbins PA, et al: Real-time ultrasonographic evaluation of normal fetal adrenal glands. *J Ultrasound Med* 1982; 1:265–270.
117. Hata K, Hata T, Kitao M: Ultrasonographic identification and measurement of the human fetal adrenal gland in utero. *Int J Gynaecol Obstet* 1985; 23:355–359.
118. Anderson ABM, Laurence KM, Davies K, et al: Fetal adrenal weight and the cause of premature delivery in human pregnancy. *J Obstet Gynaecol Br Commonwealth* 1971; 78:481–487.
119. Lawson TL, Foley WD, Berland LL, et al: Ultrasonic evaluation of fetal kidneys: Analysis of normal size and frequency of visualization as related to stage of pregnancy. *Radiology* 1981; 138:153–156.

120. Jeanty P, Dramaix-Wilmet M, Elkhazen N, et al: Measurement of fetal kidney growth on ultrasound. *Radiology* 1982; 144:159–162.
121. Grannum P, Bracken M, Silverman R, et al: Assessment of fetal kidney size in normal gestation by comparison of ratio of kidney circumference to abdominal circumference. *Am J Obstet Gynecol* 1980; 136:249–254.
122. Bertagnoli L, Lalatta F, Gallicchio R, et al: Quantitative characterization of the growth of the fetal kidney. *J Clin Ultrasound* 1983; 11:349–356.
123. Bowie JD, Rosenberg ER, Andreotti RF, et al: The changing sonographic appearance of fetal kidneys during pregnancy. *J Ultrasound Med* 1983; 2:505–507.
124. Hoddick WK, Filly RA, Mahony BS, et al: Minimal fetal renal pylectasis. *J Ultrasound Med* 1985; 4:85–89.
125. Arger PH, Coleman BG, Mintz MC, et al: Routine fetal genitourinary tract screening. *Radiology* 1985; 156:485–489.
126. Grignon A, Filion R, Filiatrault D, et al: Urinary tract dilatation in utero: Classification and clinical applications. *Radiology* 1986; 160:645–647.
127. Blane CE, Koff SA, Bowerman RA, et al: Nonobstructive fetal hydronephrosis: Sonographic recognition and therapeutic implications. *Radiology* 1983; 147:95–99.
128. Diamond DA, Sanders R, Jeffs RD: Fetal hydronephrosis: Considerations regarding urological intervention. *J Urol* 1984; 131:1155–1159.
129. Campbell S, Wladimiroff JW, Dewhurst CJ: The antenatal measurement of fetal urine production. *J Obstet Gynaecol Br Commonwealth* 1973; 80:680–686.
130. Campbell S: The assessment of fetal development by diagnostic ultrasound. *Clin Perinatol* 1974; 1:507–525.
131. Dubbins PA, Kurtz AB, Wapner RJ, et al: Renal agenesis: Spectrum of in utero findings. *J Clin Ultrasound* 1981; 9:189–193.
132. Nyberg DA, Mack LA, Patten RM, et al: Fetal bowel: Normal sonographic findings. *J Ultrasound Med* 1987; 6:3–6.

Fetal Extremity Measurements

133. Russell JGB: Radiological assessment of fetal maturity. *J Obstet Gynaecol Br Commonwealth* 1969; 76:208–219.
134. Russell JGB, Mattison AE, Easson WT, et al: Skeletal dimensions as an indication of foetal maturity. *Br J Radiol* 1972; 45:667–669.
135. Owen RH: The estimation of foetal maturity. *Br J Radiol* 1971; 44:531–534.
136. Martin RH, Higginbottom J: A clinical and radiological assessment of fetal age. *J Obstet Gynaecol Br Commonwealth* 1971; 78:155–162.
137. Queenan JT, O'Brien GD, Campbell S: Ultrasound measurement of fetal limb bones. *Am J Obstet Gynecol* 1980; 138:297–302.
138. O'Brien GD, Queenan JT, Campbell S: Assessment of gestational age in the second trimester by real-time ultrasound measurement of the femur length. *Am J Obstet Gynecol* 1981; 139:540–545.
139. Farrant P, Meire H: Ultrasound measurement of fetal limb lengths. *Br J Radiol* 1981; 54:660–664.
140. Jeanty P, Kirkpatrick C, Dramaix-Wilmet M, et al: Ultrasonographic evaluation of fetal limb growth. *Radiology* 1981; 140:165–168.
141. Goldstein RB, Filly RA, Simpson G: Pitfalls in femur length measurements. *J Ultrasound Med* 1987; 6:203–207.
142. Abrams SL, Filly RA: Curvature of the fetal femur: A normal sonographic finding. *Radiology* 1985; 156:490.
143. Warda AH, Deter RL, Rossavik IK, et al: Fetal femur length: A critical reevaluation of the relationship to menstrual age. *Obstet Gynecol* 1985; 66:69–75.
144. Chinn DH, Bolding DB, Callen PW, et al: Ultrasonographic identification of fetal lower extremity epiphyseal ossification centers. *Radiology* 1983; 147:815–818.
145. Merz E, Kim-Kern MS, Pehl S: Ultrasonic mensuration of fetal limb bones in the

second and third trimesters. *J Clin Ultrasound* 1987; 15:175–183.
146. Hadlock FP, Harrist RB, Deter RL, et al: A prospective evaluation of fetal femur length as a predictor of gestational age. *J Ultrasound Med* 1983; 2:111–112.
147. Hadlock FP, Harrist RB, Deter RL, et al: Fetal femur length as a predictor of menstrual age: Sonographically measured. *AJR* 1982; 138:875–878.
148. Wolfson RN, Peisner DB, Chik LL, et al: Comparison of biparietal diameter and femur length in the third trimester: Effects of gestational age and variation in fetal growth. *J Ultrasound Med* 1986; 5:145–149.
149. Woo JSK, Wan CW, Fang A, et al: Is fetal femur length a better indicator of gestational age in the growth-retarded fetus as compared with biparietal diameter? *J Ultrasound Med* 1985; 4:139–142.
150. Yeh MN, Bracero L, Reilly KB, et al: Ultrasonic measurement of the femur length as an index of fetal gestational age. *Am J Obstet Gynecol* 1982; 144:519–522.
151. Tse CH, Lee KW: A comparison of the fetal femur length and biparietal diameter in predicting gestational age in the third trimester. *Aust NZ J Obstet Gynaecol* 1984; 24:186–188.
152. Hohler CW, Quetel TA: Fetal femur length: Equations for computer calculation of gestational age from ultrasound measurements. *Am J Obstet Gynecol* 1982; 143:479–481.
153. Oman SD, Wax Y: Estimating fetal age by ultrasound measurements: An example of multivariate calibration. *Biometrics* 1984; 40:947–960.
154. Yagel S, Adoni A, Oman S, et al: A statistical examination of the accuracy of combining femoral length and biparietal diameter as an index of fetal gestational age. *Br J Obstet Gynaecol* 1986; 93:109–115.
155. Winter J, Kimme-Smith C, King W: Measurement accuracy of sonographic sector scanners. *AJR* 1985; 144:645–648.
156. Gamba JL, Bowie JD, Dodson WC, et al: Accuracy of ultrasound in fetal femur length determination: Ultrasound phantom study. *Invest Radiol* 1985; 20:316–323.
157. Pretorius DH, Nelson TR, Manco-Johnson ML: Fetal age estimation by ultrasound: The impact of measurement errors. *Radiology* 1984; 152:763–766.
158. Jeanty P, Beck GJ, Chervenak FA, et al: A comparison of sector and linear array scanners for the measurement of the fetal femur. *J Ultrasound Med* 1985; 4:525–530.
159. Mahoney MJ, Hobbins JC: Prenatal diagnosis of chondroectodermal dysplasia (Ellis-van Creveld syndrome) with fetoscopy and ultrasound. *N Engl J Med* 1977; 297:258–260.
160. Hobbins JC, Bracken MB, Mahoney MJ: Diagnosis of fetal skeletal dysplasias with ultrasound. *Am J Obstet Gynecol* 1982; 142:306–312.
161. Filly RA, Golbus MS, Carey JC, et al: Short-limbed dwarfism: Ultrasonographic diagnosis by mensuration of fetal femoral length. *Radiology* 1981; 138:653–656.
162. Kurtz AB, Wapner RJ: Ultrasonographic diagnosis of second-trimester skeletal dysplasias: A prospective analysis in a high-risk population. *J Ultrasound Med* 1983; 2:99–106.
163. O'Brien FD, Queenan JT: Ultrasound fetal femur length in relation to intrauterine growth retardation: Part II. *Am J Obstet Gynecol* 1982; 144:35–39.
164. Kurtz AB, Filly RA, Wapner RJ, et al: In utero analysis of heterozygous achondroplasia: Variable time of onset as detected by femur length measurements. *J Ultrasound Med* 1986; 5:137–140.
165. Roopnarinesingh S, Ramseqak S: Decreased birth weight and femur length in fetuses of patients with the sickle-cell trait. *Obstet Gynecol* 1986; 68:46–48.
166. Persson PH, Weldner BM: Normal range growth curves for fetal biparietal diameter, occipito frontal diameter, mean abdominal diameters and femur length. *Acta Obstet Gynecol Scand* 1986; 65:759–761.

167. Quinlan RW, Brumfield C, Martin M, et al: Ultrasonic measurement of femur length as a predictor of fetal gestational age. *J Reprod Med* 1982; 27:392–394.
168. Jeanty P, Dramaix-Wilmet M, Van Kerkem J, et al: Ultrasonic evaluation of fetal limb growth. *Radiology* 1982; 143:751–754.
169. Jeanty P: Fetal limb biometry. *Radiology* 1983; 147:601–602.
170. Jeanty P, Rodesch F, Delbeke D, et al: Estimation of gestational age from measurements of fetal long bones. *J Ultrasound Med* 1984; 3:75–79.
171. O'Brien GD, Queenan JT: Growth of the ultrasound fetal femur length during normal pregnancy: Part I. *Am J Obstet Gynecol* 1981; 141:833–837.
172. Shalev E, Feldman E, Weiner E, et al: Assessment of gestational age by ultrasonic measurement of the femur length. *Acta Obstet Gynecol Scand* 1985; 64:71–74.
173. Haines CJ, Langlois SLeP, Jones WR: Ultrasonic measurement of fetal femoral length in singleton and twin pregnancies. *Am J Obstet Gynecol* 1986; 155:838–841.
174. Seeds JW, Cefalo RC: Relationship of fetal limb lengths to both biparietal diameter and gestational age. *Obstet Gynecol* 1982; 60:680–685.
175. Hohler CW, Quetel TA: Comparison of ultrasound femur length and biparietal diameter in late pregnancy. *Am J Obstet Gynecol* 1981; 141:759–762.
176. Mercer BM, Sklar S, Shariatmadar A, et al: Fetal foot length as a predictor of gestational age. *Am J Obstet Gynecol* 1987; 156:350–355.
177. Gentili P, Trasimeni A, Giorlandino C: Fetal ossification centers as predictors of gestational age in normal and abnormal pregnancies. *J Ultrasound Med* 1984; 3:193–197.
178. Tabsh KMA: Correlation of ultrasonic epiphyseal centers and the lecithin:sphingomyelin ratio. *Obstet Gynecol* 1984; 64:92–96.

Other Osseous Structures

179. Yarkoni S, Schmidt W, Jeanty P, et al: Clavicular measurement: A new biometric parameter for fetal evaluation. *J Ultrasound Med* 1985; 4:467–470.

Soft Tissue Measurements

180. Russell JGB, Lewis GJ: Radiological assessment of fetal growth retardation. *Clin Radiol* 1981; 32:567–569.
181. Ogita S, Kamei T, Sugawa T: Estimation of fetal weight by fetography. *Am J Obstet Gynecol* 1977; 127:37–42.
182. Hoffbauer H, Pachaly J, Arabin B, et al: Control of fetal development with multiple ultrasonic body measures. *Contrib Gynecol Obstet* 1979; 6:147–156.
183. Vintzileos AM, Neckles S, Campbell WA, et al: Ultrasound fetal thigh-calf circumferences and gestational age-independent fetal ratios in normal pregnancy. *J Ultrasound Med* 1985; 4:287–292.
184. Jeanty P, Romero R, Hobbins JC: Fetal limb volume: A new parameter to assess fetal growth and nutrition. *J Ultrasound Med* 1985; 4:273–282.
185. Deter RL, Warda A, Rossavik IK, et al: Fetal thigh circumference: A critical evaluation of its relationship to menstrual age. *J Clin Ultrasound* 1986; 14:105–110.
186. Warda A, Deter RL, Duncan G, et al: Evaluation of fetal thigh circumference measurements: A comparative ultrasound and anatomical study. *J Clin Ultrasound* 1986; 14:99–103.
187. Benacerraf BR, Frigoletto FD Jr, Laboda LA: Sonographic diagnosis of Down syndrome in the second trimester. *Am J Obstet Gynecol* 1985; 153:49–52.
188. Benacerraf BR, Barss VA, Laboda LA: A sonographic sign for the detection in the second trimester of the fetus with Down's syndrome. *Am J Obstet Gynecol* 1985; 151:1078–1079.

Chapter 7

Combined Fetal Head and Body Measurements

In the neonatal literature, parameters have been combined in an attempt to better evaluate the newborn infant. One of the most popular is Rohrer's ponderal index, a weight-to-length ratio used to obtain a three-dimensional newborn volume.[1] This index is equal to 100 times the weight (in grams) divided by the length (in centimeters) cubed.

This same type of analysis can be performed in utero. By combining or comparing fetal parameters during one examination or by evaluating these parameters serially during gestation, attempts have been made better to understand and predict fetal growth.

FETAL MEASUREMENT COMPARISONS

Head to Abdomen

The head and body grow symmetrically through most of fetal life. Any large discrepancy often implies abnormality. If the fetal body is significantly smaller than the normal fetal head, particularly after 30 weeks, this strongly suggests asymmetric growth retardation.[2,3] Conversely, if the fetal head is significantly smaller than the normal fetal body, this suggests microcephaly or anencephaly.[4] There is always one central problem in the comparison of any two dissimilar parameters, which is normal and which is abnormal? It is therefore necessary to have a third independent variable, either another fetal measurement such as femoral length or an outside parameter such as an accurate last menstrual period. Using this third variable, it can often be determined which of the two original measurements was normal. Then the abnormal parameter can be further evaluated.

In analyzing the ratio of the head to body, linear, circumference, and area measurements have been compared. For linear measurements, the biparietal diameter and abdominal diameter at the appropriate anatomical positions were evaluated in five articles.[5–9] Gottesfeld[5] found that linear measurements of the biparietal diameter should be within ± 5 mm of the average body diameter. Sarti et al.[7] examined the AP and transverse body diameters, the average body diameter and the longitudinal body diameter, comparing each to the biparietal diameter from 12 to 26 weeks. In chart form, the best correlation was with the average and transverse body diameters. The abdominal growth during this interval of fetal life was slightly less than the biparietal diameter and was found to be linear with a slope of 0.96, approximately 1:1. Sarti et al.[7] then examined five cases of abnormal head to body ratios. In three, the head was smaller, and either microcephaly or anencephaly was detected. In the other two with the body smaller, growth retardation and triploidy were found.

The findings of Eriksen and co-workers[10] agreed with the work of Sarti et al.[7] While no ratio table of biparietal to abdominal diameters is available, a ratio of mean biparietal and average body diameters can be computed at each stage of gestation from their table[10] (Table 7–1). The ratio was approximately 1:1 throughout the second trimester, 1.12 at 13 weeks decreasing to 0.97 by 28 weeks.[10] In the third trimester, however, the body progressively enlarged in relation to the fetal head so that the ratio decreased to 0.94, 0.90, and 0.85 at 33, 37, and 40 weeks, respectively. Fescina et al.[6] computed the biparietal to abdominal diameter ratio in number form from 15 to 40 weeks. While the authors did not state how these measurements were obtained, the progression from a higher to a lower ratio was also found. Their range was wider than that found by Eriksen et al.,[10] a mean of 1.20 at 15 weeks decreasing to 0.84 at term. At a range of 2 SD the variation was even wider.

Gross et al.[8] compared the transverse and Elliott et al.[9] the average body diameter, respectively, to the biparietal diameter. Both approached their evaluation in unusual ways. Gross et al.[8] analyzed their data from 26 weeks to term and obtained an increase in body size, similar to that of Eriksen et al.,[10] as the pregnancy progressed to term. Using an equation of transverse body diameter (TBD) minus biparietal diameter (BPD), a number was obtained from 26 weeks to term which attempted to distinguish normal from growth retarded fetuses. When the BPD was equal to or less than 70 mm (a mean gestational age of up to 27.5 weeks), the TBD − BPD was ≥ −3. When the BPD was 70 to 75 mm (mean gestational ages of 27.5 to 29.5 weeks), the TBD was ≥ BPD. When the BPD was 76 to 80 mm (mean gestational ages of 30.0 to 31.6 weeks), the TBD − BPD was ≥2, and when the BPD was greater than 80 mm (a mean gestational age of greater than 31.6 weeks), the TBD − BPD was ≥4. Using these ratios, Gross et al.[8] detected asymmetric growth retardation with a sensitivity of 68%, a specificity of 69%, an accuracy of positive diagnosis of 42%, and an accuracy of negative diagnosis in 87%. They cautioned not to compress the fetal body during scanning, since this could distort the TBD measurement. Elliott et al.[9] used their comparison differently; i.e., to establish a number that would distinguish normal from large (macrosomic) fetuses. They used an average "chest" diameter minus the biparietal diameter from 35 weeks to term. In actuality, the "chest" was measured at the liver and will be considered an abdominal measurement. If the average abdominal diameter minus BPD were ≥1.4 cm, the fetal body was so large that shoulder dystocia occurred in 4 of 15 macrosomic infants from diabetic mothers. The work by both groups[8,9] appears to be of limited value in the evaluation of small and large fetuses. Both methods are

TABLE 7-1.
Comparison of Biparietal Diameter to Abdominal Diameter Table*

Gestational Age, wk	Predicted Mean Biparietal Diameter, mm	Predicted Mean Average Abdominal Diameter, mm
13	25.6	22.7
14	28.5	26.4
15	31.5	30.1
16	34.6	33.7
17	37.7	37.3
18	40.9	40.9
19	44.1	44.5
20	47.4	48.0
21	50.6	51.4
22	53.9	54.9
23	57.1	58.3
24	60.4	61.7
25	63.5	65.0
26	66.6	68.4
27	70.0	71.7
28	72.6	74.9
29	75.4	78.2
30	78.1	81.4
31	80.7	84.6
32	83.1	87.7
33	85.4	90.8
34	87.5	93.9
35	89.4	97.0
36	91.1	100.1
37	92.6	103.1
38	93.8	106.1
39	94.8	109.0
40	95.5	112.0

*From Eriksen P S, Sechor N J, Weis-Bentzon M: Normal growth of the fetal biparietal diameter and the abdominal diameter in a longitudinal study: An evaluation of the two parameters in predicting fetal weight. *Acta Obstet Gynecol Scand* 1985; 64:65–70. Used by permission.

somewhat cumbersome and do not offer increased detection rates. The work by Elliott et al.[9] is especially questionable, since an adequate analysis of shoulder dystocia would have to include a measurement of the upper chest or shoulders, not just the abdomen.

The discrepancies in this direct comparison of the mean biparietal diameter and average body diameter, without a consistent approach, are too great to recommend a table. However, these two mean numbers can be compared in another way, by analyzing the number of SD between them. Since the biparietal and average body diameters are almost the same number throughout the second and into the early third trimester, a deviation of one from the other of 2 to 3 SD would strongly suggest that one of the two measurements is abnormal. For the biparietal diameter, one article found 2 SD to be 1.4 mm,[11] 2 articles calculated 2 SD as approximately 3 mm,[7,8] and two articles determined 2 SD to be 5 mm or greater.[12-14] While these numbers are somewhat discrepant, our experience agrees with those that found each standard deviation to be 3 mm.[14] Therefore, if the biparietal diameter and average body diameter are within 6 mm (2 SD) of each other throughout the second and into the early third trimester (13 to 34 weeks) (see Table 7-1), the two are most likely normal. If, however, there is a deviation of at least 6 mm (2 SD) and definitely 9 mm (3 SD), abnormalities should be carefully sought.

This approach can be used to evaluate both an abnormally small body (most commonly seen in asymmetric growth retardation) and an abnormally small head (microcephaly). While this approach has not been adequately evaluated in the detection of growth retardation, microcephaly has been analyzed.[5,14,15] Chervenak et al.[14] in the first of two studies found that microcephaly could be diagnosed if the biparietal diameter was more than 3 SD below the norm. In a follow-up prospective study,[15] they found that to eliminate all false negative diagnoses, the occipital-frontal diameter, head circumference, and head to abdominal circumference ratio also had to be decreased by 4, 5, and 3 SD, respectively.[15] Furthermore, to eliminate all false positive diagnoses, the ratio of femur length to head circumference had to be taken into account.[15] While this approach is undoubtedly accurate, it seems cumbersome and would not have to be used in most cases of microcephaly, since, in addition to an abnormally small head, the internal brain structures are usually also grossly abnormal.[5]

The circumferences of the head and abdomen have also been compared using the same anatomical landmarks that were used for the biparietal diameter and abdominal diameter. Six articles compared the ratio of the head to abdominal circumference.[6,14,16-19] All were calculated throughout the second and third trimester, three giving numbers with the 5th and 95th percentile confidence limits[6,14,17] and three in graph form.[16,18,19] The results were similar to those found for the linear ratio of biparietal diameter and average abdominal diameter. In the early second trimester, all articles showed the head circumference to be greater than the abdominal circumference, so that the head to body ratio was slightly greater than 1. As the abdomen increased in size in the middle to late third trimester, this ratio decreased. At term, Fescina et al.,[6] Campbell and Thoms[17] and Deter et al.[16] found a reversal in the ratio to less than one, while the other three[14,18,19] showed the ratio to decrease but to still remain greater than 1. Campbell and Thoms[17] further stated that the ratio, which slowly decreased between 17 and 29 weeks, had a sharper decline to 40 weeks. Of all the circumference ratio articles, Campbell and Thoms' work[17] most closely parallels the linear head to abdomen ratio analysis of Eriksen et al.[10] and is therefore recommended (Fig 7-1); (Table 7-2).

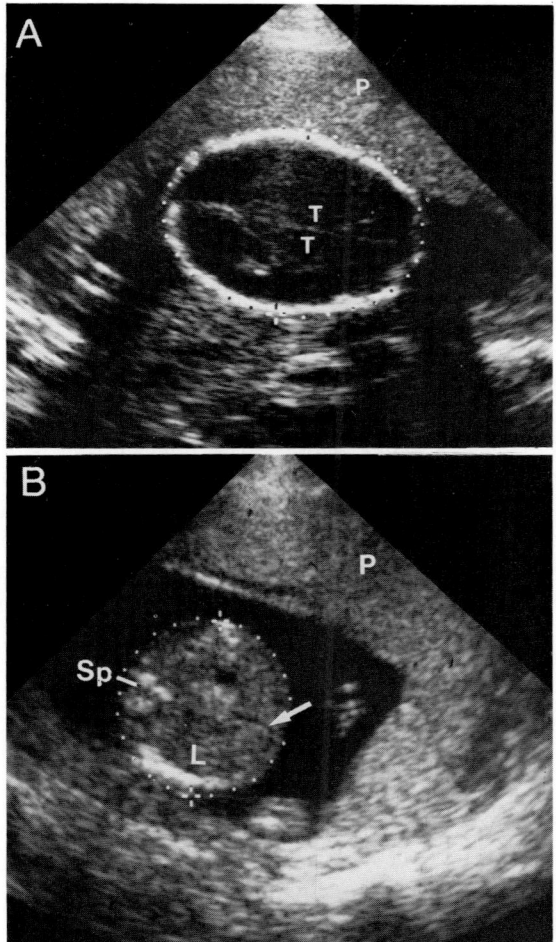

FIG 7–1.
Circumference measurements of the fetal head and abdomen. **A,** transaxial image of the head at the thalami *(T)*. With either the thalami or midbrain in the midline, the circumference is traced around the outer margin of the head with a digitizer or map reader *(dotted line)* or can be calculated from an equation. **B,** transaxial image of the upper abdomen at the region of the liver *(L)*. The umbilical portion of the left portal vein *(arrow)* is situated within the liver in the midline. The circumference is traced with a digitizer or map reader *(dotted line)* or can be calculated from an equation. *P* indicates placenta; *Sp,* spine.

In the evaluation of in utero growth retardation, Campbell and Thoms[17] found that if the ratio of the head to abdominal circumference were abnormally high, indicative of a small fetal body, it was strongly suggestive of asymmetric growth retardation. In a prospective study using the table of Campbell and Thoms, Crane and Kopta[20] evaluated 47 fetuses. When the head to abdominal circumference ratio was normal, all fetuses were found to be normal. However, when the head to abdominal circumference ratio was abnormally high, all the fetuses had asymmetric growth retardation. They therefore concluded that the head to body ratio was a sensitive indicator of asymmetric growth retardation and particularly useful as an initial determination of growth retardation when only one examination had been performed.

An additional method of evaluating the head and abdominal circumferences is to compare the two by using the number of SD between them. As stated for the linear dimensions of the biparietal diameter and average body diameter, any variation of 2 and definitely of 3 SD is strongly suggestive of an abnormality. Athey and Hadlock[21] stated that 1 SD for head a circumference was 9.5 mm and 1 SD for an abdominal circumference was 11.4 mm. The average of the two is approximately 10 mm per each SD. Therefore, if the head and abdomen circumference measurements deviate from one another by 20 mm (2 SD) and certainly by 30 mm (3 SD), this is indicative of abnormality.

In the evaluation of the ratio of the head to body, the question remains whether linear (diameters) or circumference measurements are more accurate. Persson and Marsal[22] evaluated the circumference ratios of the head and abdomen and compared them to the linear ratios of the biparietal and average body diameters. They found that the circumference ratios were wide and that differentiation could not be made between average and small-for-gestational-age (SGA) babies. This finding had also been suggested by Deter et al.[23] when they found great variability in the head to abdominal circumferences. Conversely, Persson and Marsal[22] thought that linear ratios might be more accurate, since the ratio of the biparietal to average abdominal diameter was significantly

TABLE 7–2.
Head to Abdomen Circumference Ratio Table*

Gestational Age, wk	Ratio of Head Circumference/ Abdominal Circumference	
	Mean	Range From 5th to 95th Percentile
13–14	1.23	1.14–1.31
15–16	1.22	1.05–1.39
17–18	1.18	1.07–1.29
19–20	1.18	1.09–1.39
21–22	1.15	1.06–1.25
23–24	1.13	1.05–1.21
25–26	1.13	1.04–1.22
27–28	1.13	1.05–1.21
29–30	1.10	0.99–1.21
31–32	1.07	0.96–1.17
33–34	1.04	0.96–1.11
35–36	1.02	0.93–1.11
37–38	0.98	0.92–1.05
39–40	0.97	0.87–1.06
41–42	0.96	0.93–1.00

*From Campbell S, Thoms A: Ultrasound measurement of the fetal head to abdomen circumference in the assessment of growth retardation. Br J Obstet Gynaecol 1977; 84:165–174. Used by permission.

better in differentiating small from average gestational age fetuses and was able to detect 72% of average and 75% of SGA fetuses. They found that the biparietal diameter to average abdominal diameter ratio for SGA fetuses was never greater than 1:1, while for average gestational age fetuses it was always greater than or equal to 1. Unfortunately, while a table of linear ratios would be desirable and might offer some clinical advantage over circumference ratios, none is recommended at present.

Four articles compared the head to abdominal areas,[6, 11, 13, 24] two in number form[6, 13] and two in graph form.[11, 24] All showed a decrease in the ratio from the second trimester to term, similar to linear and circumference ratios. Wladimiroff et al.[11, 13] obtained the head area by squaring the biparietal diameter and obtained the fetal body area with a digitizer. Their landmarks for the body measurement included visualization of the liver, so that, although they termed this a chest area, it will be considered instead an abdominal area. Fescina et al.[6] used two formulas, one for the head and another for the body, to obtain their areas. Varma et al.[24] used a planimeter to obtain both the head and abdomen areas. In two articles, the overall accuracy reported in the detection of asymmetric growth retarded was 76%[13] and 85%.[24] While these numbers are encouraging, they are not significantly better than those reported for linear and circumference ratios. In addition, since the use of a digitizer or formula to obtain the head and abdominal areas is not as well established as the linear or circumference techniques, there appears at present to be no benefit to the use of area ratios.

Last, a ratio of the head to abdominal volume has been proposed.[25] The volumes were computed solely from transverse images rather than by using a long-axis measurement. Nevertheless, the data in number form reveal a decreasing ratio of 2.1 at 12 weeks to 0.9 at term, with a 2 SD range. Although the decreasing ratio has also been observed with the linear and circumference ratios, the mean and range values are much larger for these volume measurements. Therefore, the linear and circumference ratios are recommended.

Femur to Head

Hohler and Quetel[26] evaluated the femoral length to biparietal diameter and found a ratio from 23 weeks to term of 79 ± 8 at the 90% confidence limits. Chervenak et al.[27] and Hadlock et al.[28] calculated the femur length to head circumference ratio from either 15 weeks[28] or 20 weeks[27] to term. They both used head circumferences instead of biparietal diameters, so that an unusually shaped head would not affect the ratio. Their numbers were in close agreement, a mean number of 18 at 20 weeks, increasing linearly to 23 at term, all at 2 SD.

These ratios may have clinical value in the detection of short-limbed dwarfism and in cases of microcephaly where the internal intracranial anatomy is normal. While more clinical evaluation is necessary, the ratios of femur length to biparietal diameter[26] and femur length to head circumference[28] are recommended (Figs 7-2 and 7-3; Tables 7-3 and 7-4).

Chest to Abdomen

Two articles compared the circumference of the chest to the circumference of the abdomen.[29, 30] In graph form, this ratio was evaluated from early second

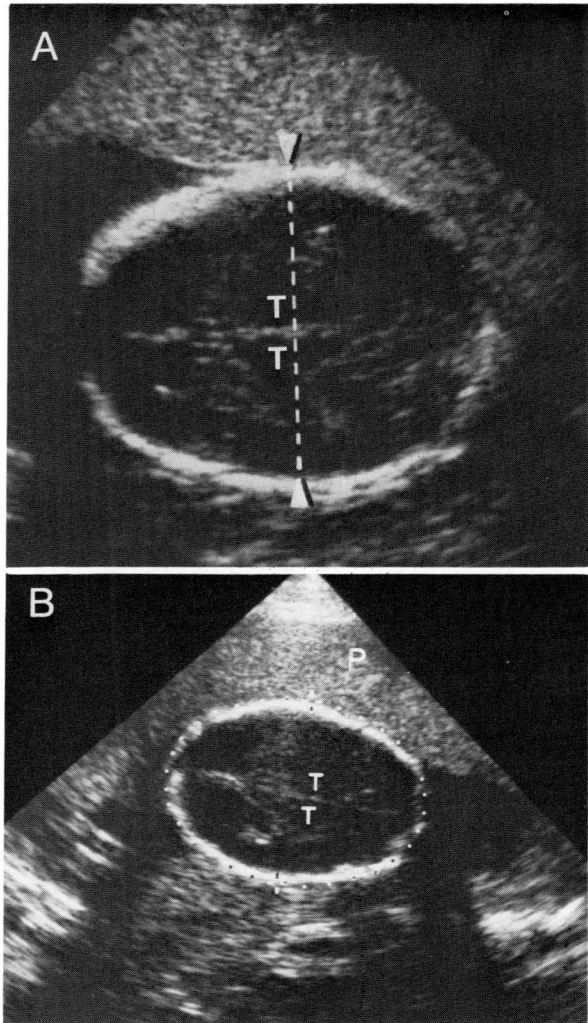

FIG 7–2.
Biparietal diameter and circumference measurements of the head. Both are taken from the transaxial image with the thalami (T) or midbrain in the midline. **A,** biparietal diameter measurement *(arrowheads* and *dotted line)* taken leading edge (outer margin) to leading edge (inner margin). **B,** head circumference measurement *(dotted line)* is traced around the outer margin of the head with a digitizer or map reader. It can also be calculated by using an equation. *P* indicates placenta.

trimester until term with a mean value and a 2 SD range. Both showed an increase in this ratio as the pregnancy progressed toward term.

This comparison is potentially important because it can be used to establish an abnormally small thorax, a finding seen in certain types of fetal skeletal dysplasias. Nevertheless, both articles have shortcomings that do not permit, at present, recommendation of this comparison. Most important, neither presented their values in number form. In addition, Skiptunas and Weiner[30] showed their graph and its use in detecting a fetus with a small thorax, citing a previous article from which the graph had been published. Unfortunately, that article did

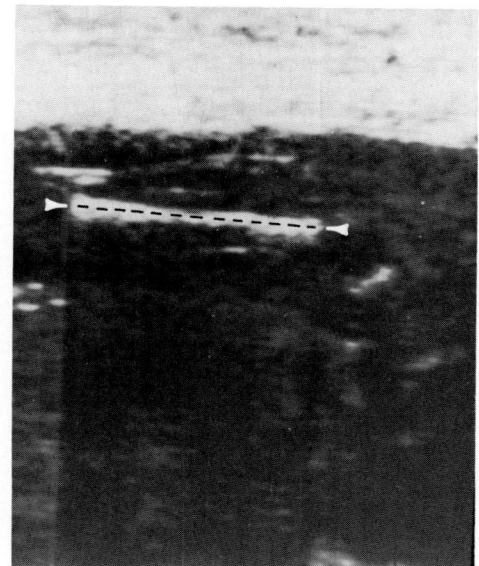

FIG 7–3.
Femur length measurement. The long axis of the hyperechoic femoral shaft is measured (*arrowheads* and *dotted line*), disregarding the hypoechoic nonossified epiphyseal cartilages.

not have the graph, but in turn referred to a scientific meeting where an abstract had been presented. Without any data on the numbers of patients and how the measurements were obtained, this graph cannot be considered further.

Femur to Abdomen

Bracero et al.[31] evaluated a ratio of the mean abdominal diameter to the femur length, attempting to detect large-for-gestational-age (LGA, or macrosomic) fetuses in a group of diabetic and nondiabetic patients. The LGA fetuses of diabetic mothers could be separated from the others if the ratio was greater than 1.385. They identified 19 of 24 large fetuses and incorrectly included 4 of 20 normal fetuses. The sensitivity, specificity, and positive predictive and negative predictive values in the prediction of large fetuses were good, 79%, 80%, 83%, and 76%, respectively. In addition, by combining these results with an abdominal to biparietal diameter ratio of greater than 1.065, they were able to lower their false negative rate to 8%.

While these results sound encouraging in the detection of LGA fetus from diabetic mothers, the authors stated that they measured the abdomen at the

TABLE 7–3.
Femur Length (FL) to Biparietal Diameter (BPD) Ratio (Range, 23 to 40 wk)*

Ratio	Mean	Range from 10th to 90th percentile
FL/BPD × 100	79	72 to 86

*Data from Hohler CW, Quetel TA: Comparison of ultrasound femur length and biparietal diameter in late pregnancy. *Am J Obstet Gynecol* 1981; 141:759–762.

level of the umbilical vein, measured an outer to inner diameter, and implied that a mean diameter was obtained from only one measurement perpendicular to the spine. There are problems with this study. First, does the umbilical vein imply the correct level of the high abdomen where the umbilical portion of the left portal vein (within the liver) is located, or a lower abdominal level where

TABLE 7–4.
Femur Length (FL) to Head Circumference (HC) Ratio Table*

Predicted Mean Gestational Age, wk	FL/HC Ratio Mean	Range, 16% to 84% (1 SD)
15	16.2	15.3–17.1
16	14.9	13.3–16.5
17	16.1	14.6–17.6
18	16.9	15.8–18.0
19	17.2	16.1–18.3
20	18.3	16.8–19.8
21	18.1	15.9–20.3
22	19.3	18.4–20.2
23	20.0	19.2–20.8
24	19.8	18.7–20.9
25	19.5	18.7–20.3
26	19.5	18.6–20.4
27	19.5	18.6–20.4
28	19.7	18.8–20.6
29	20.2	19.6–20.8
30	20.3	19.2–21.4
31	20.3	19.3–21.3
32	20.2	19.1–21.3
33	20.7	19.9–21.5
34	20.6	19.4–21.8
35	21.2	20.1–22.3
36	21.1	20.1–22.1
37	21.7	20.8–22.6
38	21.8	20.9–22.7
39	22.0	20.6–23.4
40	21.6	20.7–22.5
41	22.4	21.6–23.2
42	22.0	20.1–23.9

*From Hadlock FP, Harrist RB, Shah Y, et al: The femur length/head circumference relation in obstetric sonography. *J Ultrasound Med* 1984; 3:439–442. Used by permission.

the umbilical vein enters the abdomen? Second, there is no reproducible way of obtaining an abdominal inner measurement. Third, many abdominal shapes are ovoid, so that an average of two diameters is more accurate in determining a mean diameter. As a result, these data cannot be recommended.

Femur length has been more extensively compared to abdominal circumference. Hadlock et al.[32] evaluated the femoral length to abdominal circumference ratio from 21 weeks to term and found a ratio independent of gestational age, 22 ± 2 at 2 SD. When the ratio was greater than 23.5, they thought that it predicted asymmetric growth retardation in 63% of 30 affected fetuses.[32] This is not at all impressive, since in the same article there were much higher detection rates (true positives) with much fewer false negatives with the use of the abdominal circumference, the ratio of the head circumference to abdominal circumference, and even the estimated weight. In addition, this ratio did not detect any cases not diagnosed by the other measurements.

Ott,[33] Vintzileos et al.,[34] Brown et al.,[35] and Benson et al.[36] also evaluated the femoral length to abdominal circumference ratio. They too found the ratio to be independent of gestational age. Their mean numbers and SD, however, were somewhat different for the detection of growth retarded fetuses, 22.33 ± 1.86,[33] 22.3 ± 2.4,[34] 24.2 ± 1.6,[35] and 23.7 ± 1.4.[36] Therefore, the 23.5 value did not consistently discriminate between normal and growth retarded fetuses.

In four studies,[35-38] SGA fetuses overlapped with the normal range and showed much less of a discriminatory value than that originally reported by Hadlock et al.[32] In fact, Benson et al.[36] found such an overlap between normal (22.4 ± 1.7) and growth retarded (23.7 ± 1.4) fetuses that this ratio had no clinical value in the prediction of growth retardation. In addition, Brown et al.[35] found the abdominal circumference much more predictive of SGA than the femur length to abdominal circumference ratio. Divon et al.[37] evaluated this ratio against the rate of growth of the abdominal circumference and amniotic fluid and found that an abdominal circumference rate of growth of less than 10 mm in 14 days or a femur length to abdominal circumference of greater than 23.5 identified most SGA fetuses, the abdominal rate of growth being more sensitive. By combining the two, however, only 15% of SGA fetuses were missed. Last, Hays and Patterson[38] analyzed the same ratio, comparing it to the neonatal skinfold thickness, birth weight, and ponderal index. While they summarized their data by stating that the ratio was significantly related to these 3 newborn variables, at best their data showed a weak correlation. It is therefore thought that the femur length to abdominal circumference ratio offers nothing but another calculation in the diagnosis of growth retardation. The ratio may even be misleading, since in the original work,[32] may false negatives (missed diagnoses) occurred.

Hadlock et al.[39] employed the same formula to evaluate macrosomic, or LGA, fetuses. Using a cutoff of 20.5 or less, they were able to predict 63% of 51 large-for-date fetuses. As with growth retardation, this formula appears to be no more accurate than the other measurements. When comparing normal to LGA fetuses, the biparietal diameter and abdominal circumference were, on average, larger by 4 mm and 38 mm, respectively, for the LGA fetuses, so that a simple evaluation of the biparietal diameters and abdominal circumferences should make the diagnosis without the use of this ratio.

There was also an overlap of this ratio with that found in three other articles.[33, 34, 40] One of these, Benson et al.,[40] specifically analyzed the femur length to abdominal circumference ratio in normal fetuses and macrosomic fetuses from diabetic mothers. The ratios were 20.4 ± 1.6 and 19.5 ± 1.4, respectively, with considerable overlap and no cutoff value to give a high specificity or sensitivity. Even the positive predictive value was poor, 36%–43%, and only slightly greater than the 26% for the control group. The only possible flaw in this study (discussed by the author and thought to be insignificant) was that some of the ultrasound femoral measurements were obtained using mechanical sector scanners. Therefore, the 20.5 value does not consistently discriminate between normal and macrosomic fetuses.

Other Comparisons

The following is a list of other ratios that have been reported in the literature but without further confirmation or proved clinical utility:

1. Biparietal diameter to transverse thoracic diameter[41]
2. Biparietal diameter to thoracic circumference[42]
3. Head circumference to thoracic circumference[42]
4. Tibial length to calf circumference[43]
5. Femur length to thigh circumference[43]
6. Tibial length to abdominal circumference[44]
7. Femur and tibial length to abdominal circumference[44]
8. Thoracic circumference to femoral length[42,45]
9. Abdominal circumference to diastolic biventricular outer dimension[46]
10. Abdominal circumference to diastolic biventricular inner dimension[46]
11. Abdominal circumference to diastolic right internal dimension[46]
12. Abdominal circumference to diastolic left internal dimension[46]
13. Abdominal circumference to tricuspid valve opening excursion[46]
14. Abdominal circumference to mitral valve opening excursion[46]
15. Abdominal circumference to right wall thickness[46]
16. Abdominal circumference to left wall thickness[46]
17. Abdominal circumference to interventricular septal thickness[46]
18. Femur length to end-diastolic right ventricular dimension[47]
19. Femur length to end-diastolic left ventricular dimension[47]
20. Femur length to end-diastolic biventricular outer dimension[47]
21. Femur length to end-diastolic biventricular inner dimension[47]
22. Femur length to tricuspid valve opening excursion[47]
23. Femur length to mitral valve opening excursion[47]
24. Femur length to right ventricular thickness[47]
25. Femur length to left ventricular thickness[47]
26. Femur length to interventricular septal thickness[47]
27. Fractional spine length to abdominal circumference[48]
28. Fetal ponderal index = weight to femur length[49]
29. Cardiac circumference to biparietal diameter[50]
30. Cardiac circumference to abdominal circumference[50]
31. Cardiac circumference to femur length[50]
32. Cardiac circumference to fetal weight[50]

MULTIPLE PARAMETERS

Fetal measurements have also been added, subtracted, and multiplied together in an attempt to increase the accuracy of fetal growth and age.

Multiple Parameter Fetal Age

The combination of fetal parameters was performed in an attempt to increase the accuracy of fetal age dating.[51-55] Oman and Wax[51] claimed that a quadratic equation containing both biparietal diameter and femoral length was more accurate than either measurement alone, approximately a one-week variation throughout the second and third trimesters. These results are unusually good and as yet have not been duplicated.

Hadlock et al.[52-54] analyzed this concept in three articles, two retrospectively[52,53] and the third prospectively.[54] All three found the biparietal diameter to be increasingly inaccurate toward term, to greater than ±3 weeks after 30 weeks. Because of this, they combined the mean values for biparietal diameter, head circumference, abdominal circumference, and femoral length. This combination decreased the inaccuracy at all stages of gestation, especially after 30 weeks. From 30 to 36 and from 36 to 42 weeks, the variation was only ±2.44 and ±2.3 weeks, respectively.[53] Hadlock et al.[53] thought that this combination of mean numbers decreased a maximum error that could be created by a discrepancy in any one or two measurements. Ott,[55] using the same four parameters, substantiated this observation. He found that the simple arithmetic average of four gave the lowest systematic and random errors.

Despite these encouraging results, several aspects of the multiple-parameter concept need further investigation. The inaccuracy of their biparietal diameter measurements, particularly near term, are large. Not all previous authors found similar inaccuracies in the biparietal diameter in the third trimester.[56-58] Others have not found the biparietal diameter to be the most inaccurate (as these articles have stated) of all single parameters. In fact, two[59,60] found the biparietal diameter to be the single most reliable indicator of gestational age.

In the three articles,[52-54] the entire study group for the second and third trimester was not greater than 360 women[53] and was much smaller in the other two.[52,54] It is possible that the large standard error near term was due to the relatively small number of patients. In addition, despite the finding that the biparietal diameter was clearly the most inaccurate, a cephalic index was not performed to determine which head shapes were so abnormal that biparietal diameters should not have been used. Furthermore, all circumferences for the head and body were taken using a linear-array transducer. In the third trimester, many heads and bodies cannot be fit onto one image so that the margins have to be estimated to calculate a circumference. This could lead to significant errors.

Despite all of these misgivings, this work does appear to have clinical usefulness in eliminating a maximum error when one, or possibly two, measurements are discrepant from the others. Therefore, a table by Hadlock et al.[53] is recommended (Figs 7–4 to 7–6, Table 7–5).

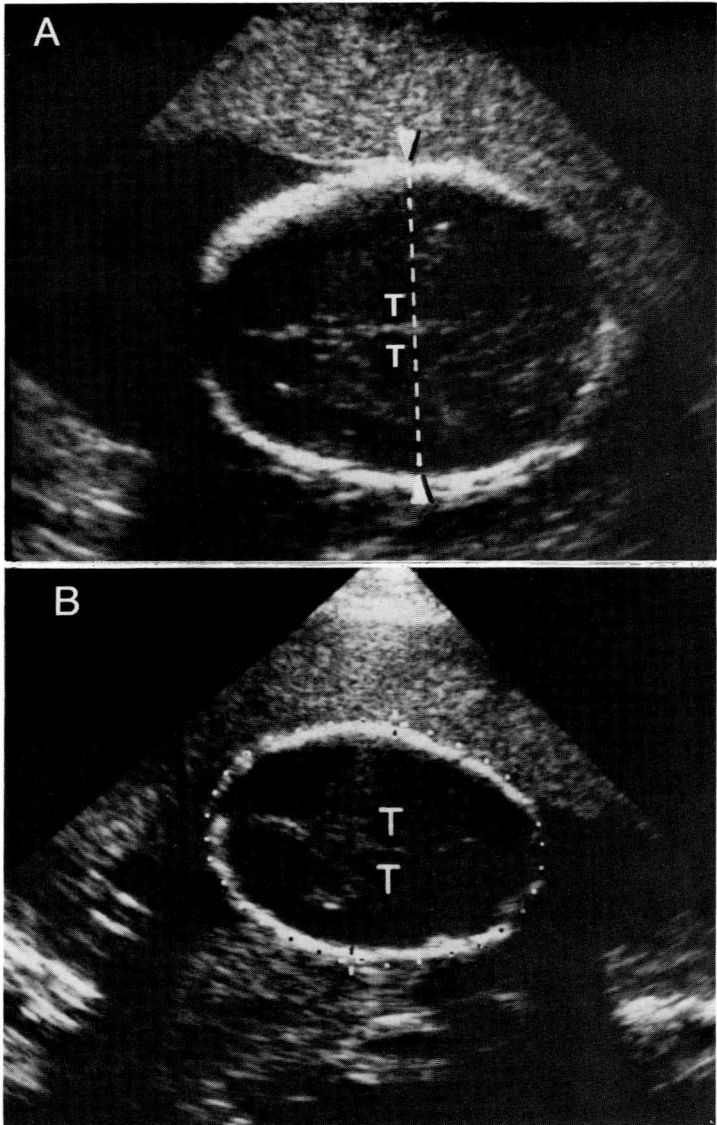

FIG 7–4.
Biparietal diameter and circumference measurements of the head. Both are taken from the transaxial image with the thalami (T) or midbrain in the midline. **A,** biparietal diameter measurement *(arrowheads* and *dotted line),* taken leading edge (outer margin) to leading edge (inner margin). **B,** head circumference measurement *(dotted line)* is traced around the outer margin of the head with a digitizer or map reader. It can also be calculated by using an equation.

Product of the Crown-Rump Length and Trunk Area

Five articles[61–65] have evaluated the product of the crown-rump length and trunk area, one from 16 weeks to term[61] and the others from 33 weeks to term. All were shown in graph form, with the measurement points obtained from static scans using a method described by Wittman et al.[62] The crown-rump length

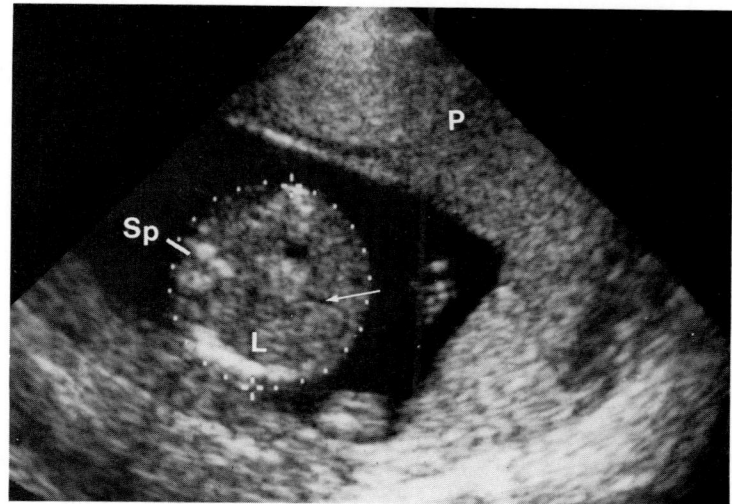

FIG 7–5.
Circumference measurement of the fetal abdomen. Transaxial image of the upper abdomen at the region of the liver (L). The umbilical portion of the left portal vein *(arrow)* is situated within the liver in the midline. The circumference is traced with a digitizer or map reader *(dotted line)* or can be calculated from an equation. P indicates placenta, Sp, spine.

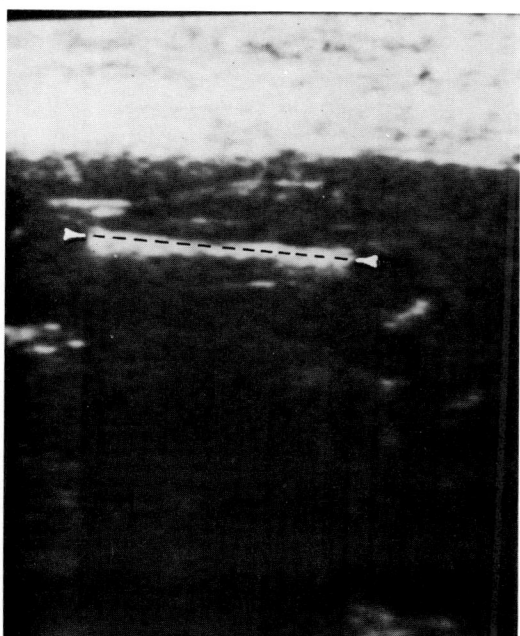

FIG 7–6.
Femur length measurement. The long axis of the hyperechoic femoral shaft is measured *(arrowheads* and *dotted line)*, disregarding the hypoechoic, nonossified epiphyseal cartilages.

TABLE 7-5
Multiple Fetal Parameters in the Assessment of Gestational Age*†

Mean Gestational Age, wk	Mean Biparietal Diameter, mm	Mean Head Circumference, mm	Mean Abdominal Circumference, mm	Mean Femur Length, mm
12.0	17	68	46	7
12.5	19	75	53	9
13.0	21	82	60	11
13.5	23	89	67	12
14.0	25	97	73	14
14.5	27	104	80	16
15.0	29	110	86	17
15.5	31	117	93	19
16.0	32	124	99	20
16.5	34	131	106	22
17.0	36	138	112	24
17.5	38	144	119	25
18.0	39	151	125	27
18.5	41	158	131	28
19.0	43	164	137	30
19.5	45	170	144	31
20.0	46	177	150	33
20.5	48	183	156	34
21.0	40	189	162	35
21.5	51	195	168	37
22.0	53	201	174	38
22.5	55	207	179	40
23.0	56	213	185	41
23.5	58	219	191	42
24.0	59	224	197	44
24.5	61	230	202	45
25.0	62	235	208	46
25.5	64	241	213	47
26.0	65	246	219	49
26.5	67	251	224	50
27.0	68	256	230	51
27.5	69	261	235	52
28.0	71	266	240	54
28.5	72	271	246	55
29.0	73	275	251	56
29.5	75	280	256	57
30.0	76	284	261	58
30.5	77	288	266	59
31.0	78	293	271	60
31.5	79	297	276	61

TABLE 7–5 (cont.).

Mean Gestational Age, wk	Mean Biparietal Diameter, mm	Mean Head Circumference, mm	Mean Abdominal Circumference, mm	Mean Femur Length, mm
32.0	81	301	281	62
32.5	82	304	286	63
33.0	83	308	291	64
33.5	84	312	295	65
34.0	85	315	300	66
34.5	86	318	305	67
35.0	87	322	309	68
35.5	88	325	314	69
36.0	89	328	318	70
36.5	89	330	323	71
37.0	90	333	327	72
37.5	91	335	332	73
38.0	92	338	336	74
38.5	92	340	340	74
39.0	93	342	344	75
39.5	94	344	348	76
40.0	94	346	353	77

*From Hadlock FP, Deter RL, Harrist RB, et al: Estimated fetal age: computer-assisted analysis of multiple fetal growth parameters. *Radiology* 1984; 152:497–501. Used by permission.
†**Instructions:** Take the mean measurements for the four parameters—biparietal diameter, head circumference, abdominal circumference, femur length. Find mean gestational ages of each, add them together, and divide by 4.

was obtained in longitudinal axis from the top of the head to the bottom of the bladder and the trunk area from an upper abdominal transaxial image. All showed an increase in the product of the fetal length times trunk area as the fetus enlarged to term.

The data claimed in one article[61] that this product correlated well with fetal weight and in three others[63–65] with the detection of in utero growth retardation in up to 94% of cases. This measurement is time-consuming and requires static scans. It may, however, offer information that other measurements do not. More work is needed, including the availability of numbers, before this product can be recommended.

INTERVAL GROWTH

Interval growth of the fetus can be analyzed when serial ultrasound examinations are performed during the pregnancy. Since the early 1970s, this concept has been used to determine the appropriate growth of the fetal head.[66, 67] The biparietal diameter was found to have an expected growth at each stage of gestation in millimeters per week.[66] This growth decreased linearly from the early second trimester until term.[66] When normal, 83% of fetuses were found to be normal at birth; when slow, 68% were small-for-dates.[67] Interval growth was carried one step further by noting that most normal fetal biparietal diameters could be separated into one of three percentile rankings: large (above the 75th percentile), average (25th to 75th percentile), and small (below the 25th percentile).[68] When 142 fetuses were evaluated, the biparietal diameter maintained the same percentile from 20 to 40 weeks in 128 cases (90%), and all were normal at birth. Of the remaining 14 fetuses, 11 showed a drop from the initial percentile rank to the next lower, and 5 of these had low birth weight. The remaining three showed an increase in percentile rank to the next higher, and all were normal at birth. Therefore, from these studies, it was determined that (1) the fetal head is expected to grow at a certain rate in millimeters per week throughout the second and third trimester, decreasing linearly from the early second trimester until term, and (2) most fetuses maintain a certain percentile growth throughout the pregnancy.[66-68] It would be expected (and discussed later in this section), based on the close relationship between the head, body, and extremity growth, that the same concept could be used to evaluate interval growth of other body parts.[69]

Since at least two examinations are needed to evaluate interval growth, it was initially suggested that the two be performed at specific times in the gestation, one prior to 26 weeks and the other between 30 and 33 weeks.[70-72] In two articles by the same group,[71, 72] it was stated that these two measurements, termed the *growth-adjusted sonographic age* (GASA), could do three things: determine the fetal growth in the correct percentile ranking, detect growth retardation, and date the fetus to within ±1 to 3 days. An additional study found that any two biparietal diameter measurements taken between 19 and 30 weeks, with at least a three-week interval between examinations, was as accurate as GASA in predicting the fetal age.[73] More recently, however, the accuracy of GASA has come into question. It has been shown that either a first trimester crown-rump length or a biparietal diameter measured up to 24 weeks is as accurate as GASA and that this accuracy was not 1 to 3 days, as initially reported, but rather ±5 to 7 days.[74, 75] In addition, an accurate menstrual history is as correct as the first and second trimester measurement in establishing fetal age.[74, 75]

Despite the inability of GASA or of any two readings between 19 and 30 weeks to narrow the estimated date of confinement to less than 5 to 7 days, the concept of interval growth is very important, since it allows assessment of fetal growth.[76, 77] There have been discrepancies among articles as to both the correct millimeters per week of growth at each stage of gestation and the shape of the growth curve. Two articles determined that the interval growth of the fetus had two slopes, initially fast at 3.0–3.2 mm per week until 31 to 33 weeks, then decreasing to 1.8 mm per week until term.[78, 79] Hohler et al.[79] reviewed an additional five studies and agreed that between 34 and 40 weeks the mean growth rate of the biparietal diameter was between 1.35 and 1.91 mm/week. Another study, however, contradicted both the slope of the curve and the mean fetal growth near term by finding that the normal growth was linear, at 2.6 mm per week from 18 to 38 weeks.[80] An additional article determined that the biparietal diameter growth rate was triphasic, 3 mm per week in the first trimester, 3.5 mm per week in the second trimester, and 2 mm per week throughout the third trimester.[81] Last, an article in graph and equation form,[82] without giving numbers, found a growth from 12 weeks to term to be slightly curvilinear. For simplicity, because of the discrepancies among studies, it will be assumed that the growth of the biparietal diameter decelerates linearly in the second and third trimester.

Eight articles have been published giving specific numbers for the biparietal diameter in millimeters per week of growth,[66, 69, 83–88] seven throughout the second and third trimesters,[66, 69, 83, 85–88] with the last from 24 weeks to term.[84] All showed a somewhat linear decrease in the biparietal diameter growth throughout the second and third trimester with four of the articles having a biphasic configuration, initially fast until 30 to 34 weeks and then slower to term.[66, 83, 85, 86] At 20 weeks, the interval growth from seven articles[66, 69, 83, 85–88] ranged from 2.63 to 3.4 mm, decreasing in all eight articles from 2.3 to 2.63 mm by 30 weeks and from 0.98 to 1.71 mm at term. In addition to the mean values, six gave percentile ratings, two at the 10th and 90th percentile,[83, 85] two at the 5th and 95th percentile (2 SD),[66, 69] two at the 1st and 99th percentile (3 SD).[87, 88]

The determination of which table to use was based on sample size, statistical analysis and range around the mean. While Levi and Smets[83] and Campbell and Newman[66] were both acceptable, the sample size of Levi and Smets[83] was much larger and is therefore recommended (Fig 7–7; Table 7–6). An example of how to use Table 7–6 is as follows: A pregnant woman is examined twice. On the first study, the fetus was found to have a biparietal diameter measuring 50 mm. Ten weeks later, the woman was reexamined, and a biparietal diameter of 80 mm was obtained. The interval change between the two examinations is 80 mm − 50 mm = 30 mm. The average rate of growth in millimeters per week is 30 mm/10 weeks = 3 mm/week. Since the growth decelerates linearly from early second to late third trimester, the mean point of growth is halfway between the two numbers. In this case, the halfway point between 50 and 80 mm is 65 mm. Along the 65-mm line, a 3 mm/week growth is found to be normal at an 80% growth rate.

The use of interval growth has been carefully evaluated in only one article.[87] Five types of fetal growth patterns were described in an attempt to determine the probability that growth retardation would occur. Although the series of 121 patients with serial measurements was relatively small, a normal interval growth or a growth which initially started low and then rose into the normal range was found in 95 fetuses. At birth, 92 (97%) were normal and the other 3 growth retarded. In a much smaller subgroup of nine patients, the growth was initially normal and then fell below normal. While this pattern would theoretically seem to portend growth retardation, only one of these nine were growth retarded at birth. The two most diagnostic patterns for growth retardation were found to be a single subnormal growth or a uniformly low profile, with growth never rising above the lower 10th percentile. In these patterns, 8 of 17 fetuses (47%) had growth retardation at birth.

Interval growth has also been analyzed in the first trimester. In 53 normal gestations, Nyberg et al.[89] found that between 4.5 and 11 gestational weeks, the average gestational sac size grew at a constant rate, at a mean of 1.13 mm/day (range, 0.71 to 1.75 mm/day). Evaluating an additional 30 abnormal gestations,

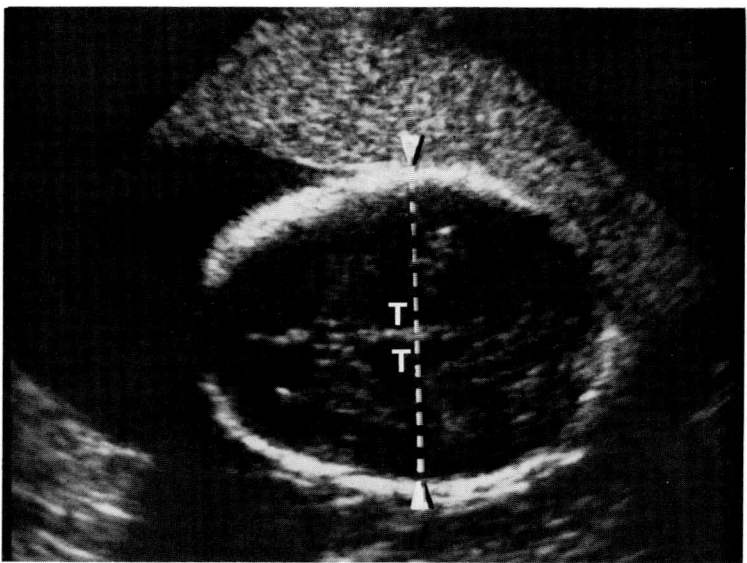

FIG 7–7.
The biparietal diameter measurement is taken in transaxial view with the thalamus (T) or midbrain in the midline. The measurement *(arrowheads* and *dotted line),* is taken leading edge (outer margin) to leading edge (inner margin).

24 demonstrated a slower mean growth of 0.70 mm/day (range, 0.14 to 1.71 mm/day). The authors therefore concluded that a gestational sac growth rate less than or equal to 0.6 mm/day is evidence of abnormal growth.[89] Crown-rump length has been evaluated in graph and equation form,[82] but no conclusion of the type of curve or rate of growth could be determined because the sample size was too small. Further work on both gestational sac and crown-rump length is needed. The work on the gestational sac is particularly interesting, since the sac can be imaged approximately 2 weeks earlier than the embryo. To avoid potential measurement errors, which can be as large as 1 to 2 mm for each study or 2 to 4 mm for two studies, a growth of at least 4 mm is needed. Using the authors' criterion of a minimum growth of 0.6 mm/day, 7 days between studies is therefore needed to be certain of adequate growth.

Interval growth has also been used to evaluate other fetal parameters. In the head, the interval growth of the fronto-occipital diameter, the head circumference, and the head area have been tabulated as numbers,[69] with the fronto-occipital diameter and head circumference also analyzed in graph and equation.[82, 90] In the body, the weekly growth of the chest area was analyzed in one article[84] and the abdominal AP, transverse, circumference, and area in three.[69, 90, 91] In one[91] it was found that within 2 weeks of delivery, the abdominal circumference should grow at greater than or equal to 10 mm/14 days, a number close to the growth of the biparietal diameter near term. In addition, Fescina et al.[69] found that the incremental growth of the abdominal diameters, both AP and transverse, was also similar to that of the biparietal diameter. This finding suggests that the use of the table of interval growth of the biparietal diameter could possibly be used in the evaluation of incremental growth of the abdominal diameter. In symmetric growth retardation, where both the fetal head and body

TABLE 7-6.
Biparietal Diameter Growth Rate Table*

Gestational Age, wk	Mean Biparietal Diameter, mm‡	Predicted Interval Growth, mm/wk†				
		Percentiles				
		10th	20th	50th	80th	90th
15	32	—	—	3.88	—	—
16	36	—	—	3.20	—	—
17	39	—	2.86	3.20	3.44	—
18	41	—	2.85	3.05	3.85	—
19	44	—	2.80	3.25	3.90	—
20	48	2.56	2.69	3.15	3.33	3.63
21	50	2.56	2.70	3.10	3.70	3.89
22	54	2.50	2.78	3.09	3.43	3.90
23	57	2.31	2.58	2.85	3.31	3.49
24	59	2.32	2.56	2.85	3.20	3.47
25	63	2.41	2.55	2.74	3.06	3.36
26	66	2.26	2.34	2.58	3.01	3.21
27	68	2.16	2.33	2.57	2.97	3.22
28	71	2.12	2.25	2.47	2.76	3.06
29	75	2.06	2.17	2.42	2.68	2.93
30	78	1.86	2.00	2.30	2.64	2.90
31	80	1.69	1.87	2.16	2.42	2.68
32	82	1.56	1.78	2.02	2.37	2.61
33	84	1.17	1.45	1.92	2.32	2.56
34	85	1.15	1.39	1.85	2.23	2.60
35	87	0.95	1.21	1.67	1.95	2.25
36	89	0.90	1.10	1.56	1.95	2.44
37	90	0.76	0.91	1.40	1.91	2.25
38	92	0.69	0.89	1.45	1.92	2.36
39	93	0.43	0.85	1.38	1.94	2.88
40	94	0.57	0.87	1.38	2.35	2.91
41	94	0.63	0.87	1.57	2.86	2.93
42	95	0.62	0.87	1.38	1.91	1.95
43	95	—	—	—	—	—

*From Levi S, Smets P: Intrauterine fetal growth studied by ultrasonic biparietal measurements. *Acta Obstet Gynecol Scand* 1973; 52:193–198. Used by permission.
†Data from Table I in original article.
‡Data from Table II in original article.

are equally affected,[76, 77] one would expect both to have similar decrease in interval growth. In asymmetric growth retardation,[76, 77] however, the initial finding would be a decrease in the interval growth of the body, with the fetal head remaining relatively normal. Only in the late stages of severe asymmetric growth retardation would the growth of both the head and body be equally affected.

The interval growth of the femoral length has also been examined, first in a clinical-radiographic study[92] and then by ultrasound.[90, 93] The clinical-radiographic study, performed from 30 to 43 weeks on newborn children, showed the length of the thigh to grow at a linear rate of 3 mm per week.[92] In utero radiographs were then evaluated and the gestational age predicated by the measurement of the femur to within 2 weeks.[92] The in utero ultrasound study found different results.[93] At 14 weeks, the femoral length grew at 3.15 mm per week, slowly decreasing to 1.55 mm per week at term. This type of growth would be more consistent with the ultrasound in utero growth of the biparietal diameter and body diameter.[69, 83] The growth of all the long bones can be affected, as can the fetal head and body, by various negative maternal effects, such as smoking.[90]

At present, not enough data are available for recommendation of interval growth of any fetal parameter other than the biparietal diameter (see Table 7–6).

FETAL WEIGHT

The weight of live infants born between 20 and 48 gestational weeks has been extensively studied in the pediatric and obstetrical literature.[94–103] All except one series[94] weighed more than 10,000 infants, with this last analyzing less than 4,000. In addition, aborted fetuses from 8 to 26 weeks[99, 104, 105] were weighed in much smaller series, 170 to 1,800 fetuses. The combination of these studies permitted an understanding of fetal weight throughout gestational life. Almost all of the articles showed an "S"-shaped fetal weight growth curve, with the fastest linear growth occurring in the second and early third trimester and slower curvilinear growth at both ends. The numbers were found to group closely together. At 25 weeks, 5 studies[96, 99, 101, 102, 105] were within 150 gm, while from 30 weeks until term, 10 articles[94–103] were within 250 gm. These articles showed a slight difference in the weight between blacks and whites and between males and females, with whites and males slightly heavier at term. The same linear growth and weight difference was confirmed in an ultrasound study in the second and early third trimester, where gestational age was established by an early second trimester biparietal diameter measurement.[106] While it could be suggested that some of the preterm infants evaluated in these studies might have been growth retarded with decreased weight and abnormal growth curve, all of the series had large numbers and used care in establishing gestational age. The weights and growth curves are therefore undoubtedly valid for normal fetuses.

Knowing the weight of a fetus at time of birth is important, particularly in very large and very small fetuses. It has been estimated that after 36 gestational weeks, poor perinatal outcome occurs in 3.9% of fetuses and tends to occur at the extremes of birth weight.[107] In low-birth-weight infants, defined as below 2,500 gm,[108] and in very-low-birth-weight infants, defined as below 1,500 gm,[109] morbidity and mortality increases. Although it is difficult to separate all of the complications of the low- from very-low-birth-weight infants, major neurodevelopmental handicaps including cerebral palsy, seizure disorders, and congenital anomalies have been noted, particularly in the very-low-birth-weight infants. Lower respiratory tract difficulties are seen in low birth rate infants, with 8% of very-low-birth-weight infants having chronic pulmonary changes, usually secondary to treatment after birth. Large fetuses, termed macrosomic and defined as greater than 4,000 gm at birth, have other problems[110–112] particularly related to difficulty during delivery. These include perinatal asphyxia and trauma, with trauma further divided into brachial palsy, fractured clavicle, and shoulder dystocia. The incidence of shoulder dystocia appears to be higher with increased fetal weight and to be more of a problem in diabetic than in nondiabetic fetuses, presumably due to a different distribution of weight to the upper extremities in diabetic fetuses.[111, 112]

Fetal weight is not an absolute predictor of the outcome of a pregnancy. Nevertheless, in one series, the newborn outcome was normal in 98% of babies born between the 10th and 90th percentile.[107] As a result, attempts have been made to accurately determine fetal weight prior to delivery. Initially studies were performed with radiographs of the pregnant uterus.[113, 114] At first the volume of the fetal head was measured with an error of one pound (455 gm) or less in 60% of cases.[113] Later, the skull (both the biparietal diameter and the fronto-occipital diameter) and the uterine lengths were added together, giving an accuracy of ±10% in 72% of patients. Obviously, because of difficulty in obtaining the correct plane of section and because of the use of ionizing radiation, this radiographic approach was only of academic interest and not routinely used in pregnant women. With the advent of ultrasound, however, the possibility of obtaining accurate fetal weights became more feasible.

To date, there have been 57 published analyses of fetal weight. Furthermore, 27 of these 57 articles and an additional 12 studies compared and reevaluated these fetal weight articles. The studies of fetal weight can be subdivided by the types of measurements used to obtain the weight. Eleven, in some of the earliest work from 1967 to 1978, measured only the fetal head. Six, from 1975 through 1979, analyzed only the fetal body, while 26 articles, most from 1976 to the present, used a combined head and body measurement to obtain fetal weight. More recently, nine articles from 1984 to the present incorporated the femur with measurements of the fetal body and fetal head to obtain fetal weight. Last, in 5 articles, fetal volumes have been calculated to estimate fetal weight.

Despite these approaches, some quite novel, the overall accuracy of fetal weight has not significantly increased. Almost all articles claimed an accuracy in fetal weight detection of between ±10% and ±15%. While some in the initial study stated much better accuracies, as low as ±2% to 3%, later works could not substantiate these claims.

The 11 articles that obtained fetal weight by using the biparietal diameter,[115–125] all presenting their results as equations, with 2 also giving numbers.[119, 123] Six calculated an SD.[115–117, 119, 120, 122] The mean error varied, but in general was ±12% to 16%. While all the reasons for the inaccuracies are not known, the errors seem to be primarily caused by changes in either head shape[126] or failure to take into account the fetal body.[127] It was found, for instance, that in women with premature rupture of the membranes, the biparietal diameter measurement, even when incorporated with abdominal circumference, underestimated actual birth weight by 12.4%.[126] Since the head shape can be significantly distorted by lack of amniotic fluid, it is likely that the alternative use of the head circumference measurement would have been more accurate. It has also been noted that different body shapes markedly changed fetal weight, despite close grouping of biparietal diameter measurements.[127] When the biparietal diameters measured between 95 and 99 mm, for example, three babies weighed from 2,200 gm to 4,830 gm.

The fetal body was used to establish fetal weight in six articles,[128-133] three with SD.[129, 131, 133] Four of the articles used abdominal circumference,[129-132] one used abdominal area,[128] and the last used a combination of abdominal circumference and fetal body length.[133] Four of the articles published their values in equation form, with one[129] presenting numbers and one[132] using a graph. Abdominal areas were suggested as the appropriate body measurement in cases where an ellipse formula could not provide an adequate approximation of the fetal abdomen.[134] The overall accuracies of these articles was ±10% to 20%, including the article that used abdominal area measurements. Higginbottom et al.[132] initially claimed in an evaluation of 50 fetuses to have an accuracy of ±2% to 3% in 94% of cases. While these results were impressive, their work was disputed by Finikiotis et al.,[135] who compared the Higginbottom and co-workers[132] results to an additional 115 fetuses and found an accuracy of only ±10%, with many less accurate, in 56% of all births.

The largest group of fetal weight articles evaluated a combination of head and body parameters. There were 26 articles published,[136-161] 16 presenting their results in equation form. Of the remaining 10, five gave numbers[137-141] and five showed only graphs.[136, 142-144, 160] The type of head and body parameters varied from study to study. The majority, 13 articles, used a combination of biparietal diameter and abdominal circumference.[139-141, 143-147, 154, 156, 157, 159, 160] Seven used a combination of biparietal diameter and thoracic diameter, either transverse or AP.[137, 138, 142, 148-151] The remaining six articles used the following: biparietal diameter and thoracic circumference,[136] head and thoracic areas,[152] head and abdominal areas,[153] biparietal and abdominal diameters,[161] biparietal diameter, fronto-occipital diameter, and abdominal diameter,[158] and biparietal diameter, thoracic diameter, and abdominal area.[155] All except four[138, 142, 144, 158] gave standard deviations.

To prove that combined head and body measurement were more accurate than either a head or body measurement alone, Thompson et al.[136, 142] calculated a decreased SD error when this combined approach was employed. In one of their articles, Thompson and Makowski[142] found the SD for the combined measurements to be ±290 gm as opposed to SD of ±350 gm and 364 gm for the biparietal diameter and the AP chest diameter, respectively. Despite this finding, the use of combined head and body parameters did not significantly affect the predictive accuracy of fetal weight. In general, the mean SD was still ±10% to 15%. Several articles, however, claimed greater accuracy. Birnholz[158] and Jordaan[157] thought that they could predict the fetal weight to within ±2% to 3%. This high accuracy could not be substantiated. Sampson et al.,[159] using his own and Birnholz's equation, found the latter to be ±8% if the fetus weighed less than 2,500 gm and at least ±10% if the fetus weighed greater than 2,500 gm. Weiner et al.[162] evaluated Jordaan's work[157] and found accuracies approached only ±15% in over half the cases.

Some observers had suggested that the reason for persistent inaccuracies in fetal weight was the failure to take into account the length of the fetus. Since it had been shown that the fetal femur length closely correlated with the neonatal crown-heel length,[163, 164] nine articles[164–172] added femoral length measurements to the head and body parameters in the hope that greater fetal weight accuracy would occur. All of the articles presented their data in equation form, with three giving additional numbers.[165, 170, 171] The articles used a combination of from two to four parameters, all with SD. Campbell et al.[166] and Warsof et al.[171] used the femoral length and abdominal circumference. Hadlock et al. in two articles[165, 167] combined the femur length and abdominal circumference with the head circumference, while Hill et al.,[168] Woo et al. in two articles[169, 170] and Benson et al.[172] combined these two parameters with the biparietal diameter measurement. Last, Roberts et al.[164] combined the femoral length and abdominal circumference with two parameters, the biparietal diameter and head circumference. The accuracy of the studies ranged from ±6.8% to 13%. Hadlock et al. in two articles[165, 167] claimed an accuracy of ±7.5% but with only a modest statistical significance of $P \leq .05$. Two other authors confirmed this small increase in accuracy when the femoral length was combined with other parameters to estimate fetal weight.[164, 168] Four other studies, however, did not. One found no statistical difference[169] and the other three,[164, 171, 173] reexamining Hadlock and co-workers' work,[165, 167] determined an accuracy of at best ±10%.

Last, five articles[174–178] formulated a fetal volume to determine fetal weight, all using different approaches. Picker and Saunders[174] took a biparietal diameter and a long axis measurement of the fetus, using the formula for a cylinder. Morrison and McLennan[175] performed transverse parallel scans at 2-cm intervals, adding up all of the areas to equal a volume. Thompson and Manning[176] took volume measurements of the fetal head, using a combination of biparietal diameter and fronto-occipital diameter, and the volume of the fetal body and extremities, using the formula for a cylinder. Brinkley et al.,[177] using a computer system, combined 19 fetal measured variables. Rossavik et al.[178] used an equation with the head and body cubed. All of the articles except one[178] gave equations with SD. While the accuracy ranged from ±7% to 14%, none of this work has been duplicated and therefore will not be considered further.

Two types of variations can occur in the evaluation of fetal weight: the variation within a study (intrapopulation) that causes approximately a ±10% to 15% error and the variation between studies (interpopulation). While not a great deal is known about either, it has been suggested that the intrapopulation variation may be caused by a number of factors.[157] It may be due to variance in sampling error if the sample is not representative of the general population. It may be due to variations in fetal anthropometry or dysmorphic growth, the latter a consequence of different growth patterns for the head (the growth of the brain) and for the body (somatic growth). None of these, however, fully explains the variation of approximately 10% to 15% that exists within all studies. Even the use of femoral length does not increase this accuracy. It is possible, however, that the femur length is not truly representative of the length of the fetus and that another measurement of the fetal long axis is needed.

The interpopulation variation is even less understood.[157] This type of variation can be best appreciated by Table 7–7. Using previous tables, the idealized numbers at 25, 30, 35, and 40 gestational weeks were calculated for biparietal

TABLE 7-7.
Comparison of Fetal Weight Tables

Gestational Age, wk	Ideal Fetal Measurements, mm*					
	BPD	FOD	HC	AD	AC	FL
25	63	80	225	65	205	45
30	76	96	275	79	260	57
35	87	110	315	95	310	69
40	95	120	350	110	360	80

Gestational Age, wk	Articles (Parameters Measured)				Average Newborn Weight (4 articles), gm
	Campbell & Wilkins[129] (AC)	Shephard et al.[139] (BPD, AC)	Jordaan[157] (HC, AC)	Birnholz[158] (BPD, FOD, AC)	Hadlock et al.[165] (HC, AC, FL)	
	Fetal Weights (gm)					
25	900	790	915	928	783	808
30	1,690	1,533	1,790	1,438	1,544	1,446
35	2,690	2,554	2,767	2,264	2,641	2,530
40	3,640	3,791	3,728	2,850	4,031	3,346

*BPD = biparietal diameter; FOD = fronto-occipital diameter; HC = head circumference; AD = abdominal diameter; AC = abdominal circumference; FL = femur length.

diameter, head circumference, body diameter, abdominal circumference, and femoral length. In addition, the fronto-occipital diameter was calculated using an ideal cephalic index of 0.78. Newborn weights at each gestational age were included for comparison. At 25 weeks, there was greater than a 130–gm variation between the studies, increasing to over 1,100 gm at term. In addition, studies that had given low fetal weights early in gestation gave high fetal weights near term and vice versa.

As a result, the choice of which weight tables to recommend is difficult. It would be useful, however, to have more than one table, using different parameters. There are occasions when a certain parameter cannot be adequately measured so that a specific weight table may not be of value. There are also certain weight ranges where specific tables may be more accurate. Because the tables all have an approximate inaccuracy of ±10% to 15%, the choice of which to recommend has been determined not only from the original article but also from the works substantiating it. In addition to the 27 original articles on fetal weight that have compared their work to others, there are 12 more articles[173, 179–189] published solely to evaluate the weight tables.

Shepard et al.[139] and Warsof et al.[140] will be considered together, since Shepard et al.[139] is a modification of the original work by Warsof et al.[140] In addition to these original two articles, 18 articles have reevaluated this head and body technique and found it to be accurate to within ±10% to 15%, and to be particularly accurate in very low and low birth weight infants.[135, 146, 159, 162, 166, 168, 173, 179–189] As a result, the work by Shepard et al.[139] using the biparietal diameter and abdominal circumference (Figs 7–8 and 7–9) is recommended (Table 7–8). The work of Campbell and Wilkin[129] using the abdominal circumference has also been reevaluated in 6 additional articles[159, 168, 180, 185, 187, 188] with fairly consistent results, variations no greater than ±10% to 12% and it, too, is recommended (see Fig 7–9; Table 7–9).

Last, the work incorporating femoral length by Hadlock et al.[165] has been reevaluated in seven additional articles[165, 167, 171–173, 186, 189] and found to be as accurate as weight tables using the biparietal diameter and abdominal circumference measurements,[171–173] with one[186] suggesting that it was more consistent than other weight formulas in larger fetuses. As a result, while more work is needed to determine if a weight table incorporating a femur has an advantage over other weight tables, the work by Hadlock et al.[165] is also recommended, particularly for normal (2,500 to 3,999 gm) and for macrosomic (>4,000 gm) fetuses. A problem arises, however, as to which equation from their article is the most accurate. An equation using three variables, head circumference (HC), abdominal circumference (AC), and femur length (FL), was proposed since the authors thought that it was the most accurate, minimizing errors due to anatomical extremes[165] (Figs 7–9 to 7–11; Table 7–10). However, since a three-variable equation cannot be presented in table form, they also recommended a slightly less preferable equation using only two of the variables, abdominal circumference and femur length (see Figs 7–9 and 7–11; Table 7–11). Two other articles have analyzed both the three-variable[173] and two-variable[171] approach of Hadlock et al.[165] While both articles found the two-variable approach to be good, Yarkoni et al.[173] thought the combined use of all three was better. Since the three-variable equation is cumbersome, however, both are recommended.

152 Second and Third Trimester Obstetrical Measurements

TABLE 7-8.
Estimated Fetal Weight (Grams) Based on Biparietal Diameter (BPD) and Abdominal Circumference (AC)*†

BPD, mm	AC, mm												
	155	160	165	170	175	180	185	190	195	200	205	210	215
31	224	234	244	255	267	279	291	304	318	332	346	362	378
32	231	241	251	263	274	286	299	312	326	340	355	371	388
33	237	248	259	270	282	294	307	321	335	349	365	381	397
34	244	255	266	278	290	302	316	329	344	359	374	391	408
35	251	262	274	285	298	311	324	338	353	368	384	401	418
36	259	270	281	294	306	319	333	347	362	378	394	411	429
37	266	278	290	302	315	328	342	357	372	388	404	422	440
38	274	286	298	310	324	337	352	366	382	398	415	432	451
39	282	294	306	319	333	347	361	376	392	409	426	444	462
40	290	303	315	328	342	356	371	386	403	419	437	455	474
41	299	311	324	338	352	366	381	397	413	430	448	467	486
42	308	320	333	347	361	376	392	408	424	442	460	479	498
43	317	330	343	357	371	387	402	419	436	453	472	491	511
44	326	339	353	367	382	397	413	430	447	465	484	504	524
45	335	349	363	377	393	408	425	442	459	478	497	517	538
46	345	359	373	386	404	420	436	454	472	490	510	530	551
47	355	369	384	399	415	431	448	466	484	503	524	544	565
48	366	380	395	410	426	443	460	478	497	517	537	558	580
49	376	391	406	422	438	455	473	491	510	530	551	572	594
50	387	402	418	434	451	468	486	505	524	544	565	587	610
51	399	414	430	446	463	481	499	518	538	559	580	602	625
52	410	426	442	459	476	494	513	532	552	573	595	618	641
53	422	438	455	472	489	508	527	547	567	589	611	634	657
54	435	451	468	485	503	522	541	561	582	604	627	650	674
55	447	464	481	499	517	536	556	577	598	620	643	667	691
56	461	477	495	513	532	551	571	592	614	636	660	684	709
57	474	491	509	527	547	566	587	608	630	653	677	701	727
58	488	505	524	542	562	582	603	625	647	670	695	719	745
59	502	520	539	558	578	598	619	642	664	688	713	738	764
60	517	535	554	573	594	615	636	659	682	706	731	757	784
61	532	550	570	590	610	632	654	677	700	725	750	777	804
62	547	566	586	606	627	649	672	695	719	744	770	797	824
63	563	583	603	624	645	667	690	714	738	764	790	817	845
64	580	600	620	641	663	686	709	733	758	784	811	838	867
65	597	617	638	659	682	705	728	753	778	805	832	860	889

Combined Fetal Head and Body Measurements

66	614	635	656	678	701	724	748	773	799	826	853	882	911
67	632	653	675	697	720	744	769	794	820	848	876	905	935
68	651	672	694	717	740	765	790	816	842	870	898	928	958
69	670	691	714	737	761	786	811	838	865	893	922	952	983
70	689	711	734	758	782	807	833	860	888	916	946	976	1,008
71	709	732	755	779	804	830	856	883	912	941	971	1,002	1,033
72	730	753	777	801	827	853	880	907	936	965	996	1,027	1,060
73	751	775	799	824	850	876	904	932	961	991	1,022	1,054	1,087
74	773	797	822	847	874	901	928	957	987	1,017	1,049	1,081	1,114
75	796	820	845	871	898	925	954	983	1,013	1,044	1,076	1,109	1,143
76	819	844	870	896	923	951	980	1,009	1,040	1,072	1,104	1,137	1,172
77	843	868	894	921	949	977	1,007	1,037	1,068	1,100	1,133	1,167	1,202
78	868	894	920	947	975	1,004	1,034	1,065	1,096	1,129	1,162	1,197	1,232
79	893	919	946	974	1,003	1,032	1,062	1,094	1,126	1,159	1,193	1,228	1,264
80	919	946	973	1,002	1,031	1,061	1,091	1,123	1,156	1,189	1,224	1,259	1,296
81	946	973	1,001	1,030	1,060	1,090	1,121	1,153	1,187	1,221	1,256	1,292	1,329
82	974	1,001	1,030	1,059	1,089	1,120	1,152	1,185	1,218	1,253	1,288	1,325	1,363
83	1,002	1,030	1,059	1,089	1,120	1,151	1,183	1,217	1,251	1,286	1,322	1,359	1,397
84	1,032	1,060	1,090	1,120	1,151	1,183	1,216	1,249	1,284	1,320	1,356	1,394	1,433
85	1,062	1,091	1,121	1,151	1,183	1,216	1,249	1,283	1,318	1,355	1,392	1,430	1,469
86	1,093	1,122	1,153	1,184	1,216	1,249	1,283	1,318	1,354	1,390	1,428	1,467	1,507
87	1,125	1,155	1,186	1,218	1,250	1,284	1,318	1,354	1,390	1,427	1,465	1,505	1,545
88	1,157	1,188	1,220	1,252	1,285	1,319	1,354	1,390	1,427	1,465	1,504	1,543	1,584
89	1,191	1,222	1,254	1,287	1,321	1,356	1,391	1,428	1,465	1,503	1,543	1,583	1,625
90	1,226	1,258	1,290	1,324	1,358	1,393	1,429	1,456	1,504	1,543	1,583	1,624	1,666
91	1,262	1,294	1,327	1,361	1,396	1,432	1,468	1,506	1,544	1,584	1,624	1,666	1,708
92	1,299	1,332	1,365	1,400	1,435	1,471	1,508	1,546	1,586	1,626	1,667	1,709	1,752
93	1,337	1,370	1,404	1,439	1,475	1,512	1,550	1,588	1,628	1,668	1,710	1,753	1,796
94	1,376	1,410	1,444	1,480	1,516	1,554	1,592	1,631	1,671	1,712	1,755	1,798	1,842
95	1,416	1,450	1,486	1,522	1,559	1,597	1,635	1,675	1,716	1,758	1,800	1,844	1,889
96	1,457	1,492	1,528	1,565	1,602	1,641	1,680	1,720	1,762	1,804	1,847	1,892	1,937
97	1,500	1,535	1,572	1,609	1,647	1,686	1,726	1,767	1,809	1,852	1,895	1,940	1,986
98	1,544	1,580	1,617	1,654	1,693	1,733	1,773	1,815	1,857	1,900	1,945	1,990	2,037
99	1,589	1,625	1,663	1,701	1,740	1,781	1,822	1,864	1,907	1,951	1,996	2,042	2,089
100	1,635	1,672	1,710	1,749	1,789	1,830	1,871	1,914	1,958	2,002	2,048	2,094	2,142

(Continued.)

TABLE 7–8 (cont.).

BPD, mm	220	225	230	235	240	245	250	255	260	265	270	275	280
31	395	412	431	450	470	491	513	536	559	584	610	638	666
32	405	423	441	461	481	502	525	548	572	597	624	651	680
33	415	433	452	472	493	514	537	560	585	611	638	666	693
34	425	444	463	483	504	526	549	573	598	624	652	680	710
35	436	455	475	495	517	539	562	587	612	638	666	695	725
36	447	466	486	507	529	552	575	600	626	653	681	710	740
37	458	478	498	519	542	565	589	614	640	667	696	725	756
38	470	490	510	532	554	578	602	628	654	682	711	741	772
39	482	502	523	545	568	592	616	642	669	697	727	757	789
40	494	514	536	558	581	606	631	657	684	713	743	773	806
41	506	527	549	572	595	620	645	672	700	729	759	790	828
42	519	540	562	585	609	634	660	688	716	745	776	807	841
43	532	554	576	600	624	649	676	703	732	762	793	825	859
44	545	567	590	614	639	665	692	719	749	779	810	843	877
45	559	581	605	629	654	680	708	736	765	796	828	861	896
46	573	596	620	644	670	696	724	753	783	814	846	880	915
47	588	611	635	660	686	713	741	770	801	832	865	899	934
48	602	626	650	676	702	730	758	788	819	851	884	919	954
49	617	641	666	692	719	747	776	806	837	870	903	938	975
50	633	657	683	709	736	765	794	824	856	889	923	959	996
51	649	674	699	726	754	783	812	843	876	909	944	980	1,017
52	665	690	717	744	772	801	831	863	895	929	964	1,001	1,039
53	682	708	734	762	790	820	851	883	916	950	986	1,023	1,061
54	699	725	752	780	809	839	870	903	936	971	1,007	1,045	1,084
55	717	743	771	799	828	859	891	924	958	993	1,030	1,068	1,107
56	735	762	789	818	848	879	911	945	979	1,015	1,052	1,091	1,131
57	753	780	809	838	869	900	933	966	1,001	1,038	1,075	1,114	1,155
58	772	800	829	858	889	921	954	989	1,024	1,061	1,099	1,139	1,180
59	792	820	849	879	911	943	977	1,011	1,047	1,085	1,123	1,163	1,205
60	811	840	870	900	932	965	999	1,035	1,071	1,109	1,148	1,189	1,231
61	832	861	891	922	955	988	1,023	1,058	1,095	1,134	1,173	1,214	1,257
62	853	882	913	945	977	1,011	1,046	1,083	1,120	1,159	1,199	1,241	1,284
63	874	904	935	967	1,001	1,035	1,071	1,107	1,145	1,185	1,226	1,268	1,311
64	896	927	958	991	1,025	1,059	1,096	1,133	1,171	1,211	1,253	1,295	1,339
65	919	950	982	1,015	1,049	1,084	1,121	1,159	1,198	1,238	1,280	1,323	1,368

Combined Fetal Head and Body Measurements

66	942	973	1,006	1,039	1,074	1,110	1,147	1,185	1,225	1,266	1,308	1,352	1,397
67	965	997	1,030	1,065	1,100	1,136	1,174	1,213	1,253	1,294	1,337	1,381	1,427
68	990	1,022	1,056	1,090	1,126	1,163	1,201	1,241	1,281	1,323	1,367	1,411	1,458
69	1,015	1,048	1,082	1,117	1,153	1,190	1,229	1,269	1,310	1,353	1,397	1,442	1,489
70	1,040	1,074	1,108	1,144	1,181	1,219	1,258	1,298	1,340	1,383	1,427	1,473	1,521
71	1,066	1,100	1,135	1,171	1,209	1,247	1,287	1,328	1,370	1,414	1,459	1,505	1,553
72	1,093	1,128	1,163	1,200	1,238	1,277	1,317	1,358	1,401	1,445	1,491	1,538	1,586
73	1,121	1,156	1,192	1,229	1,267	1,307	1,348	1,390	1,433	1,478	1,524	1,571	1,620
74	1,149	1,184	1,221	1,259	1,297	1,338	1,379	1,421	1,465	1,511	1,557	1,605	1,655
75	1,178	1,214	1,251	1,289	1,328	1,369	1,411	1,454	1,499	1,544	1,592	1,640	1,690
76	1,207	1,244	1,281	1,320	1,360	1,401	1,444	1,487	1,533	1,579	1,627	1,676	1,727
77	1,238	1,275	1,313	1,352	1,393	1,434	1,477	1,522	1,567	1,614	1,663	1,712	1,764
78	1,269	1,306	1,345	1,385	1,426	1,468	1,512	1,557	1,603	1,650	1,699	1,749	1,801
79	1,301	1,339	1,378	1,418	1,460	1,503	1,547	1,592	1,639	1,687	1,737	1,787	1,840
80	1,333	1,372	1,412	1,453	1,495	1,538	1,583	1,629	1,676	1,725	1,775	1,826	1,879
81	1,367	1,406	1,446	1,488	1,531	1,575	1,620	1,666	1,714	1,763	1,814	1,866	1,919
82	1,401	1,441	1,482	1,524	1,567	1,612	1,657	1,704	1,753	1,803	1,854	1,906	1,960
83	1,436	1,477	1,518	1,561	1,605	1,650	1,696	1,744	1,793	1,843	1,895	1,948	2,002
84	1,473	1,513	1,555	1,599	1,643	1,689	1,735	1,784	1,833	1,884	1,936	1,990	2,045
85	1,510	1,551	1,594	1,637	1,682	1,728	1,776	1,825	1,875	1,926	1,979	2,033	2,089
86	1,548	1,589	1,633	1,677	1,722	1,769	1,817	1,866	1,917	1,969	2,022	2,077	2,134
87	1,586	1,629	1,673	1,717	1,764	1,811	1,859	1,909	1,960	2,013	2,067	2,122	2,179
88	1,626	1,669	1,714	1,759	1,806	1,854	1,903	1,953	2,005	2,058	2,113	2,169	2,226
89	1,667	1,711	1,756	1,802	1,849	1,897	1,947	1,998	2,050	2,104	2,159	2,216	2,274
90	1,709	1,753	1,799	1,845	1,893	1,942	1,992	2,044	2,097	2,151	2,207	2,264	2,322
91	1,752	1,797	1,843	1,890	1,938	1,988	2,039	2,091	2,144	2,199	2,255	2,313	2,372
92	1,796	1,841	1,888	1,936	1,984	2,035	2,086	2,139	2,193	2,248	2,305	2,363	2,423
93	1,841	1,887	1,934	1,982	2,032	2,083	2,135	2,188	2,242	2,298	2,356	2,414	2,475
94	1,887	1,934	1,982	2,030	2,080	2,132	2,184	2,238	2,293	2,350	2,407	2,467	2,527
95	1,935	1,982	2,030	2,080	2,130	2,182	2,235	2,289	2,345	2,402	2,460	2,520	2,582
96	1,984	2,031	2,080	2,130	2,181	2,233	2,287	2,342	2,398	2,456	2,515	2,575	2,637
97	2,033	2,082	2,131	2,181	2,233	2,286	2,340	2,396	2,452	2,510	2,570	2,631	2,693
98	2,085	2,133	2,183	2,234	2,286	2,340	2,395	2,451	2,508	2,567	2,627	2,688	2,751
99	2,137	2,186	2,237	2,288	2,341	2,395	2,450	2,507	2,565	2,624	2,684	2,746	2,810
100	2,191	2,241	2,292	2,344	2,397	2,452	2,507	2,564	2,623	2,682	2,743	2,806	2,870

(Continued.)

TABLE 7–8 (cont.).

BPD, mm	\multicolumn{13}{c}{AC, mm}
	285	290	295	300	305	310	315	320	325	330	335	340	345
31	696	726	759	793	828	865	903	943	985	1,029	1,075	1,123	1,173
32	710	742	774	809	844	882	921	961	1,004	1,048	1,094	1,143	1,193
33	725	757	790	825	861	899	938	979	1,022	1,067	1,114	1,163	1,214
34	740	773	806	841	878	916	956	998	1,041	1,087	1,134	1,183	1,235
35	756	789	823	858	896	934	975	1,017	1,061	1,107	1,154	1,204	1,256
36	772	805	840	876	913	953	993	1,036	1,080	1,127	1,175	1,226	1,278
37	788	822	857	893	931	971	1,012	1,056	1,101	1,147	1,196	1,247	1,300
38	805	839	874	911	950	990	1,032	1,076	1,121	1,168	1,218	1,269	1,323
39	822	856	892	930	969	1,009	1,052	1,096	1,142	1,190	1,240	1,292	1,346
40	839	874	911	949	988	1,029	1,072	1,117	1,163	1,212	1,262	1,315	1,369
41	857	892	929	968	1,008	1,049	1,093	1,138	1,185	1,234	1,285	1,338	1,393
42	875	911	948	987	1,028	1,070	1,114	1,159	1,207	1,256	1,308	1,361	1,417
43	893	930	968	1,007	1,048	1,091	1,135	1,181	1,229	1,279	1,331	1,385	1,442
44	912	949	987	1,027	1,069	1,112	1,157	1,204	1,252	1,303	1,355	1,410	1,467
45	932	969	1,008	1,048	1,090	1,134	1,179	1,226	1,275	1,326	1,380	1,435	1,492
46	951	989	1,028	1,069	1,112	1,156	1,202	1,249	1,299	1,351	1,404	1,460	1,518
47	971	1,010	1,049	1,091	1,134	1,178	1,225	1,273	1,323	1,375	1,430	1,486	1,545
48	992	1,031	1,071	1,113	1,156	1,201	1,248	1,297	1,348	1,401	1,455	1,512	1,571
49	1,013	1,052	1,093	1,135	1,179	1,225	1,272	1,322	1,373	1,426	1,482	1,539	1,599
50	1,034	1,074	1,115	1,158	1,203	1,249	1,297	1,347	1,399	1,452	1,508	1,566	1,626
51	1,056	1,096	1,138	1,181	1,226	1,273	1,322	1,372	1,425	1,479	1,535	1,594	1,655
52	1,078	1,119	1,161	1,205	1,251	1,298	1,347	1,398	1,451	1,506	1,563	1,622	1,683
53	1,101	1,142	1,185	1,229	1,276	1,323	1,373	1,425	1,478	1,533	1,591	1,651	1,713
54	1,124	1,166	1,209	1,254	1,301	1,349	1,399	1,452	1,506	1,562	1,620	1,680	1,742
55	1,148	1,190	1,234	1,279	1,327	1,376	1,426	1,479	1,534	1,590	1,649	1,710	1,773
56	1,172	1,215	1,259	1,305	1,353	1,402	1,454	1,507	1,562	1,619	1,678	1,740	1,803
57	1,197	1,240	1,285	1,332	1,380	1,430	1,482	1,535	1,591	1,649	1,709	1,770	1,835
58	1,222	1,266	1,311	1,358	1,407	1,458	1,510	1,564	1,621	1,679	1,739	1,802	1,866
59	1,248	1,292	1,338	1,386	1,435	1,486	1,539	1,594	1,651	1,710	1,770	1,834	1,899
60	1,274	1,319	1,366	1,414	1,464	1,515	1,569	1,624	1,682	1,741	1,802	1,866	1,932
61	1,301	1,346	1,393	1,442	1,493	1,545	1,599	1,655	1,713	1,773	1,835	1,899	1,965
62	1,328	1,374	1,422	1,471	1,522	1,575	1,630	1,686	1,745	1,805	1,868	1,932	1,999
63	1,356	1,403	1,451	1,501	1,552	1,606	1,661	1,718	1,777	1,838	1,901	1,967	2,034
64	1,385	1,432	1,481	1,531	1,583	1,637	1,693	1,751	1,810	1,872	1,935	2,001	2,069
65	1,414	1,462	1,511	1,562	1,615	1,669	1,725	1,784	1,844	1,906	1,970	2,037	2,105

Combined Fetal Head and Body Measurements

66	1,444	1,492	1,542	1,594	1,647	1,702	1,759	1,817	1,878	1,941	2,006	2,073	2,142
67	1,474	1,523	1,574	1,626	1,679	1,735	1,792	1,852	1,913	1,976	2,042	2,109	2,179
68	1,505	1,555	1,606	1,658	1,713	1,769	1,827	1,887	1,949	2,012	2,078	2,147	2,217
69	1,537	1,587	1,639	1,692	1,747	1,803	1,862	1,922	1,985	2,049	2,116	2,184	2,255
70	1,570	1,620	1,672	1,726	1,781	1,839	1,898	1,959	2,022	2,087	2,154	2,223	2,295
71	1,603	1,654	1,706	1,761	1,817	1,875	1,934	1,996	2,059	2,125	2,193	2,262	2,334
72	1,636	1,688	1,741	1,796	1,853	1,911	1,971	2,044	2,098	2,164	2,232	2,302	2,375
73	1,671	1,723	1,777	1,832	1,890	1,948	2,009	2,072	2,137	2,203	2,272	2,343	2,416
74	1,706	1,759	1,813	1,869	1,927	1,987	2,048	2,111	2,176	2,244	2,313	2,384	2,458
75	1,742	1,795	1,850	1,907	1,965	2,025	2,087	2,151	2,217	2,265	2,354	2,426	2,501
76	1,779	1,833	1,888	1,945	2,004	2,065	2,127	2,192	2,258	2,326	2,397	2,469	2,544
77	1,816	1,871	1,927	1,985	2,044	2,105	2,168	2,233	2,300	2,369	2,440	2,513	2,588
78	1,855	1,910	1,966	2,025	2,085	2,146	2,210	2,275	2,343	2,412	2,484	2,557	2,633
79	1,894	1,949	2,006	2,065	2,126	2,188	2,252	2,318	2,386	2,456	2,528	2,603	2,679
80	1,934	1,990	2,048	2,107	2,168	2,231	2,296	2,362	2,431	2,501	2,574	2,649	2,725
81	1,975	2,031	2,089	2,149	2,211	2,275	2,340	2,407	2,476	2,547	2,620	2,695	2,773
82	2,016	2,073	2,132	2,193	2,255	2,319	2,385	2,462	2,522	2,594	2,667	2,743	2,821
83	2,059	2,116	2,176	2,237	2,300	2,364	2,431	2,499	2,569	2,641	2,715	2,791	2,870
84	2,102	2,160	2,220	2,282	2,345	2,410	2,477	2,546	2,617	2,689	2,764	2,841	2,920
85	2,146	2,205	2,266	2,328	2,392	2,457	2,525	2,594	2,665	2,739	2,814	2,891	2,970
86	2,192	2,251	2,312	2,375	2,439	2,505	2,573	2,643	2,715	2,789	2,864	2,942	3,022
87	2,238	2,298	2,359	2,423	2,488	2,554	2,623	2,693	2,765	2,840	2,916	2,994	3,074
88	2,285	2,346	2,408	2,472	2,537	2,604	2,673	2,744	2,817	2,892	2,968	3,047	3,128
89	2,333	2,394	2,457	2,521	2,587	2,655	2,725	2,796	2,869	2,944	3,021	3,101	3,182
90	2,382	2,444	2,507	2,572	2,639	2,707	2,777	2,849	2,923	2,998	3,076	3,155	3,237
91	2,433	2,495	2,559	2,624	2,691	2,760	2,830	2,903	2,977	3,053	3,131	3,211	3,293
92	2,484	2,547	2,611	2,677	2,744	2,814	2,885	2,958	3,032	3,109	3,187	3,268	3,350
93	2,536	2,599	2,664	2,731	2,799	2,869	2,940	3,014	3,089	3,166	3,245	3,326	3,409
94	2,590	2,653	2,719	2,786	2,854	2,925	2,997	3,070	3,146	3,224	3,303	3,384	3,468
95	2,644	2,709	2,774	2,842	2,911	2,982	3,054	3,129	3,205	3,283	3,362	3,444	3,528
96	2,700	2,765	2,831	2,899	2,969	3,040	3,113	3,188	3,264	3,343	3,423	3,505	3,589
97	2,757	2,822	2,889	2,958	3,028	3,099	3,173	3,248	3,325	3,404	3,484	3,567	3,651
98	2,815	2,881	2,948	3,017	3,088	3,160	3,234	3,309	3,387	3,466	3,547	3,630	3,715
99	2,874	2,941	3,009	3,078	3,149	3,222	3,296	3,372	3,450	3,529	3,611	3,694	3,779
100	2,935	3,002	3,070	3,140	3,211	3,285	3,359	3,436	3,514	3,594	3,676	3,759	3,845

(Continued.)

TABLE 7-8 (cont.).

BPD, mm	AC, mm											
	350	355	360	365	370	375	380	385	390	395	400
31	1,225	1,279	1,336	1,396	1,458	1,523	1,591	1,661	1,735	1,812	1,893
32	1,246	1,301	1,358	1,418	1,481	1,546	1,615	1,686	1,761	1,838	1,920
33	1,267	1,323	1,381	1,441	1,504	1,570	1,639	1,711	1,786	1,865	1,946
34	1,289	1,345	1,403	1,464	1,528	1,595	1,664	1,737	1,812	1,891	1,973
35	1,311	1,367	1,426	1,488	1,552	1,619	1,689	1,762	1,839	1,918	2,001
36	1,333	1,390	1,450	1,512	1,577	1,645	1,715	1,789	1,865	1,945	2,029
37	1,356	1,413	1,474	1,536	1,602	1,670	1,741	1,815	1,893	1,973	2,057
38	1,379	1,437	1,498	1,561	1,627	1,696	1,768	1,842	1,920	2,001	2,086
39	1,402	1,461	1,523	1,586	1,653	1,722	1,794	1,870	1,948	2,030	2,115
40	1,426	1,486	1,548	1,612	1,679	1,749	1,822	1,898	1,977	2,059	2,145
41	1,451	1,511	1,573	1,638	1,706	1,776	1,849	1,926	2,005	2,088	2,174
42	1,475	1,536	1,599	1,664	1,733	1,804	1,878	1,954	2,035	2,118	2,205
43	1,500	1,562	1,625	1,691	1,760	1,832	1,906	1,984	2,064	2,148	2,236
44	1,526	1,588	1,652	1,718	1,788	1,860	1,935	2,013	2,094	2,179	2,267
45	1,552	1,614	1,679	1,746	1,816	1,889	1,964	2,043	2,125	2,210	2,298
46	1,579	1,641	1,706	1,774	1,845	1,918	1,994	2,073	2,156	2,241	2,330
47	1,605	1,669	1,734	1,803	1,874	1,948	2,024	2,104	2,187	2,273	2,363
48	1,633	1,697	1,763	1,832	1,904	1,976	2,055	2,136	2,219	2,306	2,396
49	1,661	1,725	1,792	1,861	1,934	2,009	2,086	2,167	2,251	2,339	2,429
50	1,689	1,754	1,821	1,891	1,964	2,040	2,118	2,200	2,284	2,372	2,463
51	1,718	1,783	1,851	1,922	1,995	2,071	2,150	2,232	2,317	2,406	2,498
52	1,747	1,813	1,882	1,953	2,027	2,103	2,183	2,266	2,351	2,440	2,532
53	1,777	1,843	1,913	1,984	2,059	2,136	2,216	2,299	2,386	2,475	2,568
54	1,807	1,874	1,944	2,016	2,091	2,169	2,250	2,333	2,420	2,510	2,604
55	1,838	1,906	1,976	2,049	2,124	2,203	2,284	2,368	2,456	2,546	2,640
56	1,869	1,938	2,008	2,082	2,158	2,237	2,319	2,403	2,491	2,582	2,677
57	1,901	1,970	2,041	2,115	2,192	2,272	2,354	2,439	2,528	2,619	2,714
58	1,934	2,003	2,075	2,150	2,227	2,307	2,390	2,475	2,564	2,657	2,752
59	1,966	2,037	2,109	2,184	2,262	2,342	2,426	2,512	2,602	2,694	2,790
60	2,000	2,071	2,144	2,219	2,298	2,379	2,463	2,550	2,640	2,733	2,829
61	2,034	2,105	2,179	2,255	2,334	2,416	2,500	2,588	2,678	2,772	2,869
62	2,069	2,140	2,215	2,291	2,371	2,453	2,538	2,626	2,717	2,811	2,909
63	2,104	2,176	2,251	2,328	2,408	2,491	2,577	2,665	2,757	2,851	2,949
64	2,140	2,213	2,288	2,366	2,446	2,530	2,616	2,705	2,797	2,892	2,991
65	2,176	2,250	2,326	2,404	2,485	2,569	2,656	2,745	2,838	2,933	3,032

66	2,213	2,287	2,364	2,443	2,524	2,609	2,696	2,786	2,879	2,975	3,075
67	2,251	2,326	2,403	2,482	2,564	2,649	2,737	2,827	2,921	3,018	3,117
68	2,290	2,365	2,442	2,522	2,605	2,690	2,778	2,869	2,964	3,061	3,161
69	2,329	2,404	2,482	2,563	2,646	2,732	2,821	2,912	3,007	3,104	3,205
70	2,368	2,444	2,523	2,604	2,688	2,774	2,863	2,955	3,050	3,149	3,250
71	2,409	2,485	2,564	2,646	2,730	2,817	2,907	2,999	3,095	3,193	3,295
72	2,450	2,527	2,607	2,689	2,773	2,861	2,951	3,044	3,140	3,239	3,341
73	2,491	2,569	2,649	2,732	2,817	2,905	2,996	3,089	3,186	3,285	3,386
74	2,534	2,612	2,693	2,776	2,862	2,950	3,041	3,135	3,232	3,332	3,435
75	2,577	2,656	2,737	2,821	2,907	2,996	3,088	3,182	3,279	3,380	3,483
76	2,621	2,700	2,782	2,866	2,953	3,042	3,134	3,229	3,327	3,428	3,531
77	2,666	2,746	2,828	2,912	3,000	3,090	3,128	3,277	3,376	3,477	3,581
78	2,711	2,792	2,874	2,959	3,047	3,137	3,230	3,326	3,425	3,526	3,631
79	2,757	2,838	2,921	3,007	3,095	3,186	3,279	3,376	3,475	3,576	3,681
80	2,804	2,886	2,969	3,056	3,144	3,235	3,329	3,426	3,525	3,627	3,733
81	2,852	2,934	3,018	3,105	3,194	3,286	3,380	3,477	3,577	3,679	3,785
82	2,901	2,983	3,068	3,155	3,244	3,336	3,431	3,529	3,629	3,732	3,838
83	2,950	3,033	3,118	3,206	3,296	3,388	3,483	3,581	3,682	3,785	3,891
84	3,001	3,084	3,169	3,257	3,348	3,441	3,536	3,634	3,735	3,839	3,945
85	3,052	3,135	3,221	3,310	3,401	3,494	3,590	3,688	3,790	3,894	4,000
86	3,104	3,188	3,274	3,363	3,454	3,548	3,644	3,743	3,845	3,949	4,056
87	3,157	3,241	3,328	3,417	3,509	3,603	3,700	3,799	3,901	4,005	4,113
88	3,210	3,295	3,383	3,472	3,565	3,659	3,756	3,855	3,958	4,063	4,170
89	3,265	3,351	3,438	3,528	3,621	3,716	3,813	3,913	4,015	4,120	4,228
90	3,321	3,407	3,495	3,585	3,678	3,773	3,871	3,971	4,074	4,179	4,287
91	3,377	3,464	3,552	3,643	3,736	3,832	3,930	4,030	4,133	4,239	4,347
92	3,435	3,522	3,611	3,702	3,795	3,891	3,989	4,090	4,193	4,299	4,408
93	3,494	3,581	3,670	3,761	3,855	3,951	4,050	4,151	4,254	4,361	4,469
94	3,553	3,641	3,738	3,822	3,916	4,013	4,111	4,213	4,316	4,423	4,532
95	3,614	3,701	3,791	3,884	3,978	4,075	4,174	4,275	4,379	4,486	4,595
96	3,675	3,763	3,854	3,946	4,041	4,138	4,237	4,339	4,443	4,550	4,659
97	3,738	3,826	3,917	4,010	4,105	4,202	4,302	4,404	4,508	4,615	4,724
98	3,802	3,890	3,981	4,074	4,170	4,267	4,367	4,469	4,573	4,680	4,790
99	3,866	3,956	4,047	4,140	4,236	4,333	4,433	4,536	4,640	4,747	4,857
100	3,932	4,022	4,113	4,207	4,303	4,400	4,501	4,603	4,708	4,815	4,924

*From Shepard MJ, Richards VA, Berkowitz RL, et al: An evaluation of two equations for predicting fetal weight by ultrasound. *Am J Obstet Gynecol* 1982; 147:47–54. Used by permission.
†Estimated fetal weights: Log (birth weight) = −1.7492 + 0.166 (BPD) + 0.046 (AC) − 2.646 (AC + BPD)/1,000.

TABLE 7–9.
Estimated Fetal Weight Based on Abdominal Circumference: Relationship Between Fetal Abdominal Circumference Measurements From 210 to 400 mm and Birth Weight Percentiles*

Abdominal Circumference, mm	Estimated Birth Weight Percentiles, gm		
	5	50	95
210	780	900	1,040
220	900	1,030	1,190
230	1,030	1,180	1,360
240	1,170	1,340	1,540
250	1,320	1,510	1,730
260	1,470	1,690	1,940
270	1,640	1,880	2,150
280	1,810	2,090	2,380
290	1,990	2,280	2,610
300	2,170	2,490	2,850
310	2,350	2,690	3,080
320	2,530	2,900	3,320
330	2,710	3,100	3,550
340	2,880	3,290	3,760
350	3,030	3,470	3,970
360	3,180	3,640	4,160
370	3,310	3,790	4,330
380	3,420	3,920	4,490
390	3,510	4,020	4,610
400	3,570	4,100	4,720

*From Campbell S, Wilkin D: Ultrasonic measurement of fetal abdominal circumference in estimation of fetal weight. Br J Obstet Gynaecol 1975; 82:689–697. Used by permission.

TABLE 7–10.
Equation With Three Variables to Compute Fetal Weight*†

$$\text{Log}_{10}\ BW = 1.5662 - 0.0108\ (HC) + 0.0468\ (AC) \\ + 0.171\ (FL) + 0.00034\ (HC)^2 - \\ 0.003685\ (AC \times FL)$$

*From Hadlock FP, Harrist RB, Carpenter RJ, et al: Sonographic estimation of fetal weight, the value of femur length in addition to head and abdomen measurements. *Radiology* 1984; 150:535–540. Used by permission.
†BW = body weight in gm; HC = head circumference; AC = abdominal circumference; FL = femur length. HC, AC, and FL given in centimeters.

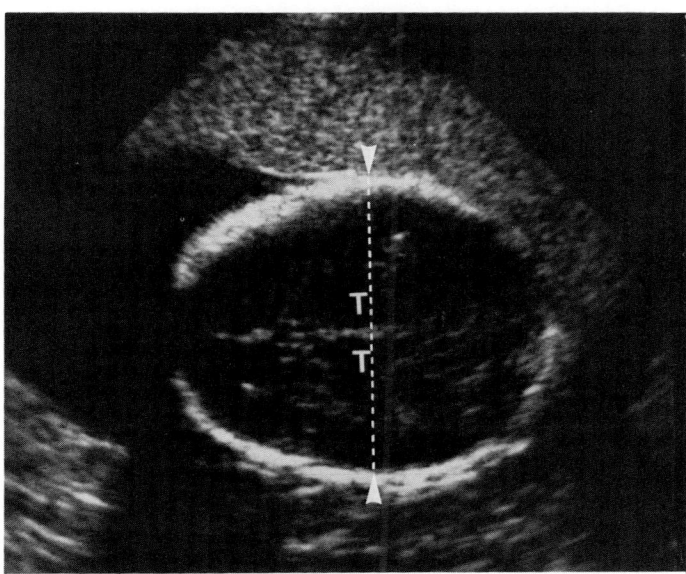

FIG 7–8.
Biparietal diameter measurement is taken in transaxial view with the thalamus *(T)* or midbrain in the midline. The measurement *(arrowheads* and *dotted line)* is taken leading edge (outer margin) to leading edge (inner margin).

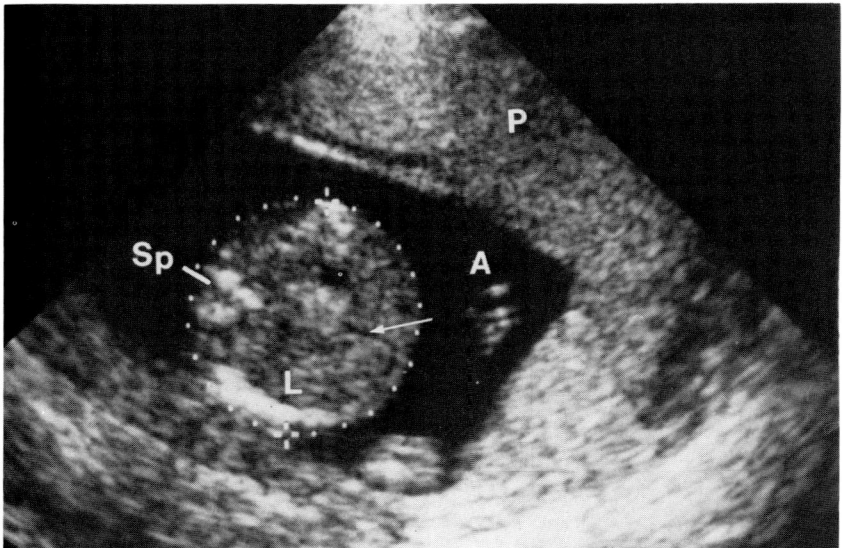

FIG 7–9.
Abdominal circumference. Transaxial image of the upper abdomen at the region of the liver (L). The umbilical portion of the left portal vein *(arrow)* is situated within the liver in the midline. The circumference is traced with a digitizer or map reader *(dotted line)* or can be calculated from an equation. P indicates placenta; *Sp*, spine; *A*, amniotic fluid.

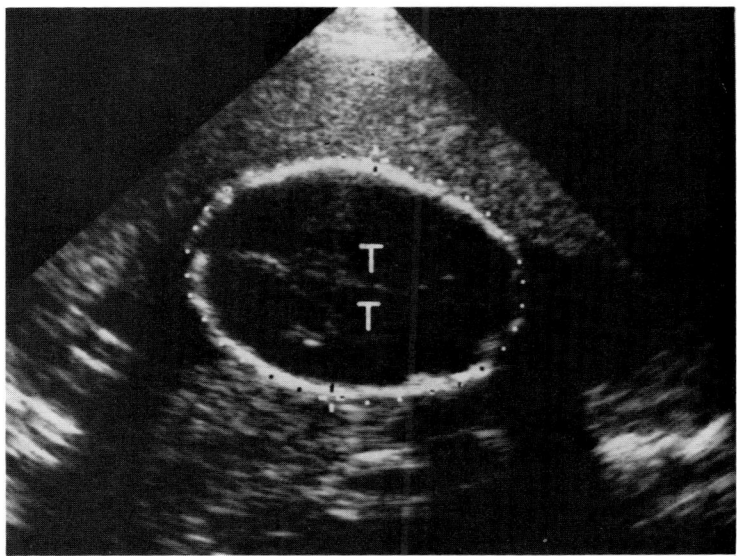

FIG 7–10.
Head circumference. Transaxial image of the head at the thalami *(T)*. With either the thalami or midbrain in the midline, the circumference is traced around the outer margin of the head with a digitizer or map reader *(dotted line)* or can be calculated from an equation.

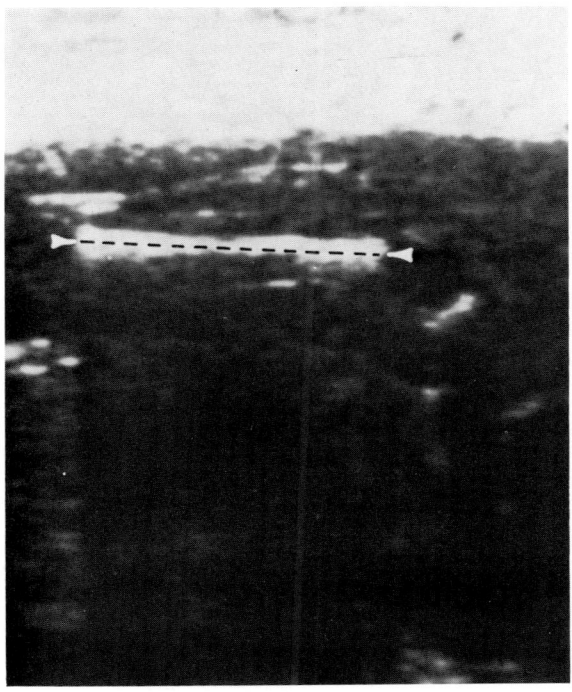

FIG 7–11.
Femoral length measurement. The long axis of the hyperechoic femoral shaft is measured, denoted by arrowheads and dotted line, disregarding the hypoechoic nonossified epiphyseal cartilages.

TABLE 7-11.
Estimated Fetal Weight (gm) Based on Abdominal Circumference (AC) and

FL, mm	AC, mm									
	200	205	210	215	220	225	230	235	240	245
40	663	691	720	751	783	816	851	887	925	964
41	680	709	738	769	802	836	871	907	946	986
42	697	726	757	788	821	855	891	928	967	1,007
43	715	745	776	808	841	875	912	949	988	1,029
44	734	764	795	827	861	896	933	971	1,010	1,051
45	753	783	815	847	882	917	954	993	1,033	1,074
46	772	803	835	868	903	939	976	1,015	1,056	1,098
47	792	823	856	889	924	961	999	1,038	1,079	1,122
48	812	844	877	911	947	984	1,022	1,062	1,103	1,146
49	833	865	899	933	969	1,007	1,046	1,086	1,128	1,171
50	855	887	921	956	993	1,031	1,070	1,111	1,153	1,197
51	877	910	944	980	1,016	1,055	1,095	1,136	1,179	1,223
52	899	933	967	1,004	1,041	1,080	1,120	1,162	1,205	1,250
53	922	956	992	1,028	1,066	1,105	1,146	1,188	1,232	1,277
54	946	981	1,016	1,053	1,091	1,131	1,172	1,215	1,259	1,305
55	971	1,005	1,041	1,079	1,118	1,158	1,199	1,242	1,287	1,333
56	995	1,031	1,067	1,105	1,144	1,185	1,227	1,271	1,316	1,362
57	1,021	1,057	1,094	1,132	1,172	1,213	1,255	1,299	1,345	1,392
58	1,047	1,084	1,121	1,160	1,200	1,242	1,285	1,329	1,375	1,422
59	1,074	1,111	1,149	1,188	1,229	1,271	1,314	1,359	1,406	1,454
60	1,102	1,139	1,178	1,217	1,258	1,301	1,345	1,409	1,437	1,485
61	1,130	1,168	1,207	1,247	1,289	1,331	1,376	1,421	1,469	1,518
62	1,160	1,198	1,237	1,278	1,319	1,363	1,408	1,454	1,501	1,551
63	1,189	1,228	1,268	1,309	1,351	1,395	1,440	1,487	1,535	1,585
64	1,220	1,259	1,299	1,341	1,384	1,428	1,473	1,520	1,569	1,619

Femur Length (FL)*†

\	\	\	\	\	AC, mm	\	\	\	\	\
250	255	260	265	270	275	280	285	290	295	300
1,006	1,048	1,093	1,139	1,188	1,239	1,291	1,346	1,403	1,463	1,525
1,027	1,070	1,115	1,162	1,211	1,262	1,315	1,371	1,429	1,489	1,551
1,049	1,093	1,138	1,186	1,235	1,287	1,340	1,396	1,454	1,515	1,578
1,071	1,116	1,162	1,209	1,259	1,311	1,365	1,422	1,480	1,541	1,605
1,094	1,139	1,185	1,234	1,284	1,336	1,391	1,448	1,507	1,568	1,632
1,118	1,163	1,210	1,259	1,309	1,362	1,417	1,474	1,534	1,596	1,660
1,142	1,187	1,235	1,284	1,335	1,388	1,444	1,501	1,561	1,623	1,688
1,166	1,212	1,260	1,310	1,316	1,415	1,471	1,529	1,589	1,652	1,717
1,191	1,237	1,286	1,336	1,388	1,442	1,498	1,557	1,618	1,681	1,746
1,216	1,263	1,312	1,363	1,415	1,470	1,527	1,585	1,647	1,710	1,776
1,243	1,290	1,339	1,390	1,443	1,498	1,555	1,615	1,676	1,740	1,806
1,269	1,317	1,367	1,418	1,471	1,527	1,584	1,644	1,706	1,770	1,837
1,296	1,344	1,395	1,447	1,500	1,556	1,614	1,647	1,737	1,801	1,868
1,324	1,373	1,423	1,476	1,530	1,586	1,645	1,705	1,768	1,833	1,900
1,352	1,401	1,452	1,505	1,560	1,617	1,675	1,736	1,799	1,865	1,933
1,418	1,431	1,482	1,535	1,591	1,648	1,707	1,768	1,832	1,897	1,966
1,411	1,461	1,513	1,566	1,622	1,679	1,739	1,801	1,864	1,931	1,999
1,441	1,491	1,544	1,598	1,654	1,712	1,772	1,834	1,898	1,964	2,033
1,472	1,523	1,575	1,630	1,686	1,744	1,805	1,867	1,932	1,999	2,068
1,503	1,555	1,608	1,663	1,719	1,778	1,839	1,902	1,966	2,034	2,103
1,535	1,587	1,641	1,696	1,753	1,812	1,873	1,936	2,002	2,069	2,139
1,568	1,620	1,674	1,730	1,788	1,847	1,908	1,972	2,038	2,105	2,175
1,602	1,654	1,709	1,765	1,823	1,882	1,944	2,008	2,074	2,142	2,212
1,636	1,689	1,744	1,800	1,858	1,919	1,981	2,045	2,111	2,180	2,250
1,671	1,724	1,779	1,836	1,895	1,956	2,018	2,082	2,149	2,218	2,289

(Continued.)

TABLE 7–11 (cont.).
Estimated Fetal Weight (gm) Based on Abdominal Circumference (AC) and

FL, mm	AC, mm									
	200	205	210	215	220	225	230	235	240	245
65	1,251	1,291	1,332	1,373	1,417	1,461	1,507	1,555	1,604	1,655
66	1,284	1,324	1,365	1,407	1,451	1,496	1,542	1,590	1,640	1,691
67	1,317	1,357	1,399	1,441	1,486	1,531	1,578	1,626	1,676	1,728
68	1,351	1,391	1,433	1,477	1,521	1,567	1,615	1,663	1,713	1,765
69	1,385	1,427	1,469	1,513	1,558	1,604	1,652	1,701	1,752	1,804
70	1,421	1,463	1,506	1,550	1,595	1,642	1,690	1,740	1,791	1,843
71	1,458	1,500	1,543	1,588	1,633	1,681	1,729	1,779	1,830	1,883
72	1,495	1,538	1,581	1,626	1,673	1,720	1,769	1,819	1,871	1,924
73	1,534	1,577	1,621	1,666	1,713	1,761	1,810	1,861	1,913	1,966
74	1,573	1,616	1,661	1,707	1,754	1,802	1,852	1,903	1,955	2,009
75	1,614	1,657	1,702	1,749	1,796	1,845	1,895	1,946	1,999	2,053
76	1,655	1,699	1,745	1,791	1,839	1,888	1,939	1,990	2,043	2,098
77	1,698	1,742	1,788	1,835	1,883	1,933	1,983	2,035	2,089	2,144
78	1,741	1,786	1,833	1,880	1,928	1,978	2,029	2,082	2,135	2,191
79	1,786	1,832	1,878	1,926	1,975	2,025	2,076	2,129	2,183	2,238
80	1,832	1,878	1,925	1,973	2,022	2,073	2,124	2,177	2,232	2,287
81	1,879	1,926	1,973	2,021	2,071	2,121	2,173	2,227	2,281	2,337
82	1,928	1,974	2,022	2,070	2,120	2,171	2,224	2,277	2,332	2,388
83	1,978	2,024	2,072	2,121	2,171	2,223	2,275	2,329	2,384	2,440

Femur Length (FL)*†

					AC, mm						
250	255	260	265	270	275	280	285	290	295	300
1,707	1,760	1,816	1,873	1,932	1,993	2,056	2,121	2,188	2,256	2,328
1,743	1,797	1,853	1,911	1,970	2,031	2,094	2,160	2,227	2,296	2,367
1,780	1,835	1,891	1,949	2,009	2,070	2,134	2,199	2,267	2,336	2,408
1,819	1,873	1,930	1,988	2,048	2,110	2,174	2,240	2,307	2,377	2,449
1,857	1,913	1,970	2,028	2,089	2,151	2,215	2,281	2,348	2,418	2,490
1,897	1,953	2,010	2,069	2,130	2,192	2,256	2,322	2,391	2,461	2,533
1,938	1,994	2,051	2,110	2,171	2,234	2,299	2,365	2,433	2,504	2,576
1,979	2,035	2,093	2,153	2,214	2,277	2,342	2,408	2,477	2,547	2,620
2,021	2,078	2,136	2,196	2,258	2,321	2,386	2,453	2,521	2,592	2,665
2,065	2,122	2,180	2,240	2,302	2,365	2,431	2,498	2,566	2,637	2,710
2,109	2,166	2,225	2,285	2,347	2,411	2,476	2,543	2,612	2,683	2,756
2,154	2,211	2,270	2,331	2,393	2,457	2,523	2,590	2,659	2,730	2,803
2,200	2,258	2,317	2,378	2,440	2,504	2,570	2,638	2,707	2,778	2,851
2,247	2,305	2,365	2,426	2,488	2,553	2,618	2,686	2,755	2,827	2,899
2,295	2,353	2,413	2,474	2,537	2,602	2,668	2,735	2,805	2,876	2,949
2,344	2,403	2,463	2,524	2,587	2,652	2,718	2,785	2,855	2,926	2,999
2,394	2,453	2,513	2,575	2,638	2,702	2,769	2,837	2,906	2,977	3,050
2,446	2,504	2,565	2,626	2,690	2,754	2,821	2,889	2,958	3,029	3,102
2,498	2,557	2,617	2,679	2,743	2,807	2,874	2,942	3,011	3,082	3,155

(Continued.)

TABLE 7–11.
Estimated Fetal Weight (gm) Based on Abdominal Circumference (AC) and

FL, mm	AC, mm									
	305	310	315	320	325	330	335	340	345	350
40	1,590	1,658	1,729	1,802	1,879	1,959	2,042	2,129	2,220	2,314
41	1,617	1,685	1,756	1,830	1,907	1,987	2,071	2,158	2,249	2,344
42	1,644	1,712	1,783	1,858	1,935	2,016	2,100	2,187	2,279	2,373
43	1,671	1,740	1,812	1,886	1,964	2,054	2,129	2,217	2,308	2,404
44	1,699	1,768	1,840	1,915	1,993	2,075	2,159	2,247	2,339	2,434
45	1,727	1,797	1,869	1,944	2,023	2,105	2,189	2,278	2,370	2,465
46	1,756	1,826	1,898	1,974	2,053	2,135	2,220	2,309	2,401	2,497
47	1,785	1,855	1,928	2,004	2,084	2,166	2,251	2,340	2,432	2,528
48	1,814	1,885	1,959	2,035	2,115	2,197	2,283	2,372	2,464	2,560
49	1,845	1,916	1,990	2,066	2,146	2,229	2,315	2,404	2,497	2,593
50	1,875	1,947	2,021	2,098	2,178	2,261	2,347	2,437	2,530	2,626
51	1,906	1,978	2,053	2,130	2,210	2,294	2,380	2,470	2,563	2,659
52	1,938	2,010	2,085	2,163	2,243	2,327	2,413	2,503	2,597	2,693
53	1,970	2,043	2,118	2,196	2,277	2,360	2,447	2,537	2,631	2,728
54	2,003	2,076	2,151	2,229	2,311	2,395	2,482	2,572	2,665	2,762
55	2,036	2,109	2,185	2,264	2,345	2,429	2,516	2,607	2,700	2,797
56	2,070	2,143	2,220	2,298	2,380	2,464	2,552	2,642	2,736	2,833
57	2,104	2,178	2,254	2,333	2,415	2,500	2,587	2,678	2,772	2,869
58	2,139	2,213	2,290	2,369	2,451	2,536	2,624	2,714	2,808	2,905
59	2,175	2,249	2,326	2,405	2,488	2,573	2,660	2,751	2,845	2,942
60	2,211	2,286	2,363	2,442	2,525	2,610	2,698	2,789	2,883	2,980
61	2,248	2,323	2,400	2,480	2,562	2,647	2,736	2,837	2,921	3,018
62	2,285	2,360	2,438	2,518	2,600	2,686	2,774	2,865	2,959	3,056
63	2,323	2,398	2,476	2,556	2,639	2,725	2,813	2,904	2,998	3,095
64	2,362	2,437	2,515	2,595	2,678	2,764	2,852	2,943	3,037	3,134

Femur Length (FL)*†

				AC, mm					
355	360	365	370	375	380	385	390	395	400
2,413	2,515	2,622	2,734	2,850	2,972	3,098	3,230	3,367	3,511
2,442	2,545	2,652	2,764	2,880	3,002	3,128	3,260	3,397	3,540
2,472	2,575	2,683	2,794	2,911	3,032	3,159	3,290	3,427	3,570
2,503	2,606	2,713	2,825	2,942	3,063	3,189	3,321	3,458	3,600
2,533	2,637	2,744	2,856	2,973	3,094	3,220	3,352	3,488	3,630
2,565	2,668	2,776	2,888	3,004	3,125	3,251	3,383	3,519	3,661
2,596	2,700	2,807	2,919	3,036	3,157	3,283	3,414	3,550	3,692
2,628	2,732	2,840	2,952	3,068	3,189	3,315	3,446	3,582	3,723
2,660	2,764	2,872	2,984	3,100	3,221	3,347	3,478	3,613	3,754
2,693	2,797	2,905	3,017	3,133	3,254	3,380	3,510	3,645	3,786
2,726	2,830	2,938	3,050	3,166	3,287	3,412	3,542	3,677	3,818
2,760	2,864	2,972	3,084	3,200	3,320	3,445	3,575	3,710	3,850
2,794	2,898	3,006	3,117	3,234	3,354	3,479	3,608	3,743	3,882
2,828	2,932	3,040	3,152	3,268	3,388	3,513	3,642	3,776	3,915
2,863	2,967	3,075	3,186	3,302	3,422	3,547	3,676	3,809	3,948
2,898	3,002	3,110	3,221	3,337	3,457	3,581	3,710	3,843	3,981
2,933	3,038	3,145	3,257	3,372	3,492	3,616	3,744	3,877	4,015
2,970	3,074	3,181	3,293	3,408	3,527	3,651	3,779	3,911	4,048
3,006	3,110	3,218	3,329	3,444	3,563	3,686	3,814	3,946	4,082
3,043	3,147	3,254	3,366	3,480	3,599	3,722	3,849	3,981	4,117
3,080	3,184	3,292	3,403	3,517	3,636	3,758	3,885	4,016	4,151
3,118	3,222	3,329	3,440	3,554	3,673	3,795	3,921	4,052	4,186
3,157	3,260	3,367	3,478	3,592	3,710	3,832	3,957	4,087	4,222
3,195	3,299	3,406	3,516	3,630	3,747	3,869	3,994	4,124	4,257
3,235	3,338	3,445	3,555	3,668	3,785	3,906	4,031	4,160	4,293

(Continued.)

TABLE 7–11 (cont.).
Estimated Fetal Weight (gm) Based on Abdominal Circumference (AC) and

FL, mm	AC, mm									
	305	310	315	320	325	330	335	340	345	350
65	2,401	2,477	2,555	2,635	2,718	2,804	2,892	2,983	3,077	3,174
66	2,441	2,517	2,595	2,675	2,759	2,844	2,933	3,024	3,118	3,215
67	2,481	2,557	2,636	2,716	2,800	2,885	2,974	3,065	3,159	3,256
68	2,523	2,599	2,677	2,758	2,841	2,927	3,016	3,107	3,200	3,297
69	2,564	2,641	2,719	2,800	2,884	2,969	3,058	3,149	3,242	3,339
70	2,607	2,683	2,762	2,843	2,927	3,012	3,101	3,192	3,285	3,381
71	2,650	2,727	2,806	2,887	2,970	3,056	3,144	3,235	3,328	3,424
72	2,694	2,771	2,850	2,931	3,014	3,100	3,188	3,279	3,372	3,468
73	2,739	2,816	2,895	2,976	3,059	3,145	3,233	3,323	3,416	3,512
74	2,785	2,861	2,940	3,021	3,105	3,190	3,278	3,369	3,461	3,557
75	2,831	2,908	2,987	3,068	3,151	3,236	3,324	3,414	3,507	3,602
76	2,878	2,955	3,034	3,115	3,198	3,283	3,371	3,461	3,553	3,648
77	2,926	3,003	3,081	3,162	3,245	3,331	3,418	3,508	3,600	3,694
78	2,974	3,051	3,130	3,211	3,294	3,379	3,466	3,555	3,647	3,741
79	3,024	3,100	3,179	3,260	3,343	3,427	3,514	3,604	3,695	3,789
80	3,074	3,151	3,229	3,310	3,392	3,477	3,564	3,653	3,744	3,837
81	3,125	3,202	3,280	3,360	3,443	3,527	3,614	3,702	3,793	3,886
82	3,177	3,253	3,332	3,412	3,494	3,578	3,664	3,752	3,843	3,935
83	3,230	3,306	3,384	3,464	3,546	3,630	3,716	3,803	3,893	3,985

*From Hadlock FP, Harrist RB, Carpenter RJ, et al: Sonographic estimation of fetal weight: The value of femur
†Based on regression model: $\log_{10}$ body weight = 1.3598 + 0.051 (AC) + 0.1844 (FL) − 0.0037 (AC × FL).

Femur Length (FL)*†

					AC, mm				
355	360	365	370	375	380	385	390	395	400
3,274	3,378	3,484	3,594	3,707	3,824	3,944	4,069	4,197	4,329
3,315	3,418	3,524	3,633	3,746	3,863	3,983	4,106	4,234	4,366
3,355	3,458	3,564	3,673	3,786	3,902	4,021	4,144	4,271	4,402
3,397	3,499	3,605	3,714	3,862	3,941	4,060	4,183	4,309	4,439
3,438	3,541	3,646	3,754	3,866	3,981	4,100	4,222	4,347	4,477
3,481	3,583	3,688	3,796	3,907	4,022	4,140	4,261	4,386	4,514
3,523	3,625	3,730	3,838	3,948	4,062	4,180	4,300	4,425	4,552
3,567	3,668	3,772	3,880	3,990	4,104	4,220	4,340	4,464	4,591
3,610	3,712	3,816	3,922	4,032	4,145	4,261	4,381	4,503	4,629
3,655	3,756	3,859	3,966	4,075	4,187	4,303	4,421	4,543	4,668
3,700	3,800	3,903	4,009	4,118	4,230	4,344	4,462	4,583	4,708
3,745	3,845	3,948	4,053	4,161	4,272	4,387	4,504	4,624	4,747
3,791	3,891	3,993	4,098	4,205	4,316	4,429	4,545	4,665	4,787
3,838	3,937	4,039	4,143	4,250	4,360	4,472	4,588	4,706	4,827
3,885	3,984	4,085	4,188	4,295	4,404	4,515	4,630	4,748	4,868
3,933	4,031	4,131	4,234	4,340	4,448	4,559	4,673	4,790	4,909
3,981	4,079	4,179	4,281	4,386	4,493	4,604	4,716	4,832	4,950
4,030	4,127	4,226	4,328	4,432	4,539	4,648	4,760	4,875	4,992
4,080	4,176	4,275	4,376	4,479	4,585	4,693	4,804	4,918	5,034

length in addition to head and abdomen measurements. *Radiology* 1984; 150:535–540. Used by permission.

REFERENCES

Head and Body Measurements
1. Lubchenco LO, Hansmann C, Boyd E: Intrauterine growth in length and head circumference as estimated from live births at gestational ages from 26 to 42 weeks. *Pediatrics* 1966; 37:403–408.

Fetal Measurement Comparisons
2. Campbell S: The assessment of fetal development by diagnostic ultrasound. *Clin Perinatol* 1974; 1:507–525.
3. Hobbins JC, Berkowitz RL: Ultrasonography in the diagnosis of intrauterine growth retardation. *Clin Obstet Gynecol* 1977; 20:957–968.
4. Kurtz AB, Wapner RJ, Rubin CS, et al: Ultrasound criteria for in utero diagnosis of microcephaly. *J Clin Ultrasound* 1980; 8:11–16.
5. Gottesfeld KR: Ultrasound in obstetrics and gynecology. *Semin Roentgenol* 1975; 10:305–313.
6. Fescina RH, Ucieda FJ, Cordano MC, et al: Ultrasonic patterns of intrauterine fetal growth in a Latin American country. *Early Hum Dev* 1982; 6:239–248.
7. Sarti DA, Crandall BF, Winter J, et al: Correlation of biparietal and fetal body diameters: 12–26 weeks gestation. *AJR* 1981; 137:87–91.
8. Gross BH, Callen PW, Filly RA: The relationship of fetal transverse body diameter and biparietal diameter in the diagnosis of intrauterine growth retardation. *J Ultrasound Med* 1982; 1:361–365.
9. Elliott JP, Garite TJ, Freeman RK, et al: Ultrasonic prediction of fetal macrosomia in diabetic patients. *Obstet Gynecol* 1982; 60:159–162.
10. Eriksen PS, Secher NJ, Weis-Bentzon M: Normal growth of the fetal biparietal diameter and the abdominal diameter in a longitudinal study. *Acta Obstet Gynecol Scand* 1985; 64:65–70.
11. Wladimiroff JW, Bloemsma CA, Wallenburg HCS: Ultrasonic assessment of fetal growth. *Acta Obstet Gynecol Scand* 1977; 56:37–42.
12. Levi S, Smets P: Intrauterine fetal growth studied by ultrasonic biparietal measurements: The percentiles of biparietal distribution. *Acta Obstet Gynecol Scand* 1973; 52:193–198.
13. Wladimiroff JW, Bloemsma CA, Wallenburg HCS: Ultrasonic assessment of fetal head and body sizes in relation to normal and retarded fetal growth. *Am J Obstet Gynecol* 1978; 131:857–860.
14. Chervenak FA, Jeanty P, Cantraine F, et al: The diagnosis of fetal microcephaly. *Am J Obstet Gynecol* 1984; 149:512–517.
15. Chervenak FA, Rosenberg J, Brightman RC, et al: A prospective study of the accuracy of ultrasound in predicting fetal microcephaly. *Obstet Gynecol* 1987; 69:908–910.
16. Deter RL, Harrist RB, Hadlock FP, et al: The use of ultrasound in the assessment of normal fetal growth: A review. *J Clin Ultrasound* 1981; 9:481–493.
17. Campbell S, Thoms A: Ultrasound measurement of the fetal head to abdomen circumference ratio in the assessment of growth retardation. *Br J Obstet Gynaecol* 1977; 84:165–174.
18. Kurjak A, Breyer B: Estimation of fetal weight by ultrasonic abdominometry. *Am J Obstet Gynecol* 1976; 125:962–965.
19. Hadlock FP, Harrist RB, Shah Y, et al: The femur length/head circumference relation in obstetric sonography. *J Ultrasound Med* 1984; 3:439–442.
20. Crane JP, Kopta MM: Prediction of intrauterine growth retardation via ultrasonically measured head/abdominal circumference ratios. *Obstet Gynecol* 1979; 54:597–601.
21. Athey PA, Hadlock FP: in Harshberger SE (ed): *Ultrasound in Obstetrics and Gynecology*. St Louis, CV Mosby, 1981, p 269.

22. Persson PH, Marsal K: Monitoring of fetuses with retarded BPD growth. *Acta Obstet Gynecol Scand* 1978; 78:49–55.
23. Deter RL, Harrist RB, Hadlock FP, et al: Longitudinal studies of fetal growth with the use of dynamic image ultrasonography. *Am J Obstet Gynecol* 1982; 143:545–554.
24. Varma TR, Taylor H, Bridges C: Ultrasound assessment of fetal growth. *Br J Obstet Gynaecol* 1979; 86:623–632.
25. Rossavik IK, Deter RL: Mathematical modeling of fetal growth: II. Head cube (A), abdominal cube (B) and their ratio (A/B). *J Clin Ultrasound* 1984; 12:535–545.
26. Hohler CW, Quetel TA: Comparison of ultrasound femur length and biparietal diameter in late pregnancy. *Am J Obstet Gynecol* 1981; 141:759–762.
27. Chervenak FA, Jeanty P, Cantraine F, et al: The diagnosis of fetal microcephaly. *Am J Obstet Gynecol* 1984; 149:512–517.
28. Hadlock FP, Harrist RB, Shah Y, et al: The femur length/head circumference relation in obstetric sonography. *J Ultrasound Med* 1984; 3:439–442.
29. DeVore GR, Horenstein J, Platt LD: Fetal echocardiography: VI. Assessment of cardiothoracic disproportion—A new technique for the diagnosis of thoracic hypoplasia. *Am J Obstet Gynecol* 1986; 155:1066–1071.
30. Skiptunas SM, Weiner S: Early prenatal diagnosis of asphyxiating thoracic dysplasia (Jeune's syndrome): Value of fetal thoracic measurement. *J Ultrasound Med* 1987; 6:41–43.
31. Bracero LA, Baxi LV, Rey HR, et al: Use of ultrasound in antenatal diagnosis of large-for-gestational age infants in diabetic gravid patients. *Am J Obstet Gynecol* 1985; 152(1):43–47.
32. Hadlock FP, Deter RL, Harrist RB, et al: A date-independent predictor of intrauterine growth retardation: Femur length/abdominal circumference ratio. *AJR* 1983; 141:979–984.
33. Ott WJ: Fetal femur length, neonatal crown-heel length, and screening for intrauterine growth retardation. *Obstet Gynecol* 1985; 65:460–464.
34. Vintzileos AM, Neckles S, Campbell WA, et al: Three fetal ponderal indexes in normal pregnancy. *Obstet Gynecol* 1985; 6:807–811.
35. Brown HL, Miller JM Jr, Gabert HA, et al: Ultrasonic recognition of the small-for-gestational-age fetus. *Obstet Gynecol* 1987; 69:631–635.
36. Benson CB, Doubilet PM, Saltzman DH, et al: FL/AC ratio: Poor predictor of intrauterine growth retardation. *Invest Radiol* 1985; 20:727–730.
37. Divon MY, Chamberlain PF, Sipos L, et al: Identification of the small for gestational age fetus with the use of gestational age-independent indices of fetal growth. *Am J Obstet Gynecol* 1986; 155:1197–2101.
38. Hays D, Patterson RM: A comparison of fetal biometric ratios to neonatal morphometrics. *J Ultrasound Med* 1987; 6:71–73.
39. Hadlock FP, Harrist RB, Fearneyhough TC, et al: Use of femur length/abdominal circumference ratio in detecting the macrosomic fetus. *Radiology* 1985; 154:503–505.
40. Benson CB, Doubilet PM, Saltzman DH, et al: Femur length/abdominal circumference ratio: Poor predictor of macrosomic fetuses in diabetic mothers. *J Ultrasound Med* 1986; 5:141–144.
41. Pap G, Szoke J, Pap L: Intrauterine growth retardation: Ultrasonic diagnosis. *Acta Paediatr Hung* 1983; 24:7–15.
42. DeVore GR, Horenstein J, Platt LD: Fetal echocardiography: VI. Assessment of cardiothoracic disproportion—A new technique for the diagnosis of thoracic hypoplasia. *Am J Obstet Gynecol* 1986; 155:1066–1071.
43. Vintzileos AM, Neckles S, Campbell WA, et al: Ultrasound fetal thigh-calf circumferences and gestational age-independent fetal ratios in normal pregnancy. *J Ultrasound Med* 1985; 4:287–292.

44. Vintzileos AM, Neckles S, Campbell WA, et al: Three fetal ponderal indexes in normal pregnancy. *Obstet Gynecol* 1985; 6:807–811.
45. Hays D, Patterson RM: A comparison of fetal biometric ratios to neonatal morphometrics. *J Ultrasound Med* 1987; 6:71–73.
46. DeVore GR, Siassi B, Platt LD: The use of the abdominal circumference as a means of assessing M-mode ventricular dimensions during the second and third trimesters of pregnancy in the normal human fetus. *J Ultrasound Med* 1985; 4:175–182.
47. DeVore GR, Siassi B, Platt LD: Use of femur length as a means of assessing M-mode ventricular dimensions during second and third trimesters of pregnancy in normal fetus. *J Clin Ultrasound* 1985; 13:619–625.
48. Li DFH, Woo JSK: Fractional spine length: A new parameter for assessing fetal growth. *J Ultrasound Med* 1986; 5:379–383.
49. Vintzileos AM, Lodeiro JG, Feinstein SJ, et al: Value of fetal ponderal index in predicting growth retardation. *J Ultrasound Med* 1986; 5:379–383.
50. Jordaan HVF: Cardiac size during prenatal development. *Obstet Gynecol* 1987; 69:854–858.

Multiple Parameters

51. Oman SD, Wax Y: Estimating fetal age by ultrasound measurements: An example of multivariate calibration. *Biometrics* 1984; 40:947–960.
52. Hadlock FP, Deter RL, Harrist RB, et al: Computer assisted analysis of fetal age in the third trimester using multiple fetal growth parameters. *J Clin Ultrasound* 1983; 11:313–316.
53. Hadlock FP, Deter RL, Harrist RB, et al: Estimating fetal age: Computer-assisted analysis of multiple fetal growth parameters. *Radiology* 1984; 152:497–501.
54. Hadlock FP, Harrist RB, Shah YP, et al: Estimating fetal age using multiple parameters: A prospective evaluation in a racially mixed population. *Am J Obstet Gynecol* 1987; 156:955–957.
55. Ott WJ: Accurate gestational dating. *Obstet Gynecol* 1985; 66:311–315.
56. Smazal SF, Weisman LE, Hoppler KD, et al: Comparative analysis of ultrasonographic methods of gestational age assessment. *J Ultrasound Med* 1983; 2:147–150.
57. Wiener SN, Flynn MJ, Kennedy AW, et al: A composite curve of ultrasonic biparietal diameters for estimating gestational age. *Radiology* 1977; 122:781–786.
58. Kurtz AB, Wapner RJ, Kurtz RJ, et al: Analysis of biparietal diameter as an accurate indicator of gestational age. *J Clin Ultrasound* 1980; 8:319–326.
59. Levi S, Erbsman F: Antenatal fetal growth from the nineteenth week: Ultrasonic study of 12 head and chest dimensions. *Am J Obstet Gynecol* 1975; 121:262–268.
60. Weinraub Z, Schneider D, Langer R, et al: Ultrasonographic measurement of fetal growth parameters for estimation of gestational age and fetal weight. *Isr J Med Sci* 1979; 15:829–832.
61. Parker AJ, Davies P, Mayho AM, et al: The ultrasound estimation of sex-related variations of intrauterine growth. *Am J Obstet Gynecol* 1984; 149:665–669.
62. Wittman BK, Robinson HP, Aitchison T, et al: The value of diagnostic ultrasound as a screening test for intrauterine growth retardation: Comparison of nine parameters. *Am J Obstet Gynecol* 1979; 134:30.
63. Neilson JP, Whitfield CR, Aitchison TC: Screening for the small-for-dates fetus: A two-stage ultrasonic examination schedule. *Br Med J* 1980; 280:1203–1206.
64. Neilson JP, Munjanja SP, Whitfield CR: Screening for small for dates fetuses: A controlled trial. *Br Med J* 1984; 289:1179–1182.
65. Neilson JP, Munjanja SP, Mooney R, et al: Product of fetal crown-rump length and trunk area: Ultrasound measurement in high-risk pregnancies. *Br J Obstet Gynaecol* 1984; 91:756–761.

Interval Growth

66. Sabbagha RE, Turner H, Rockett H, et al: Sonar BPD and fetal age: Definition of the relationship. *Obstet Gynecol* 1974; 43:7–14.
67. Campbell S, Dewhurts CJ: Diagnosis of the small-for-dates fetus by serial ultrasonic cephalometry. *Lancet* 1971; 2:1002–1006.
68. Sabbagha RE, Barton BA, Barton FA, et al: Sonar biparietal diameter: II. Predictive of the three fetal growth patterns leading to a closer assessment of gestational age and neonatal weight. *Am J Obstet Gynecol* 1976; 126:485–490.
69. Fescina RH, Ucieda FJ, Cordano MC, et al: Ultrasonic patterns of intrauterine fetal growth in a Latin American country. *Early Hum Dev* 1982; 6:239–248.
70. Persson PH, Grennert L, Gennser G: Diagnosis of intrauterine growth retardation by serial ultrasonic cephalometry. *Acta Obstet Gynecol Scand [Suppl]* 1978; 78:40–48.
71. Sabbagha RE, Hughey M, Depp R: Growth adjusted sonographic age: A simplified method. *Obstet Gynecol* 1978; 51:383–386.
72. Sabbagha RE: Intrauterine growth retardation: Antenatal diagnosis by ultrasound. *Obstet Gynecol* 1978; 52:252–256.
73. Kopta MM, Tomich PG, Crane JP: Ultrasonic methods of predicting the estimated date of confinement. *Obstet Gynecol* 1981; 57:657–660.
74. Dubowitz LMS, Goldberg C: Assessment of gestation by ultrasound in various stages of pregnancy in infants differing in size and ethnic origin. *Br J Obstet Gynaecol* 1981; 88:255–259.
75. Simon NV, Levisky JS, Siegle JC, et al: Evaluation of the dating of gestation via the growth adjusted sonographic age method. *J Clin Ultrasound* 1984; 12:195–199.
76. Arias F: The diagnosis and management of intrauterine growth retardation. *Obstet Gynecol* 1977; 49:293–298.
77. Crane JP, Kopta MM, Welt SI, et al: Abnormal fetal growth patterns: Ultrasonic diagnosis and management. *Obstet Gynecol* 1977; 50:205–211.
78. Persson PH, Grennert L, Gennser G, et al: Normal range curves for the intrauterine growth of the biparietal diameter. *Acta Obstet Gynecol Scand* 1978; 78:15–20.
79. Hohler CW, Inglis J, Collins H, et al: Ultrasound biparietal diameter defining relationships in normal pregnancy. *NY State J Med* 1976; 76:373–376.
80. Queenan JT, Kubarych SF, Cook LN, et al: Diagnostic ultrasound for detection of intrauterine growth retardation. *Am J Obstet Gynecol* 1976; 124:865–873.
81. Yiu-Chiu V, Chiu L: Ultrasonographic evaluation of normal fetal anatomy and congenital malformations. *J Comput Tomogr* 1981; 5:367–381; 508–509.
82. Deter RL, Harrist RB, Hadlock FP, et al: Longitudinal studies of fetal growth with the use of dynamic image ultrasonography. *Am J Obstet Gynecol* 1982; 143:545–554.
83. Levi S, Smets P: Intra-uterine fetal growth studied by ultrasonic biparietal measurements: The percentiles of biparietal distribution. *Acta Obstet Gynecol Scand* 1973; 52:193–198.
84. Wladimiroff JW, Bloemsma CA, Wallenburg HCS: Ultrasonic assessment of fetal head and body sizes in relation to normal and retarded fetal growth. *Am J Obstet Gynecol* 1978; 131:857–860.
85. Varma TR: Prediction of delivery date by ultrasound cephalometry. *J Obstet Gynaecol Br Commonwealth* 1973; 80:316–319.
86. Osefo NJ, Chukudebelu WO: Sonar cephalometry and fetal age relationship in the Nigerian woman. *East Afr Med J*, Feb 1983, pp. 98–102.
87. Sholl JS, Woo D, Rubin JM, et al: Intrauterine growth retardation risk detection for fetuses of unknown gestational age. *Am J Obstet Gynecol* 1982; 144:709–714.
88. Santos-Ramos R, Deunhoelter JH, Reisch JS, et al: Reliability of sonar fetal cephalometry in the estimation of gestational age and in the diagnosis of fetal growth retardation. *Ultrasound Med* 1977; 4:247–251.

89. Roopnarinesing S, Ramseqak S: Decreased birth weight and femur length in fetuses of patients with the sickle-cell trait. *Obstet Gynecol* 1986; 68:46–48.
90. Jeanty P, Cousaert E, deMaertelaer V, et al: Sonographic detection of smoking-related decreased fetal growth. *J Ultrasound Med* 1987; 6:13–18.
91. Divon MY, Chamberlain PF, Sipos L, et al: Identification of the small for gestational age fetus with the use of gestational age-independent indices of fetal growth. *Am J Obstet Gynecol* 1986; 155:1197–2101.
92. Martin RH, Higginbottom J: A clinical and radiological assessment of fetal age. *J Obstet Gynaecol Br Commonwealth* 1971; 78:155–162.
93. O'Brien GD, Queenan JT: Growth of the ultrasound fetal femur length during normal pregnancy: Part I. *Am J Obstet Gynecol* 1981; 141:833–837.

Fetal Weight

94. Usher R, McLean F: Intrauterine growth of live-born Caucasian infants at sea level: Standards obtained from measurements in 7 dimensions of infants born between 25 and 44 weeks of gestation. *Pediatrics* 1969; 74:901–910.
95. Babson SG, Benda GI: Growth graphs for the clinical assessment of infants of varying gestational age. *Pediatrics* 1976; 89:814–820.
96. Lubchenco LO, Hansman C, Dressler M, et al: Intrauterine growth as estimated from liveborn birth-weight data at 24 to 42 weeks of gestation. *Pediatrics* 1963; 32:793–800.
97. Gruenwald P: Growth of the human fetus, parts I & II. *Am J Obstet Gynecol* 1966; 94:1112–1132.
98. Thomson AM, Billewicz WZ, Hytten FE: The assessment of fetal growth. *J Obstet Gynaecol Br Commonwealth* 1968; 75:903–916.
99. Brenner WE, Edelman D, Hendricks CH: A standard of fetal growth for the United States of America. *Am J Obstet Gynecol* 1976; 126:555–564.
100. Naeye RL, Dixon JB: Distortions in fetal growth standards. *Pediatr Res* 1978; 12:987–991.
101. Freeman MG, Graves WL, Thompson AB: Indigent Negro and Caucasian birth weight-gestational age tables. *Pediatrics* 1970; 46:9–15.
102. Williams RL, Creasy RK, Cunningham GC, et al: Fetal growth and perinatal viability in California. *Obstet Gynecol* 1982; 59:624–632.
103. Wong KS, Scott KE: Fetal growth at sea level. *Biol Neonate* 1972; 20:175–188.
104. Hern WA: Correlation of fetal age and measurements between 10 and 26 weeks of gestation. *Obstet Gynecol* 1984; 63:26–32.
105. Golbus MS, Berry LC Jr: Human fetal development between 90 and 170 days postmenses. *Teratology* 1976; 15:103–108.
106. Secher NJ, Hansen PK, Lenstrup C, et al: Birthweight-for-gestational age charts based on early ultrasound estimation of gestational age. *Br J Obstet Gynaecol* 1986; 93:128–134.
107. Patterson RM, Prihoda TJ, Gibbs CE, et al: Analysis of birth weight percentile as a predictor of perinatal outcome. *Obstet Gynecol* 1986; 68:459–463.
108. McMormick MC: The contribution of low birth weight to infant mortality and childhood morbidity. *N Engl J Med* 1985; 312:82–89.
109. Kitchen WH, Yu VYH, Orgill AA, et al: Collaborative study of very-low-birth-weight infants. *Am J Dis Child* 1983; 137:555–559.
110. Boyd ME, Usher RH, Mclean FH: Fetal macrosomia: Prediction, risks, proposed management. *Obstet Gynecol* 1983; 61:715–722.
111. Acker DB, Sachs BP, Freidman EA: Risk factors for shoulder dystocia. *Obstet Gynecol* 1985; 66:762–768.
112. Deter RL, Hadlock FP: Use of ultrasound in the detection of macrosomia: A review. *J Clin Ultrasound* 1985; 13:519–524.

113. Donaldson SW, Cheney W: Prenatal estimation of birth weight by pelvicephalometry. *Radiology* 1948; 50:666–667.
114. Stockland L, Stanton AM: A new method of fetal weight determination. *Am J Roent Rad Theo Nucl Med* 1961; 86:425–431.
115. Kohorn EI: An evaluation of ultrasonic fetal cephalometry. *Am J Obstet Gynecol* 1967; 97:553–559.
116. Campbell S, Newman GB: Growth of the fetal biparietal diameter during normal pregnancy. *J Obstet Gynaecol Br Commonwealth* 1971; 78:518–519.
117. Bartolucci L: Biparietal diameter of the skull and fetal weight in the second trimester: An allometric relationship. *Am J Obstet Gynecol* 1975; 122:439–445.
118. Ojala A, Ylostalo P, Jouppila P, et al: Fetal cephalometry by ultrasound in normal and complicated pregnancy. *Ann Chir Gynaecol Fenniae* 1970; 59:71–75.
119. Pathak DR, Skipper BE, Munsick RA: Estimation of fetal or neonatal weight from the biparietal diameter. *J Reprod Med* 1977; 18:87–89.
120. Stocker J, Mawad R, Deleon A, et al: Ultrasonic cephalometry: Its use in estimating fetal weight. *Obstet Gynecol* 1975; 45:275–278.
121. Ianniruberto A, Gibbons JM: Predicting fetal weight by ultrasonic b-scan cephalometry: An improved technic with disappointing results. *Obstet Gynecol* 1971; 37:689–694.
122. Jordaan HVF: Fetal biparietal diameter and birth weight: An interpopulation comparison. *S Afr Med J* 1976; 50:1166–1170.
123. Sabbagha RE, Turner JH: Methodology of b-scan sonar cephalometry with electronic calipers and correlation with fetal birth weight. *Obstet Gynecol* 1972; 40:74–81.
124. Gonzales AC, Dale E, Byers RH, et al: Limitations in predictions of gestational age and birth weight by ultrasonographic methods. *J Clin Ultrasound* 1978; 6:233–238.
125. Jordaan HVF: Biological variation in the biparietal diameter and its bearing on clinical ultrasonography. *Am J Obstet Gynecol* 1978; 131:53–59.
126. Divon MY, Chamberlain MC, Sipos L, et al: Underestimation of fetal weight in premature rupture of membranes. *J Ultrasound Med* 1984; 3:529–531.
127. Kosar WP, Steer CM: The relation of body weight to the biparietal diameter in the newborn. *Am J Obstet Gynecol* 1956; 71:1232–1234.
128. Weinraub Z, Schneider D, Langer R, et al: Ultrasonographic measurement of fetal growth parameters for estimation of gestational age and fetal weight. *Isr J Med Sci* 1979; 15:829–832.
129. Campbell S, Wilkin D: Ultrasonic measurement of fetal abdomen circumference in the estimation of fetal weight. *Br J Obstet Gynaecol* 1975; 82:689–697.
130. Kurjak A, Breyer B: Estimation of fetal weight by ultrasonic abdominometry. *Am J Obstet Gynecol* 1976; 125:962–965.
131. Poll V, Kasby CB: An improved method of fetal weight estimation using ultrasound measurements of fetal abdominal circumference. *Br J Obstet Gynaecol* 1979; 86:922–928.
132. Higgingbottom J, Slater J, Porter G, et al: Estimation of fetal weight from ultrasonic measurement of trunk circumference. *Br J Obstet Gynaecol* 1975; 82:698–701.
133. McCallum WD, Brinkley JF: Estimation of fetal weight ultrasonic measurements. *Am J Obstet Gynecol* 1979; 133:195–200.
134. Rossavik IK, Deter RL: The effect of abdominal profile shape changes on the estimation of fetal weight. *J Clin Ultrasound* 1984; 12:57–59.
135. Finikiotis F, MacLennan AH, Verco PW, et al: An evaluation of two methods of antenatal ultrasonic fetal weight estimation. *Aust NZ J Obstet Gynaecol* 1980; 20:135–138.

136. Thompson HE, Holmes JH, Gottesfeld KR, et al: Fetal development as determined by ultrasonic pulse echo techniques. *Am J Obstet Gynecol* 1965; 92:44–52.
137. Pap G, Pap L: Ultrasonic estimation of gestational age and fetal weight. *Paediatr Acad Sci Hung* 1979; 20:119–135.
138. Hansmann M: A critical evaluation of the performance of ultrasonic diagnosis in present-day obstetrics. *Gynakologe* 1974; 7:26–35.
139. Shepard MJ, Richard VA, Berkowitz RL, et al: An evaluation of two equations for predicting fetal weight by ultrasound. *Am J Obstet Gynecol* 1982; 142:47–54.
140. Warsof SL, Gohari P, Berkowitz RL, et al: The estimation of fetal weight by computer-assisted analysis. *Am J Obstet Gynecol* 1977; 128:881–892.
141. Jeanty P, Cantraine F, Romero R, et al: A longitudinal study of fetal weight growth. *J Ultrasound Med* 1984; 3:321–328.
142. Thompson HE, Makowski EL: Estimation of birth weight and gestational age. *Obstet Gynecol* 1971; 37:44–47.
143. Timor-Tritsch IE, Itskovitz J, Brandes JM: Estimation of fetal weight by real-time sonography. *Obstet Gynecol* 1981; 57:653–656.
144. Ott WH, Doyle S: Ultrasonic diagnosis of altered fetal growth by use of a normal ultrasonic fetal weight curve. *Obstet Gynecol* 1984; 63:201–204.
145. Ott WJ: Clinical application of fetal weight determination by real-time measurements. *Obstet Gynecol* 1981; 57:758–762.
146. Weinberger E, Cyr DR, Jirsch JH, et al: Estimating fetal weights less than 2000 g: An accurate and simple method. *AJR* 1984; 141:937–977.
147. Tamura RK, Sabbagha RE, Dooley SL, et al: Real-time ultrasound estimations of weight in fetuses of diabetic gravid women. *Am J Obstet Gynecol* 1985; 153:57–60.
148. Eik-Nes SH, Grottum P, Andersson NJ: Clinical evaluation of two formulas for ultrasonic estimation of fetal weight. *Acta Obstet Gynecol Scand* 1981; 60:567–573.
149. Eik-Nes SH, Grottum P: Estimation of fetal weight by ultrasound measurement: Development of a new formula. *Acta Obstet Gynecol Scand* 1982; 61:299–305.
150. Eik-Nes SH, Grottum P, Andersson NJ: Estimation of fetal weight by ultrasound measurement: Clinical application of a new formula. *Acta Obstet Gynecol Scand* 1982; 61:307–312.
151. Eik-Nes SH, Persson PH, Grottum P, et al: Prediction of fetal growth deviation by ultrasonic biometry: Clinical application. *Acta Obstet Gynecol Scand* 1983; 62:117–123.
152. Lunt R, Chard T: A new method for estimation of fetal weight in late pregnancy by ultrasonic scanning. *Br J Obstet Gynaecol* 1976; 83:1–5.
153. Rossavik IK, Bjoro K: The prenatal determination of fetal weight by dynamic scanning. *Early Hum Dev* 1981; 5:133–138.
154. Thurnau GR, Tamura RK, Sabbagha R, et al: A simple estimated fetal weight equation based on real-time ultrasound measurements of fetuses less than thirty-four weeks' gestation. *Am J Obstet Gynecol* 1983; 145:557–561.
155. Campogrande M, Todros T, Brizzolara M: Prediction of birth weight by ultrasound measurements of the fetus. *Br J Obstet Gynaecol* 1977; 84:175–178.
156. Jordaan HVF, Clark WB: Prenatal determination of fetal brain and somatic weight by ultrasound. *Am J Obstet Gynecol* 1980; 138:54–59.
157. Jordaan HVF: Estimation of fetal weight by ultrasound. *J Clin Ultrasound* 1983; 11:59–66.
158. Birnholz JC: Ultrasound characterization of fetal growth. *Ultrason Imaging* 1980; 2:135–149.
159. Sampson MB, Thomason JL, Kelly SL, et al: Prediction of intrauterine fetal weight using real-time ultrasound. *Am J Obstet Gynecol* 1982; 142:554–556.
160. Dornan KJ, Hansmann M, Redord DHA, et al: Fetal weight estimation by real-time ultrasound measurement of biparietal and transverse diameter. *Am J Obstet Gynecol* 1982; 142:652–657.

161. Secher NJ, Djursing H, Hansen PK, et al: Estimation of fetal weight in the third trimester by ultrasound. *Eur J Obstet Gynecol Reprod Biol* 1987; 24:1–11.
162. Weiner CP, Sabbagha RE, Vaisrub N, et al: Ultrasonic fetal weight prediction: Role of head circumference and femur length. *Obstet Gynecol* 1985; 65:812–816.
163. Hadlock FP, Deter RL, Roecker E, et al: Relation of fetal femur length to neonatal crown-heel length. *J Ultrasound Med* 1984; 3:1–3.
164. Roberts AV, Lee AJ, James AG: Ultrasonic estimation of fetal weight: A new predictive model incorporating femur length for the low-birth-weight fetus. *J Clin Ultrasound* 1985; 13:555–559.
165. Hadlock FP, Harrist RB, Carpenter RJ, et al: Sonographic estimation of fetal weight: The valve of femur length in addition to head and abdomen measurements. *Radiology* 1984; 150:535–540.
166. Campbell WA, Vintzileos AM, Neckkles S, et al: Use of the femur length to estimate weight in premature infants: Preliminary results. *J Ultrasound Med* 1985; 4:583–590.
167. Hadlock FP, Harrist RB, Sharman RS, et al: Estimation of fetal weight with the use of head, body, and femur measurements—a prospective study. *Am J Obstet Gynecol* 1985; 151:333–337.
168. Hill LM, Breckle R, Gehrking WC, et al: Use of femur length in estimation of fetal weight. *Am J Obstet Gynecol* 1985; 152:847–852.
169. Woo JSK, Wan CW, Cho KM: Computer-assisted evaluation of ultrasonic fetal weight prediction using multiple regression equations with and without the fetal femur length. *J Ultrasound Med* 1985; 4:65–67.
170. Woo JSK, Wan MCW: An evaluation of fetal weight prediction using a simple equation containing the fetal femur length. *J Ultrasound Med* 1986; 5:453–457.
171. Warsof SL, Wolf P, Coulehan J, et al: Comparison of fetal weight estimation formulas with and without head measurements. *Obstet Gynecol* 1986; 67:569–573.
172. Benson CB, Doubilet PM, Saltzman DH: Sonographic determination of fetal weights in diabetic pregnancies. *Am J Obstet Gynecol* 1987; 156:441–444.
173. Yarkoni S, Reece A, Wan M, et al: Intrapartum fetal weight estimation: A comparison of three formulae. *J Ultrasound Med* 1986; 5:707–710.
174. Picker RH, Saunders DM: A simple geometric method for determining fetal weight in utero with the compound gray scale ultrasonic scan. *Am J Obstet Gynecol* 1976; 124:493–494.
175. Morrison J, McLennan MJ: The theory, feasibility and accuracy of an ultrasonic method of estimating fetal weight. *Br J Obstet Gynaecol* 1976; 83:833–837.
176. Thompson TR, Manning FA: Estimation of volume and weight of the perinate: Relationship to morphometric measurement by ultrasonography. *J Ultrasound Med* 1983; 2:113–116.
177. Brinkley JF, McCallum WD, Muramatsu SK, et al: Fetal weight estimation from lengths and volumes found by three-dimensional ultrasonic measurements. *J Ultrasound Med* 1984; 3:163–168.
178. Rossavik IK, Torjusen GO, Deter RL, et al: Efficacy of mathematical methods for ultrasound examinations in diabetic pregnancies. *Am J Obstet Gynecol* 1986; 155:638–644.
179. Eden RD, Frederick RJ, Kodack LD, et al: Accuracy of ultrasonic fetal weight prediction in preterm infants. *Am J Obstet Gynecol* 1983; 147:43–48.
180. Deter RL, Hadlock FP, Harrist RB, et al: Evaluation of three methods for obtaining fetal weight estimates using dynamic image ultrasound. *J Clin Ultrasound* 1981; 9:421–425.
181. Chervenak FA, Romero R, Berkowitz RL, et al: Use of sonographic estimated fetal weight in the prediction of intrauterine growth retardation. *Am J Perinatol* 1984; 1:298–301.
182. Ott WJ, Doyle S: Ultrasonic diagnosis of altered fetal growth by use of a normal ultrasonic fetal weight curve. *Obstet Gynecol* 1984; 63:201–204.

183. Key RC, Dattel BJ, Resnik R: The ultrasonographic estimation of fetal weight in the very low-birth weight infant. *Am J Obstet Gynecol* 1983; 145:574–578.
184. Sampson MB, Beckmann CRB, Thomason JL, et al: Single ultrasonic estimation of fetal weight in utero compared with birth weight. *J Reprod Med* 1985; 30:28–29.
185. Patterson RM: Estimation of fetal weight during labor. *Obstet Gynecol* 1985; 65:330–332.
186. Miller JM Jr, Korndoffer FA III, Gabert HA: Fetal weight estimates in late pregnancy with emphasis on macrosomia. *J Clin Ultrasound* 1986; 14:437–442.
187. Hill LM, Breckle R, Wolfgram KR, et al: Evaluation of three methods for estimating fetal weight. *J Clin Ultrasound* 1986; 14:171–178.
188. Wong F, Rogers M, Chang A: An evaluation of three ultrasound equations for fetal weight prediction. *Aust NZ J Obstet Gynaecol* 1985; 25:271.
189. Miller JM, Kissling GE, Korndoffer FA III, et al: A cross-sectional study of in utero growth of the above average sized fetus. *Am J Obstet Gynecol* 1986; 155:1052–1055.

Chapter 8

Uterine Measurements

UTERINE VOLUME

The volume of the pregnant uterus, initially termed the *total intrauterine volume*, or TIUV, was first calculated in the late 1970s.[1-3] All three articles computed the volume using a prolated ellipse formula (TIUV = 0.523 × the maximum uterine length, width, and height), all giving their data in graph form with a standard deviation range. Gohari et al.[1] presented their data from +1 to −2 SD, Phillips et al.[2] gave a 1 SD range and showed the difference between singleton, twin, and triplet gestations, and Levine et al.[3] gave a range from the upper to the lower 2.5th percentile. All three articles showed a linear relationship with the TIUV increasing as both the weeks of gestation and biparietal diameter increased to term. The articles, however, differed markedly in their values. At 24 weeks, with a biparietal diameter of 61 mm, the TIUV ranged from 1,400 to 3,800 cc. By 40 weeks, with a biparietal diameter of 95 mm, variation was even larger, 4,200 to 7,800 cc. Despite these discrepancies, the initial success in the detection of growth retardation was found to be good, with Gohari et al.[1] reporting a sensitivity of 75%, a specificity of 100%, and a predictive accuracy of 100% when a threshold of 1.5 SD below the mean was used. This accuracy, however, could not be reproduced.[4] In a group of 252 patients, using a threshold of abnormality at the lower 10% tolerance limit, growth retardation was detected with a predictive accuracy of only 41%.

Conceptually the idea of the total uterine volume is sound. It should be a good indicator of not only the size of the pregnant uterus but also of its three main components, the fetus, the amniotic fluid, and the placenta. The reasons for the marked discrepancies between studies and the poor predictive accuracy in the detection of growth retardation are therefore puzzling. Three studies[5-7] found that the major source of error was not in the concept of uterine volume but in the use of the prolated ellipse formula for its calculation. When the uterine volume was calculated instead from a stepped area-to-volume technique with comparison to known volumes, the stepped area method was accurate to within 5% of the true volume, while the prolated ellipse method was inaccurate by as much as 55%. As a result, it was recommended that the stepped area-to-volume method be used to calculate the uterine volume[6,7] and that the name be changed from TIUV to total uterine volume (TUV), since the measurement encompassed not just the intrauterine contents but also the myometrium.[7]

One additional article suggested an entirely different method of measuring the uterus.[8] It stated that the addition of the maximum longitudinal and transverse uterine areas (LTUA) gave less of an error than the multiplication of the three linear measurements used in the prolate ellipse formula. While this may be true, and while greater reproducibility in measurements might be obtained, the two areas do not relate to uterine volumes except in very specific and unusual situations.[7] For this reason, the LTUA technique is not of clinical value.

Two different groups evaluated the stepped area-to-volume TUV technique.[9, 10] Both used similar technique with a static scanner. Transverse scans were obtained at specific intervals from the bottom to the top of the uterus. The area of each transverse image was computed from an equation for an ellipse (π D1/2 × D2/2) and all the areas added together to obtain the TUV. Geirsson et al.[10] presumably scanned at 1-cm intervals, as proposed in their previous article.[6] Kurtz et al.[9] found that obtaining scans at 3-cm intervals closely approximated the volumes obtained at 1-cm intervals, with an average error of only 3.5%.[7] Both articles[9, 10] stated their results in graph and number form. Kurtz et al.[9] presented a range of values at 200-cc increments from mean gestational ages of 15.4 to 38.7 weeks and from mean biparietal diameters of 35.3 to 91.1 mm, while Geirsson et al.[10] gave their results from 20 to 40 weeks in 5-week increments. Both had standard deviation ranges, Kurtz et al.[9] from the upper and lower first, fifth, and tenth percentile and Geirsson et al.[10] from the upper and lower third percentile. Both had reasonably sized series, Kurtz et al.[9] evaluating 260 normal pregnancies cross-sectionally, almost all patients scanned only once, while Geirsson et al.[10] examined 147 women longitudinally on four separate occasions. Geirsson et al.,[10] however, eliminated 32 patients (over 21% of their cases) for clinical reasons without stating if these fetuses were ultimately abnormal at birth. Since many of these reasons for exclusion would not be expected to affect the fetuses or the uterus, their exclusions could possibly greatly weaken their final results. Therefore this paper will not be considered further.

Kurtz et al.[9] also examined 26 abnormal cases, 14 large uteruses and 12 small uteruses. All of the large and 10 of the 12 small uteruses fell outside the upper or lower 90th percentile confidence limit. Because of the apparent clinical usefulness of their data, the two tables of TUV vs. both biparietal diameter and gestational age by Kurtz et al.[9] are recommended (Fig 8–1, Tables 8–1 and 8–2). More work is necessary for further evaluation of this technique, since only a small number of abnormal patients were studied. For the appropriate measurements to be taken, static images are necessary. Since more and more emphasis is being placed on real-time examinations and less on static scanning, it is not certain whether this technique, although presumably valuable, will ever be fully evaluated.

PLACENTA

Placental weight and thickness has been analyzed pathologically. In two series on delivered placentas,[11, 12] the weight was measured in one series from 23 to 43 weeks[11] and in the other at term.[12] The results at term matched closely, both articles finding a placental weight of approximately 420 gm. In addition, one of the articles measured the thickness of the placenta at term and found it

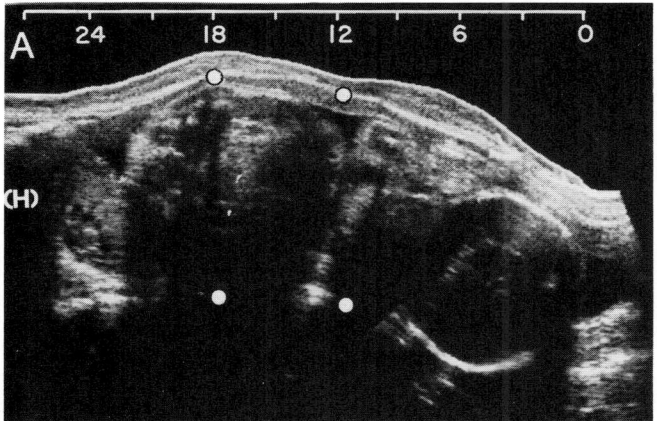
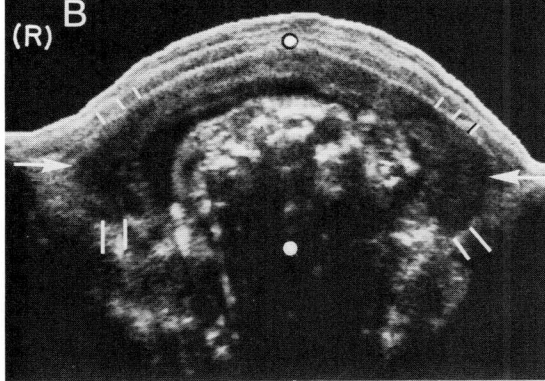
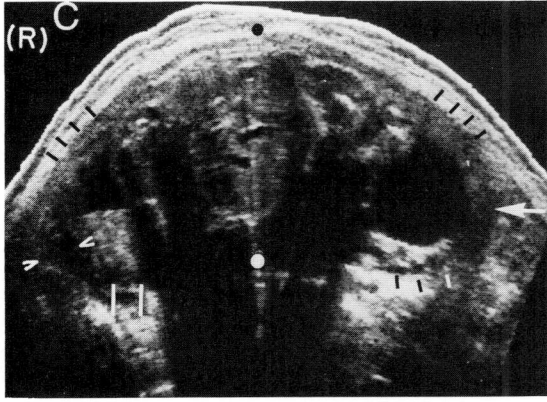

FIG 8–1.
Calculation of total uterine volume. **A**, long-axis midline static scan of the pregnant uterus. The centimeter scale *(top)* demonstrates the uterus divided into 3-cm intervals. *Dots* represent the anterior and posterior uterine margins of scans at 12 and 18 cm above the maternal bladder. Transverse static scans at 12 cm (**B**) and 18 cm (**C**) above the maternal bladder. The outer uterine walls are denoted by *dots* anteriorly and posteriorly, by *dashes* anterolaterally and posterolaterally, and by *arrows* laterally. *H* indicates toward patient's head; *R*, toward patient's right. (From Kurtz AB, Kurtz RJ, Rifkin MD, et al: Total uterine volume: A new graph and its clinical applications. *J Ultrasound Med* 1984; 3:299–308. Used by permission.)

to be 1.64 cm ± 0.5.[12] The exact place for measuring placental thickness, however, was never indicated.

Ultrasound evaluated the placental thickness and volume. Two articles[13, 14] measured placental thickness at various stages of gestation. Grannum et al.,[13] without stating where the measurement was taken, found placental thickness to decrease gradually in the middle to late third trimester. At 30 to 32, 32 to 34, and 34 to 36 weeks, the placental thickness averaged 38, 36.6, and 34.8 mm, respectively. Hoddick et al.[14] measured the midportion of the placenta with

TABLE 8−1.
Comparison of Total Uterine Volume (TUV) to the Biparietal Diameter*

	Biparietal Diameter, mm						
	Lower Percentile Limits of Normal				Upper Percentile Limits of Normal		
TUV, cc	99th	95th	90th	Mean	99th	95th	90th
600	18.9	22.8	24.8	35.3	45.7	47.8	51.7
800	23.4	27.3	29.3	39.7	50.2	52.2	56.1
1,000	27.6	31.5	33.6	44.0	54.4	56.5	60.4
1,200	31.7	35.6	37.6	48.1	58.5	60.6	64.4
1,400	35.6	39.5	41.5	52.0	62.4	64.5	68.3
1,600	39.3	43.2	45.3	55.7	66.1	68.2	72.1
1,800	42.9	46.7	48.8	59.2	69.7	71.7	75.6
2,000	46.2	50.1	52.1	62.6	73.0	75.1	79.0
2,200	49.4	53.3	55.3	65.7	76.2	78.2	82.1
2,400	52.4	56.2	58.3	68.7	79.2	81.2	85.1
2,600	55.2	59.0	61.1	71.5	82.0	84.0	87.9
2,800	57.8	61.7	63.7	74.1	84.6	86.6	90.5
3,000	60.2	64.1	66.1	76.6	87.0	89.1	93.0
3,200	62.5	66.3	68.4	78.8	89.3	91.3	95.3
3,400	64.5	68.4	70.5	80.9	91.3	93.4	97.3
3,600	66.4	70.3	72.3	82.8	93.2	95.3	99.1
3,800	68.1	72.0	74.0	84.5	95.0	97.0	100.8
4,000	69.6	73.5	75.6	86.0	96.4	98.5	102.4
4,200	71.0	74.9	76.9	87.3	97.8	99.8	103.7
4,400	72.1	76.0	78.0	88.5	98.9	101.0	104.9
4,600	73.1	77.0	79.0	89.5	99.9	101.9	105.8
4,800	73.9	77.8	80.0	90.2	100.7	102.7	106.6
5,000	74.5	78.4	80.4	90.8	101.3	103.3	107.2
5,200	74.9	78.8	80.8	91.3	101.7	103.7	107.6
5,400	75.1	79.0	81.1	91.5	101.9	104.0	107.9
5,600	75.2	79.1	81.1	91.6	102.0	104.0	107.9
5,800	75.1	78.9	81.0	91.4	101.9	103.9	107.8
6,000	74.7	78.6	80.7	91.1	101.6	103.6	107.5

*From Kurtz AB, Kurtz RJ, Rifkin MD, et al: Total uterine volume: A new graph and its clinical applications. *J Ultrasound Med* 1984; 3:299–308. Used by permission.

static scans from 10 weeks until term, excluding the myometrium and subplacental veins. Without using the umbilical cord insertion or any other anatomical landmark, they found the placenta to increase in thickness with advancing menstrual age, never exceeding 40 mm. Presenting their numbers in graph form, they found the placenta to have a mean value of 10 ± 5 mm at 10 weeks, increasing to 20 ± 10 mm at 20 weeks. At 30 and 40 weeks, respectively, the placenta measured 28 ± 6 mm and 33 ± 7 mm. These upper and lower limits could be of value in the future in evaluating small and large placentas if a landmark can be established to make the measurements reproducible. It is recommended that the umbilical cord insertion be used as the anatomical landmark, measurements taken perpendicularly from the chorionic plate to the decidua

TABLE 8–2.
Comparison of Total Uterine Volume (TUV) to the Average Gestational Age*

	Average Gestational Age, wk						
	Lower Percentile Limits of Normal				Upper Percentile Limits of Normal		
TUV, cc	99th	95th	90th	Mean	99th	95th	90
600	8.7	10.3	11.1	15.4	19.7	20.5	22.1
800	10.5	12.1	12.9	17.2	21.5	22.3	23.9
1,000	11.9	13.5	14.3	18.6	22.9	23.7	25.3
1,200	13.3	14.9	15.7	20.0	24.3	25.1	26.7
1,400	14.6	16.2	17.0	21.3	25.6	26.5	28.0
1,600	15.9	17.5	18.3	22.6	26.9	27.7	29.3
1,800	17.1	18.7	19.6	23.9	28.1	29.0	30.6
2,000	18.3	19.9	20.8	25.1	29.3	30.2	31.8
2,200	19.5	21.1	21.9	26.2	30.5	31.3	32.9
2,400	20.6	22.2	23.0	27.3	31.6	32.4	34.0
2,600	21.6	23.2	24.0	28.3	32.6	33.5	35.1
2,800	22.6	24.2	25.0	29.3	33.6	34.5	36.0
3,000	23.6	25.2	26.0	30.3	34.6	35.4	37.0
3,200	24.5	26.1	26.9	31.2	35.5	36.3	37.9
3,400	25.3	26.9	27.8	32.0	36.3	37.2	38.8
3,600	26.1	27.7	28.6	32.8	37.1	38.0	39.6
3,800	26.9	28.5	29.3	33.6	37.9	38.7	40.3
4,000	27.6	29.1	30.0	34.3	38.6	39.4	41.0
4,200	28.3	29.8	30.7	35.0	39.3	40.1	41.7
4,400	28.9	30.5	31.3	35.6	39.9	40.7	42.3
4,600	29.4	31.0	31.9	36.1	40.4	41.3	42.9
4,800	29.9	31.5	32.4	36.7	40.9	41.8	43.4
5,000	30.4	32.0	32.8	37.1	41.4	42.2	43.8
5,200	30.8	32.4	33.3	37.5	41.8	42.7	44.3
5,400	31.2	32.8	33.6	37.9	42.2	43.0	44.6
5,600	31.5	33.1	34.0	38.2	42.5	43.4	45.0
5,800	31.8	33.4	34.2	38.5	42.8	43.6	45.2
6,000	32.0	33.6	34.5	38.7	43.0	43.9	45.5

*From Kurtz AB, Kurtz RJ, Rifkin MD, et al: Total uterine volume: A new graph and its clinical applications. J Ultrasound Med 1984; 3:299–308. Used by permission.

basalis (the edge of the myometrium). While it may be difficult to identify the myometrium, neither the myometrium nor the retroplacental zone should be included in the measurement (Fig 8–2).

Three additional ultrasound articles evaluated with static scans the volumetric growth of the human placenta,[15–17] 2 giving their results in number and graph form[15, 16] and the other in graph form only.[17] Different techniques were used. Geirsson et al.,[15] scanning presumably at 1-cm intervals, calculated the placental volume in 115 pregnant women as the difference between the total uterine volume and the intra-amniotic volume. Bleker et al.[16] obtained one long axis and then three transverse scans of the placenta, approximating the area between slices and comparing it to 10 delivered placentas. While close correlation was detected, placental volume was found to decrease after birth due to the loss of the fetal blood to the neonate. Wolf et al.[17] produced transverse images at 1- to 2-cm intervals, tracing the placental outline with a digitizer to calculate an area for each slice. The volume was estimated by a modified rectangular formula. Close correlation was obtained with six placentas measured shortly after birth. While all three articles showed an initial increase in placental volume early in the pregnancy, Bleker et al.[16] stated that in 10 of 12 patients the placental volume reached its maximum by approximately 32 gestational weeks and thereafter either leveled off or decreased. Geirsson et al.[15] and Wolf et al.[17] showed an increasing placental volume throughout pregnancy, with the incremental growth either greatest prior to 35 weeks with very little additional growth thereafter[15] or increasing steadily to term.[17] Geirrson et al.[15] gave a standard deviation while the other two did not.

The numbers between studies varied considerably. Geirsson et al.[15] showed a steady increase in placental volumes from 259 to 800 ml from 20 weeks to term, while Wolf et al.[17] revealed a steady increase from 200 to greater than 1,000 ml over the same period of time. Bleker et al.[16] revealed variable numbers throughout gestation with some of their cases changing only 100 ml between 20 and 40 weeks. While the technique by Wolf et al.[17] seems to be the most accurate in measuring placental volumes, more work on a much larger group of patients is necessary to establish its validity and clinical usefulness.

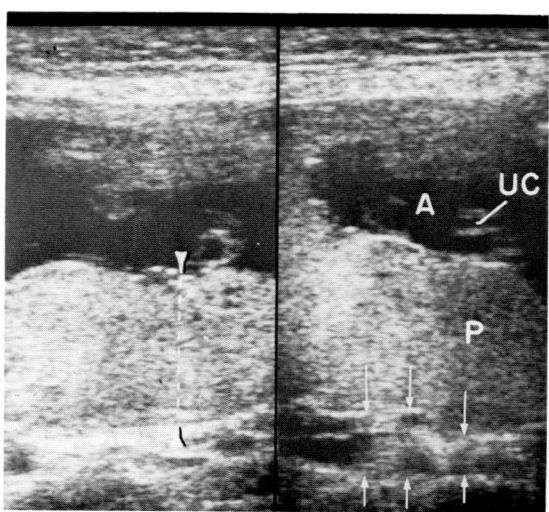

FIG 8–2.
Dual-image scan of an early third trimester uterus. **Right image,** scan of the placenta *(P)* at the point of umbilical cord *(UC)* insertion. A indicates amniotic fluid. *Arrows* denote hypoechoic retroplacental zone. **Left image,** measurement of the placenta obtained perpendicularly at the origin of the umbilical cord *(arrowheads* and *dotted line)*. Note that the measurement is taken from the thin hyperechoic chorionic plate (at the cord insertion) through the placenta, not including the retroplacental area.

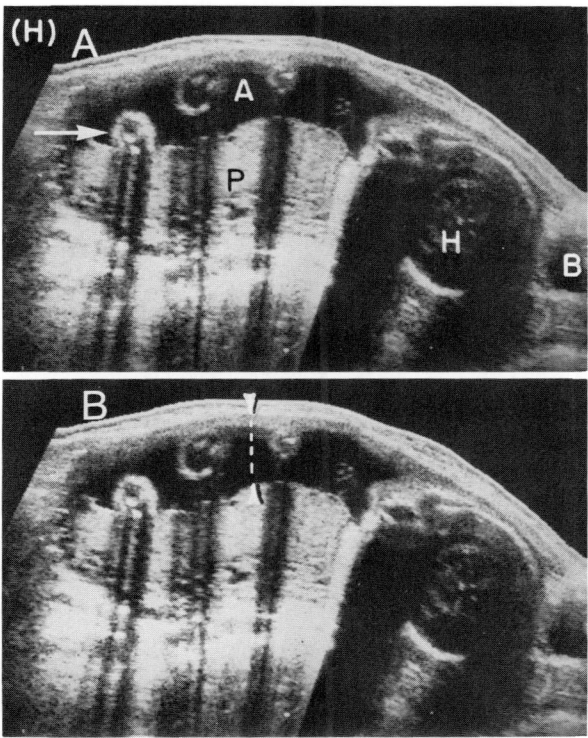

FIG 8–3.
Long-axis midline scan of a 28-week pregnancy. The amount of amniotic fluid *(A)* is normal by both objective and subjective criteria. **A,** fetus is in vertex presentation with its head *(H)* immediately superior to the maternal bladder *(B)*. *Arrow* denotes fetal limb. **B,** same image as **A** measuring an AP pocket of fluid greater than 3 cm in size *(arrowheads* and *dotted line)*. *P* indicates placenta; *(H),* toward patient's head.

AMNIOTIC FLUID

The amount of amniotic fluid surrounding the fetus is important during fetal development and affects perinatal outcome.[18] Oligohydramnios (decreased amniotic fluid) has been associated with fetal dysmaturity syndromes, fetal congenital anomalies, particularly renal abnormalities, and, if prolonged, with hypoplasia of the fetal lungs. Polyhydramnios, or hydramnios (increased amniotic fluid), has been associated with maternal factors (such as diabetes mellitus, Rh-isoimmunization) and fetal anomalies (mostly upper gastrointestinal or neurologic).

Amniotic fluid can be evaluated either qualitatively (subjectively) or quantitatively (objectively with measurements). Whether analyzed subjectively or objectively, the determination of both normal and decreased amniotic fluid was found to be accurate with little intraobserver or interobserver variation and regardless of the experience of the observer.[19] Crowley[20] further used the subjective criteria that amniotic fluid could be considered normal if it could be demonstrated between fetal limbs and the uterine wall anteriorly or between fetal limbs and the fetal trunk posteriorly (Fig 8–3). When determined to be normal, she found the incidence of meconium staining, fetal acidosis, fetal distress, and the Apgar scores were significantly reduced or nonexistent. Hashimoto et al.[21] also found that the subjective diagnosis of decreased amniotic fluid was accurate.

Four studies[18, 20-22] attempted to quantify amniotic fluid by measuring its largest pocket and setting a lower limit for normal (see Fig 8–3). Manning et al.[22] decided that the amniotic fluid could be considered normal if one pocket measured 10 mm or greater in its broadest diameter. Mercer et al.[23] defined amniotic fluid as normal if the largest pocket was greater than 10 mm in size, moderately decreased if the pocket was 5 to 10 mm in size, and markedly decreased if less than 5 mm. Chamberlain,[18] in a nonrefereed journal, used scans perpendicular to the maternal abdomen and measured both transverse and vertical pockets of fluid. He defined the amniotic fluid as decreased if the largest pocket was less than 10 mm in both vertical and transverse dimensions and marginal if between 10 and 20 mm in vertical and 10 mm in transverse dimension. Hashimoto et al.[21] measured the length, width, and depth of the largest pocket of fluid and multiplied the three numbers together. An arbitrary number of 60 was found to be the dividing line between a normal amount of amniotic fluid above and oligohydramnios below.

Manning et al.[22] found that by using his 10 mm definition, later termed the 1-cm rule, a diagnosis of normal amniotic fluid could accurately predict a normal fetus in 93.4% of cases while a diagnosis of decreased amniotic fluid meant growth-retardation in 89.9% of cases with a significant tenfold increase in perinatal morbidity. Mercer et al.,[23] using his own 5-mm rule, found that when cases of ruptured membranes were discarded, 7% of neonates with less than a 5-mm pocket of amniotic fluid had congenital malformations, lower Apgar scores at 1 and 5 minutes, increased fetal distress and meconium, and if detected prior to 27 weeks, had significantly poorer neonatal outcome. Chamberlain et al.[18] also found the same significant relationship between decreased amniotic fluid volume and the incidence of both major congenital anomalies (9.37%) and growth retardation (38.6%).

A reevaluation of the 1-cm rule was performed in two studies.[24, 25] When this rule was used as the sole criterion for the diagnosis of growth retardation,[24] only 5 of 125 small-for-date fetuses were detected, and it was concluded that the 1-cm rule was not of value in predicting growth retardation.[24] In addition, in 3 of 6 small-for-date fetuses, the correct diagnosis of oligohydramnios was made subjectively, although the largest pocket of fluid was greater than 1 cm[25] (Fig 8–4). Therefore, while it is important that decreased amniotic fluid be detected, it is not important whether this diagnosis is made qualitatively or quantitatively. Furthermore, if an observer subjectively thinks that there is decreased amniotic fluid, he should not be dissuaded from making that diagnosis on the basis of the quantitative measurement of a fluid pocket. Although not as yet proved, it would seem that the same subjective decision can be used to differentiate most cases of polyhydramnios (increased amniotic fluid) from normal (Fig 8–5). No measurements have as yet been proposed.

An attempt at determining intra-amniotic fluid volumes has also been performed. Geirsson in two articles[26, 27] measured intra-amniotic fluid volume by use of the stepped area-to-volume method. Although it is not clear from their studies, it would seem that the intra-amniotic number encompasses both the

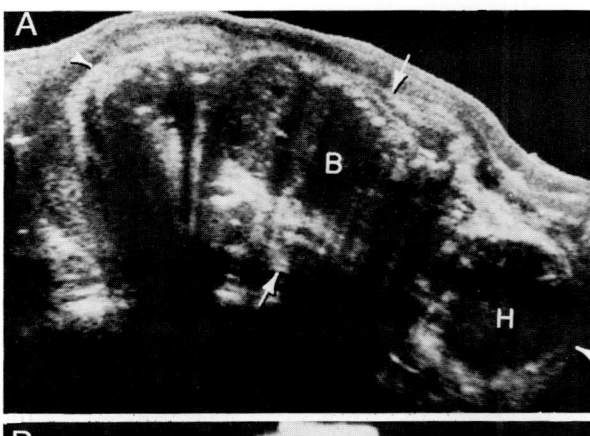
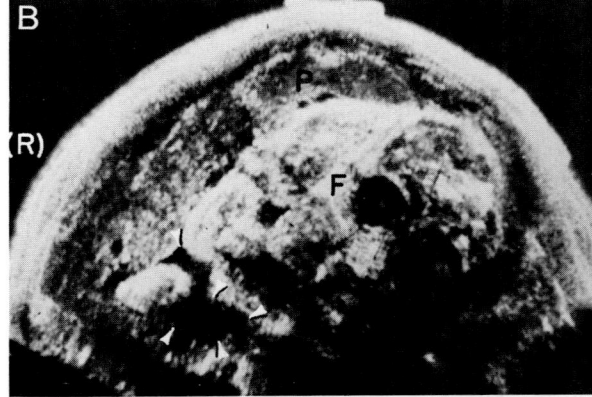
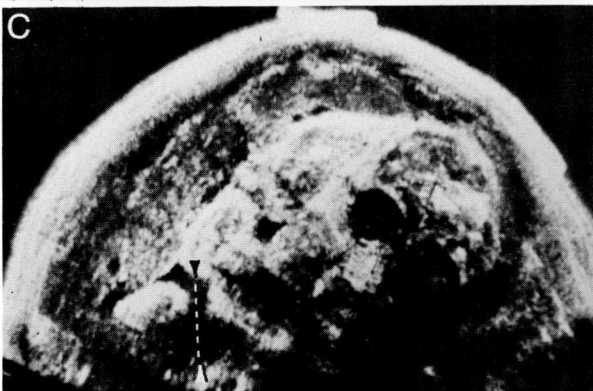

FIG 8–4.
Static scans of a 34-week fetus with subjectively marked decrease in amniotic fluid. Objectively, and incorrectly, the fluid measured within the normal range. **A,** long-axis midline scan showing the uterus (outlined by *arrows* and *arrowheads*) without any demonstrable fluid surrounding the fetus. H indicates fetal head; B, fetal body. **B,** transaxial scan at upper portion of uterus, showing the only pocket of amniotic fluid *(arrowheads)*, adjacent to the fetal body *(F)*. P indicates placenta with grade II changes. **C,** same image as **B**. The pocket of amniotic fluid measured in its broadest dimension is over 2 cm in size *(arrowheads and dotted line)*. Although objectively the fluid measures normal in amount, severe oligohydramnios is present. *(R)* indicates toward patient's right.

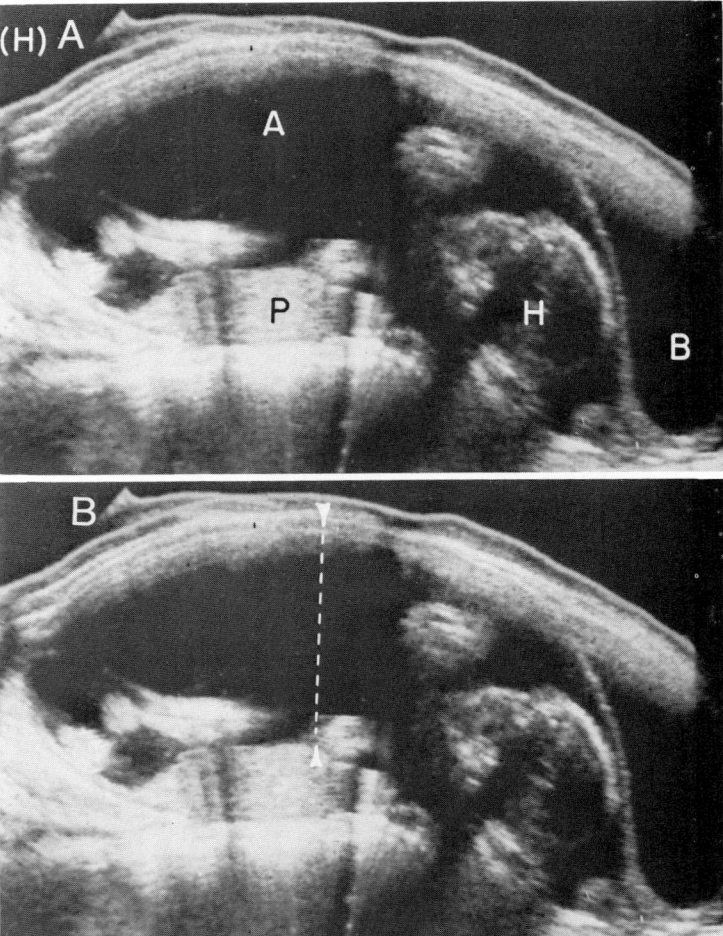

FIG 8–5.
Static scans of a 30-week pregnancy with subjectively increased amniotic fluid (polyhydramnios). No objective measurements are available at present. **A,** long-axis midline scan showing increased amniotic fluid *(A)*. *H* indicates fetal head; *P*, placenta; *B*, maternal bladder; *H*, toward patient's head. **B,** same image as **A** showing AP measurement *(arrowheads* and *dotted line)*.

fluid and the fetus. In the second and early third trimester, there is more fluid than fetus, with the reverse near term. While specific numbers were given and there was correlation with dye dilution techniques performed on the amniotic fluid, this method does not seem to offer any more information than the amniotic fluid analyses described above.

UMBILICAL CORD AND UMBILICAL VEIN

Studies have been performed on newborn infants, born prematurely from as early as 20 weeks until term, to evaluate the length and width of the umbilical cord.[28–32] The normal umbilical cord was found to increase in length from the early gestational age to term, a mean and 1 SD of 32 ± 8 mm at 20 weeks to 60 ± 13 mm at 40 weeks.[28] The width has also been measured and at term found to have a mean number of 14 mm in preterm and 16 mm in term gestations.[28] While it has been determined that a short umbilical cord is associated with psychomotor abnormalities from either early intrauterine constraint or fetal-limb dysfunction,[29, 30] there is a low predictive value in determining fetal abnormality, because the normal cord length has such a wide range of normal values.

The number and size of the blood vessels within the umbilical cord has also been studied in newborn infants.[33, 34] While there are usually one vein and two arteries, occasionally only one vein and one artery are detected. This finding of a single umbilical artery has been extensively reviewed in an autopsy series.[34] In singleton gestations, a single artery has been found in 20% of cases and, when detected, coexists with a higher incidence of fetal malformations (approximately 20%, many major and multiple), stillbirths, spontaneous abortions, and increased perinatal mortality. It should be remembered, however, that while abnormalities are high, 80% of fetuses with a single umbilical artery are still normal. Of interest is the additional finding that a single umbilical artery occurs much more commonly in twin gestations and that in this setting does not have any increased incidence of malformations or mortality. To detect a single umbilical artery, multiple places along the cord should be evaluated.[34] Particularly at the distal end, where the cord inserts into the placenta, two umbilical arteries may normally fuse into a single trunk. In another article,[33] the mean and minimum diameter of the umbilical artery and veins were evaluated at time of delivery. Within 5 seconds after delivery, the mean and minimum diameter measurements of the vein were 6.6 and 2.4 mm and of the artery 5.4 and 1.1 mm.

To date there have been no ultrasound studies of the umbilical cord. It would be difficult to evaluate the length of the umbilical cord because of the cord's variable placement and coiled configuration within the amniotic fluid (Fig 8–6).

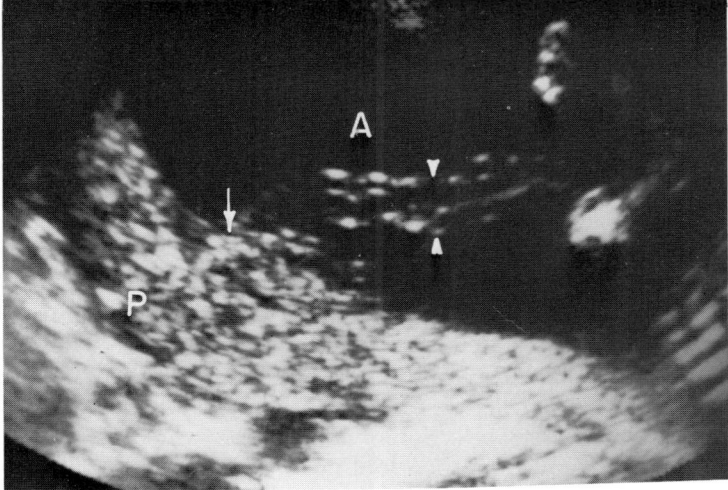

FIG 8–6.
Ultrasound scan of a 36-week pregnancy showing an 8-cm portion of the umbilical cord *(arrowheads)* from its insertion *(arrow)* into the placenta *(P)*. Due to the coiled configuration of the cord within the amniotic fluid *(A)*, it would be very difficult to measure its full length.

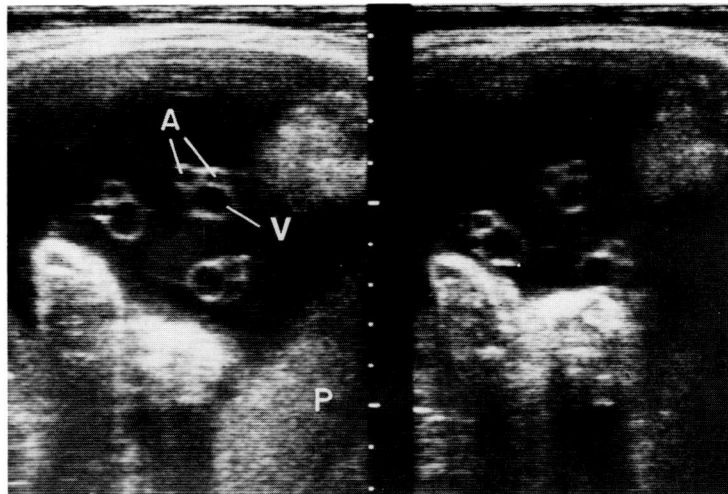

FIG 8–7.
Ultrasound dual image of a 30-week pregnancy showing multiple cross sections of the umbilical cord. The labeled scan on the left shows the normal two arteries (A) and one vein (V) of each segment. Note that the vein is slightly larger than the arteries. P indicates placenta.

Nevertheless, an umbilical cord of less than 30 mm would be strongly suggestive of abnormal shortening. In addition, it would not be easy to image multiple places along the cord to evaluate for the number of umbilical arteries (Fig 8–7). Even if a single artery were diagnosed, however, the finding would have limited value, since the fetus would most likely still be normal.

It has been suggested in two articles from the same institution[35, 36] that the size of the umbilical vein may be of value in the detection of Rh isoimmunization. These articles found that the umbilical vein diameters were normally slightly different in the amniotic fluid and within the liver and at different times in gestational life. From 18 to 37 weeks, the diameters were shown to slightly increase in the amniotic fluid from 7 to 11.6 mm and within the liver from 6.6 to 10 mm. When larger diameters were detected, both articles stated that this was strongly suggestive of Rh sensitization. While the authors of both articles thought that the umbilical vein within the cord had more of a tendency to dilate than that within the liver, both were found to be increased in a small but significant number of Rh-isoimmunized fetuses. In fact, they stated that this dilatation sometimes preceded the optical density changes of the amniotic fluid. However, in two more recent articles,[37, 38] the umbilical vein diameter was found to be relatively insensitive. Vintzileos et al.[39] detected an increase in the vein diameter in only 1 of 16 cases (8 of which were severe) of isoimmunized fetuses. Witter and Graham[38] evaluated 24 fetuses with Rh-isoimmunization and found all cases to overlap the normal range. Therefore, while the umbilical vein diameter is an interesting measurement, it does not appear to be as promising as originally proposed for the detection of affected Rh-isoimmunized fetuses, even when severe. At present, it is therefore not recommended.

THE CERVIX

In the pregnant uterus, the exact location of the cervix, and in particular the internal cervical os, is important. When a low-lying placenta is detected, it allows for a determination of whether the placenta covers the internal cervical os, termed a placenta previa. The overall length and width of the cervix is also helpful in diagnosing effacement due to either an incompetent cervix or premature onset of labor.

There have been four ultrasound articles that have evaluated the cervical dimensions,[39-41] two by the same group of authors.[40, 41] Three[39-41] were performed using static scanners, most of the images produced while the maternal urinary bladder was markedly distended. The last[42] employed real-time ultrasound with the maternal bladder at first completely or partially filled and then after emptying. In the three articles performed with static scans,[39-41] the area of the external cervical os was defined. While the endocervical canal could not be imaged, it was claimed that the area of the internal cervical os could be identified by an "isthmus," a point of narrowing at the upper part of the cervix. This particular landmark is questionable and is probably due to distortion of the cervix by its compression between the distended bladder and the sacrum. As confirmation of this, images within these same articles with the bladder partially empty did not show the same narrowing. Nevertheless, it was stated that the normal cervix in a pregnant woman should not be greater than 60 mm in length[39] and that the normal mean cervical width at the internal cervical os should measure 16 to 18 mm $\pm$ 6 mm (Fig 8–8). Patients with incompetent cervixes had an internal cervical os statistically widened to 25 or 26 mm $\pm$ 3 mm[40, 41] (Fig 8–9).

The major problems with these studies are twofold: (a) the use of a distended maternal urinary bladder can narrow and distort both the cervix and lower uterine segment, and (b) the inability to consistently identify both the internal cervical os and the endocervical canal leads to uncertainty about a possible placenta previa or an incompetent cervix. Bowie et al.,[42] using a real-time scanner and different degrees of maternal bladder distension, were able to detect the endocervical canal as either a hyperechoic or hypoechoic band within the cervix and define the internal cervical os as either flat or very slightly funnel-shaped (without an "isthmus") (Fig 8–8,A). In a group of 50 pregnant patients, 30 (60%) could be visualized. This visualization varied with the stage of gestation, caused by differences in the size and position of the fetus relative to the cervix. Prior to 20 weeks, the cervix could be clearly imaged in 100% of patients, decreasing to 68% between 20 and 30 weeks and 18% between 30 weeks and term. When the urinary bladder was partially distended, the mean cervix and its endocervical canal measured 46 mm, with a range of 34 to 61 mm (see Fig 8–8). This corresponded to the previous work of Zemlyn.[39] When the urinary bladder was emptied, however, the mean length of the cervix was significantly decreased to 32.5 mm, with a range of 23 to 45 mm (Fig 8–10). The number of previous pregnancies did not cause a difference in the cervical length. Width measurements were not taken.

From these articles, when the endocervical canal is identified, a mean and maximum cervical length of 46 and 60 mm can occur when the maternal bladder is filled, decreasing to a mean and maximum length of 32.5 and 45 mm when the bladder is emptied (Table 8–3). While cervical width measurements had been taken with the bladder distended, these are not recommended, since the degree of bladder filling seems directly to affect the width measurements. This cannot be controlled in a clinical setting. While width measurements might be of value with the bladder empty, these are not currently available.

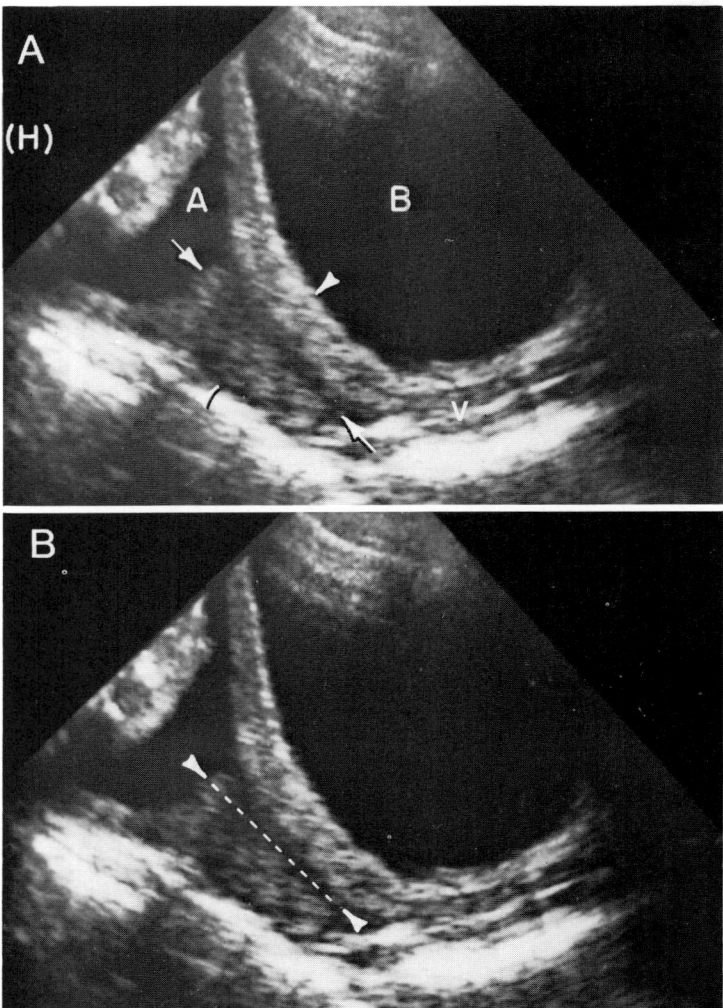

FIG 8–8.
Real-time long-axis midline scan of the normal lower uterine segment performed through a partially distended maternal urinary bladder (B). **A,** the cervix is defined in length (arrows) from the external cervical os to the flattened internal cervical os, the latter toward the patient's head (H). Note the hypoechoic endocervical canal between the two arrows. The cervical width denoted by arrowheads. V indicates vagina; A, amniotic fluid. **B,** same image as **A** showing the length measurement of the cervix and its endocervical canal (arrowheads and dotted lines).

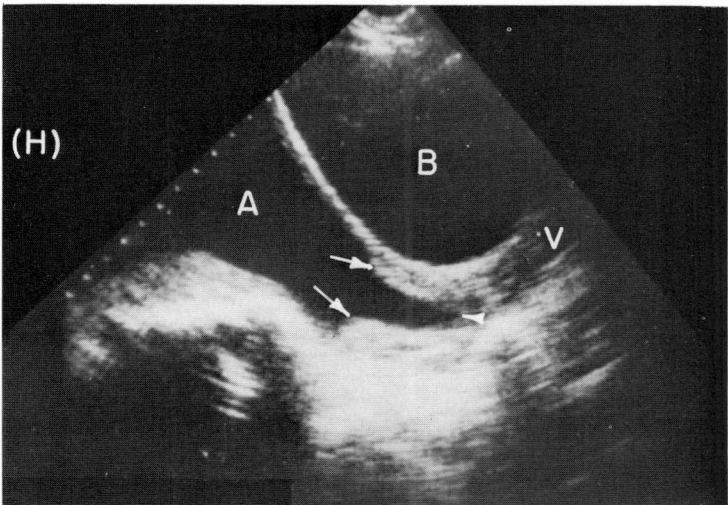

FIG 8–9.
Incompetent cervix. Real-time long-axis midline scan of the lower uterine segment performed through a distended maternal urinary bladder (B) showing an open endocervical canal from the internal cervical os (arrows) to the external cervical os (arrowhead). The overall width of the cervix, especially at the level of the internal os, is markedly enlarged. A indicates amniotic fluid; V, vagina; (H), toward patient's head.

TABLE 8–3.
Length of the Cervix and Cervical Canal in Pregnancy

Maternal Bladder	Mean Length, mm	Range, mm
Distended*† (partially or fully)	46	34–61
Empty*	32.5	23–45

*Data from Bowie JD, Andreotti RF, Rosenberg ER: Sonographic appearance of the uterine cervix in pregnancy: The vertical cervix. *AJR* 1983; 140:737–740.
†Data from Zemlym S: The length of the uterine cervix and its significance. *J Clin Ultrasound* 1981; 9:267–296.

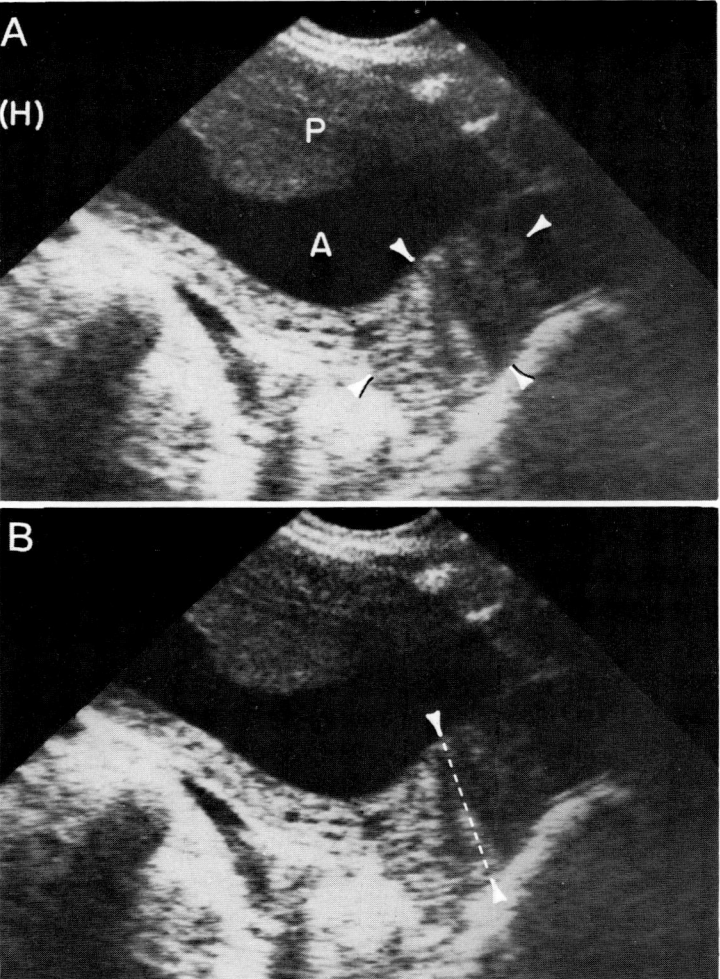

FIG 8–10.
Real-time long-axis midline scan of the lower uterine segment. **A,** the maternal urinary bladder is completely empty so that the image is obtained by scanning through the amniotic fluid *(A)*. Arrowheads outline the cervix, which is much more squared off than when distorted by a distended bladder. *P* indicates placenta; *(H),* toward patient's head. **B,** same image as **A.** The hyperechoic endocervical canal is positioned more anteroposteriorly when the bladder is empty. Both the endocervical and cervical measurement are denoted by *arrowheads* and *dotted line.*

REFERENCES

Uterine Volume
1. Gohari P, Berkowitz RL, Hobbins JC: Prediction of intrauterine growth retardation by determination of total intrauterine volume. *Am J Obstet Gynecol* 1977; 127:255–260.
2. Phillips JF, Goodwin DW, Thomason SB, et al: The volume of the uterus in normal and abnormal pregnancy. *J Clin Ultrasound* 1976; 5:107–110.
3. Levine SC, Filly RA, Creasy RK: Identification of fetal growth retardation by ultrasonographic estimation of total intrauterine volume. *J Clin Ultrasound* 1979; 7:21–26.
4. Chinn DH, Filly RA, Callen PW: Prediction of intrauterine growth retardation by sonographic estimation of total intrauterine volume. *J Clin Ultrasound* 1981; 9:175–179.
5. Grossman M, Flynn JJ, Aufrichtig D, et al: Pitfalls in ultrasonic determination of total intrauterine volume. *J Clin Ultrasound* 1982; 10:17–20.
6. Geirsson RT, Christie AD, Patel N: Ultrasound volume measurements comparing a prolate ellipsoid method with a parallel planimetric area method against a known volume. *J Clin Ultrasound* 1982; 10:329–332.
7. Kurtz AB, Shaw WM, Kurtz RJ, et al: The inaccuracy of total uterine volume measurements: Sources of error and a proposed solution. *J Ultrasound Med* 1984; 3:289–297.
8. Middleton WD, Bowie JD, Welt SI: LTUA—a new and more reproducible method of estimating intrauterine size. *J Ultrasound Med* 1982; 1:123–127.
9. Kurtz AB, Kurtz RJ, Rifkin MD, et al: Total uterine volume: A new graph and its clinical applications. *J Ultrasound Med* 1984; 3:299–308.
10. Geirsson RT, Ogston SA, Patel NB, et al: Growth of total intrauterine, intra-amniotic and placental volume in normal singleton pregnancy measured by ultrasound. *Br J Obstet Gynaecol* 1985; 92:46–53.

Placenta
11. Molteni RA, Stys SJ, Battaglia FC: Relationship of fetal and placental weight in human beings: Fetal/placental weight ratio at various gestational ages and birth weight distributions. *J Reprod Med* 1978; 21:327–334.
12. Younosazai MK, Haworth JC: Placental dimensions and relations in preterm, term, and growth-retarded infants. *Am J Obstet Gynecol* 1969; 103:265–271.
13. Grannum PAT, Berkowitz RL, Hobbins JC: The ultrasonic changes in the maturing placenta and their relation to fetal pulmonic maturity. *Am J Obstet Gynecol* 1979; 133:915–922.
14. Hoddick WK, Mahony BS, Callen PW, et al: Placental thickness. *J Ultrasound Med* 1985; 4:479–482.
15. Geirsson RT, Ogston SA, Patel NB, et al: Growth of total intrauterine, intra-amniotic and placental volume in normal singleton pregnancy measured by ultrasound. *Br J Obstet Gynaecol* 1985; 92:46–53.
16. Bleker OP, Kloosterman GJ, Breur W, et al: The volumetric growth of the human placenta: A longitudinal ultrasonic study. *Am J Obstet Gynecol* 1977; 127:657–661.
17. Wolf H, Oosting H, Treffers PE: Placental volume measurement by ultrasonography: Evaluation of the method. *Am J Obstet Gynecol* 1987; 156:1191–1194.

Amniotic Fluid
18. Chamberlain P: Amniotic fluid volume: Ultrasound assessment and clinical significance. *Semin Perinatol* 1985; 9:163–167.
19. Halperin ME, Fong KW, Zalev AH, et al: Reliability of amniotic fluid volume estimation from ultrasonograms: Intraobserver and interobserver variation before and after the establishment of criteria. *Am J Obstet Gynecol* 1985; 153:264–267.

20. Crowley P: Non quantitative estimation of amniotic fluid volume in suspected prolonged pregnancy. *J Perinat Med* 1980; 8:249–251.
21. Hashimoto B, Filly RA, Belden C, et al: Objective method of diagnosing oligohydramnios in postterm pregnancies. *J Ultrasound Med* 1987; 6:81–84.
22. Manning FA, Hill LM, Platt LD: Qualitative amniotic fluid volume determination by ultrasound: Antepartum detection of intrauterine growth retardation. *Am J Obstet Gynecol* 1981; 139:254–258.
23. Mercer LJ, Brown LG, Petres RE, et al: A survey of pregnancies complicated by decreased amniotic fluid. *Am J Obstet Gynecol* 1984; 149:355–361.
24. Hoddick WK, Callen PW, Filly RA, et al: Ultrasonographic determination of qualitative amniotic fluid volume in intrauterine growth retardation: Reassessment of the 1cm rule. *Am J Obstet Gynecol* 1984; 149:758–762.
25. Hill LM, Breckle R, Wolfgram KR, et al: Oligohydramnios: Ultrasonically detected incidence and subsequent fetal outcome. *Am J Obstet Gynecol* 1983; 147:407–410.
26. Geirsson RT, Ogston SA, Patel NB, et al: Growth of total intrauterine, intra-amniotic and placental volume in normal singleton pregnancy measured by ultrasound. *Br J Obstet Gynaecol* 1985; 92:46–53.
27. Geirsson RT, Patel NB, Christie AD: In-vivo accuracy of ultrasound measurements of intrauterine volume in pregnancy. *Br J Obstet Gynaecol* 1984; 91:37–40.

Umbilical Cord and Umbilical Vein

28. Younoszai MK, Haworth JC: Placental dimensions and relations in preterm, term, and growth-retarded infants. *Am J Obstet Gynecol* 1969; 103:265–271.
29. Naeye RL: Umbilical cord length: Clinical significance. *J Pediatr* 1985; 107:278–281.
30. Miller ME, Higginbottom M, Smith DW: Short umbilical cord: Its origin and relevance. *Pediatrics* 1981; 67:618–621.
31. Malpas P: Length of the human umbilical cord at term. *Br Med J* 1964; 1:673–674.
32. Walker CW, Pye BG: The length of the human umbilical cord: A statistical report. *Br Med J* 1960; 1:546–548.
33. Moinian M, Meyer WW, Lind J: Diameters of umbilical cord vessels and the weight of the cord in relation to clamping time. *Am J Obstet Gynecol* 1969; 105:604–611.
34. Heifetz SA: Single umbilical artery: A statistical analysis of 237 autopsy cases and review of the literature. *Perspect Pediatr Pathol* 1984; 8:345–378.
35. Mayden KL: The umbilical vein diameter in Rh isoimmunization. *Med Ultrasound* 1980; 4:119–125.
36. DeVore GR, Mayden K, Tortora M, et al: Dilation of the fetal umbilical vein in rhesus hemolytic anemia: A predictor of severe disease. *Am J Obstet Gynecol* 1981; 141:464–466.
37. Vintzileos AM, Campbell WA, Storlazzi E, et al: Fetal liver ultrasound measurements in isoimmunized pregnancies. *Obstet Gynecol* 1986; 68:162–167.
38. Witter FR, Graham D: The utility of ultrasonically measured umbilical vein diameters in isoimmunized pregnancies. *Am J Obstet Gynecol* 1983; 146:225–226.

The Cervix

39. Zemlyn S: The length of the uterine cervix and its significance. *J Clin Ultrasound* 1981; 9:267–269.
40. Brook I, Feingold M, Schwartz A, et al: Ultrasonography in the diagnosis of cervical incompetence in pregnancy—a new diagnostic approach. *Br J Obstet Gynaecol* 1981; 88:640–643.
41. Feingold M, Brook I, Zakut H: Detection of cervical incompetence by ultrasound. *Acta Obstet Gynecol Scand* 1984; 63:407–410.
42. Bowie JD, Andreotti RF, Rosenberg ER: Sonographic appearance of the uterine cervix in pregnancy: The vertical cervix. *AJR* 1983; 140:737–740.

Chapter 9

Mathematical Growth Models

Recently, a number of authors have mathematically analyzed fetal growth. By the use of equations that were linear, quadratic, cubic, or even more complicated, fetal parameters have been studied in small populations of fetuses. While some of the theoretical approaches are novel, none appears to offer practical advantages over existing tables. Nevertheless, the fetal parameters that have been evaluated and the articles that have studied them are listed in Table 9–1.

TABLE 9–1.
Evaluation of Fetal Parameters

Parameter	Reference Data	No. of Articles
Biparietal diameter	Adam et al.[1]; Deter et al.[2]; Wexler et al.[3]; Todros et al.[4]; Deter et al.[5]	5
Head circumference	Adam et al.[1]; Deter et al.[2]; Todros et al.[4]; Deter et al.[5]	4
Head area	Deter et al.[5]; Rossavik et al.[6]	2
Head volume	Deter et al.[5]; Rossavik et al.[7]; Deter et al.[8]	3
Abdominal circumference	Adam et al.[1]; Deter et al.[2]; Todros et al.[4]; Deter et al.[5]	4
Abdominal area	Deter et al.[5]; Rossavik et al.[9]	2
Abdominal volume	Deter et al.[5]; Rossavik et al.[7]; Deter et al.[8]	3
Femur length	Deter et al.[10]	1
Head-to-abdominal volume ratio	Rossavik and Deter[8]	1
Total fetal volume	Deter al et.[11]	1
Fetal weight	Deter et al.[2]; Rossavik et al.[12]	2

REFERENCES

1. Adam AH, Robinson HP, Dunlop C: A comparison of crown-rump length measurements using a real-time scanner in an antenatal clinic and a conventional B-scanner. *Br J Obstet Gynaecol* 1979; 86:521–524.
2. Deter RL, Harrist RB, Hadlock FP, et al: Longitudinal studies of fetal growth with the use of dynamic image ultrasonography. *Am J Obstet Gynecol* 1982; 143:545.
3. Wexler S, Fuchs C, Golan A, et al: Tolerance intervals for standards in ultrasound measurements: Determination of BPD standards. *J Clin Ultrasound* 1986; 14:243–250.
4. Todros T, Ferrazzi E, Groli C, et al: Fitting growth curves to head and abdomen measurements of the fetus: A multicentric study. *J Clin Ultrasound* 1987; 15:95–105.
5. Deter RL, Rossavik IK, Harrist RB, et al: Mathematic modeling of fetal growth: Development of individual growth curve standards. *Obstet Gynecol* 1986; 68:156–161.
6. Rossavik IK, Deter RL, Hadlock FP: Mathematical modeling of fetal growth: III. Evaluation of head growth using the head profile area. *J Clin Ultrasound* 1987; 15:23–30.
7. Rossavik IK, Deter RL: Mathematical modeling of fetal growth: I. Basic principles. *J Clin Ultrasound* 1984; 12:529–533.
8. Rossavik IK, Deter RL: Mathematical modeling of fetal growth: II. Head cube (A), abdominal cube (B) and their ratio (A/B). *J Clin Ultrasound* 1984; 12:535–545.
9. Rossavik IK, Deter RL, Hadlock FP: Mathematical modeling of fetal growth: IV. Evaluation of trunk growth using the abdominal profile area. *J Clin Ultrasound* 1987; 15:31–35.
10. Deter RL, Rossavik IK, Hill RM, et al: Longitudinal studies of femur growth in normal fetuses. *J Clin Ultrasound* 1987; 15:299–305.
11. Deter RL, Harrist RB, Hadlock FP, et al: Longitudinal studies of fetal growth using volume parameters determined with ultrasound. *J Clin Ultrasound* 1984; 12:313–324.
12. Rossavik IK, Torjusen GO, Deter RL, et al: Efficacy of mathematical methods for ultrasound examinations in diabetic pregnancies. *Am J Obstet Gynecol* 1986; 155:638–644.

PART 3

Multiple Gestations

Chapter 10

Twins

Many articles have been published evaluating twin gestations. At birth, the mean weight and duration of the gestations are lower for twin than for singleton pregnancies,[1, 2] with birth weights and pregnancy durations even shorter for triplet and quadruplet pregnancies. Twins occur approximately one in every 85 births, varying in incidence in different racial groups and in different nations. The incidence of triplet and quadruplet pregnancies are much more uncommon, one in 7,600 and one in 670,000, respectively. The remainder of this chapter will therefore be confined to the analysis of twin gestations, since adequate series have not been compiled on larger-sized multiple pregnancies.

There are two types of twinning, dizygotic and monozygotic. The dizygotic twins occur in about 80% of cases and are caused by the production of two ova and their subsequent fertilization. Monozygotic twins arise from the division of one ovum after fertilization. This occurs in the remaining 20% of cases. Twinning can be evaluated in another way; i.e., by the type of membranes separating the twins. In dizygotic twins, each fetus is in a totally separate sac surrounded by its own chorion and amnion, therefore termed dichorionic-diamniotic. In a certain percentage of monozygotic twins, approximately 20% to 30%, the ovum divides within the first day after fertilization. This division is early enough so that these twins also are in their own separate sacs and also are dichorionic-diamniotic. Most monozygotic twins, however, are not. In about 70% to 75% of cases, the ovum divides between the first and seventh days and, while the twins are in their own amniotic sac, they share a common chorionic sac and are called monochorionic-diamniotic twins. A smaller percentage, approximately 3%, divide even later, 7 to 13 days after fertilization, so that the twins are within the same sac, share the same amnion and chorion, and are termed monochorionic-monoamniotic. Rarely, if the division is after the 13th day, the twins only partially separate, a situation leading to conjoined or siamese twinning.

The type of twinning is important. All twins have the same increased complication rate of prematurity and smallness in size, and all have the same problems at birth, with the second born twin having increased perinatal mortality, usually from anoxia and prolapsed cord.[3] In addition, the monochorionic twins, whether in 1 or 2 amniotic sacs, have further potential complications.[4] They may have a twin-twin transfusion caused by placental vascular shunting which can lead to one small growth retarded and one plethoric hydropic fetus. In addition monochorionic-monoamniotic twins may be further complicated by umbilical cord entanglement.

The purpose of the ultrasound evaluation of twin gestations is to establish whether there are multiple gestations, to analyze the gestational age of the twins, and to determine whether physical and growth abnormalities exist. While physical abnormalities are the same as those in singleton gestations and will not be discussed further, the in utero growth of twin gestations is unique.

In addition to the number of pregnancies, the determination of dichorionicity and monochorionicity is of predictive value in the assessment of the potential risk factors described above. Two recent articles[5,6] have stated that separate placentas and different fetal genders assure dichorionicity. In addition, a thick separation membrane composed of two layers of chorion and two layers of amnion would favor the same diagnosis, while a thin membrane of two layers of amnion would favor the diagnosis of monochorionic-diamniotic twinning[6,7] (Fig 10–1). If a membrane cannot be identified, even when good technique has been used, monochorionic-monoamniotic twinning is probable.

The most common measurement for twin gestations, as with singleton gestations, has been the biparietal diameter, which has been evaluated in 12 articles.[8-19] Eight presented numbers,[8-14,19] all except 1[13] giving a standard deviation and all except another[8] also showing their results in graph form. Two articles[15,16] presented their results only in graph form, one giving an SD.[16] The last 2 articles[17,18] stated their results only in their conclusions, without giving any numbers or graphs. These last 2 articles will therefore not be considered further in the analysis of the biparietal diameters.

Of the remaining 10,[8-16,19] eight also evaluated the biparietal diameter growth of the twin gestations in comparison to similar growth for singleton gestations.[9-12,14-16,19] In addition 4 of the articles evaluated the biparietal diameter growth of one twin against the other.[8,13-15] From these articles, it can be stated that the growth of the biparietal diameter of both twins closely parallels the biparietal diameter growth of singleton gestations until at least 28 to 30 weeks. After that time, there is some decrease in the growth of the biparietal diameters, with most articles still showing an overlap with singleton gestations at 2 SD, even as late as 38 weeks. As a result, the biparietal diameter measurement tables of singleton gestations can be used for twin gestations until at least the mid-third trimester. A table of biparietal diameter measurements in twin gestations is presented[19] (Fig 10–2; Table 10–1). While it is based on much smaller numbers and therefore has a large standard deviation, its mean values are accurate. This table serves as a reminder of the slowing in biparietal diameter growth after 30 weeks.

The growth of the biparietal diameter of each twin closely paralleled the other. Approximately 1–3 mm may normally separate the two biparietal diameters throughout gestation.[8,9,13,14,16,20,21] Two of these articles considered the twins normal even when the biparietal diameters were 5 mm different.[13,16] There were, however, discrepancies between studies. Authors disagreed on whether the biparietal diameter growth is similar for both dichorionic and monochorionic twins. Two articles found dichorionic twins to be larger,[15,17] with

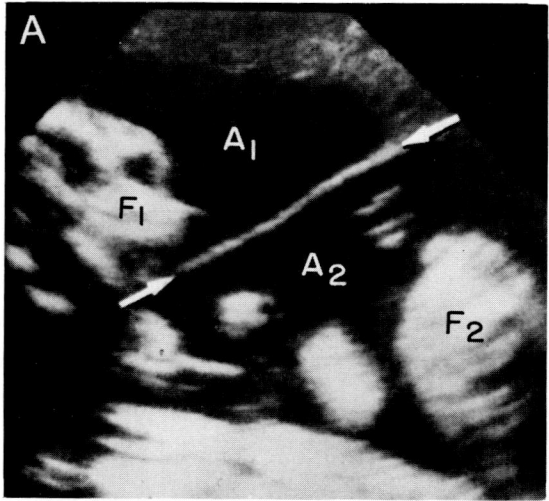
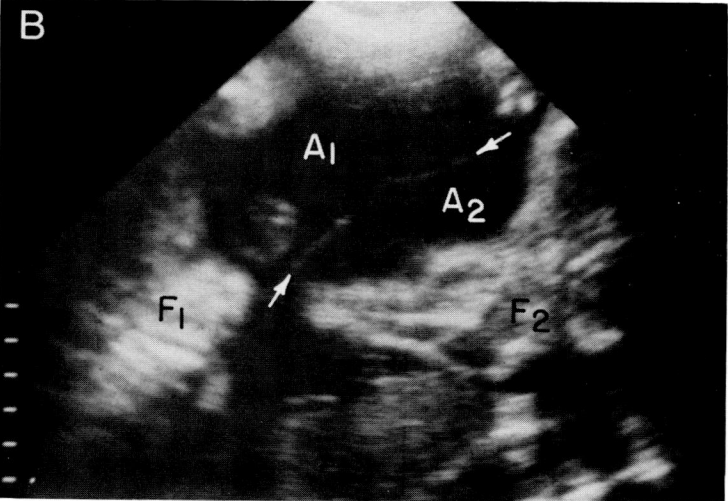

FIG 10–1.
Membrane characteristics separating twin gestations. **A,** dichorionic-diamniotic membrane *(arrows)* is thick and well-defined. One fetus (F_1) and its amniotic fluid (A_1) is separated from the other fetus (F_2) and its amniotic fluid (A_2). **B,** monochorionic-diamniotic membrane *(arrows)* is much thinner and "wispy" in appearance. The fetuses $(F_1$ and $F_2)$ and their amniotic fluid $(A_1$ and $A_2)$ are separate.

one study finding them equal in size.[10] It is possible that the discrepancies in head size may be related to unusual-shaped heads caused by the crowding of the twins against each other rather than true differences in growth. Although this cannot be proved, since no articles measured the fronto-occipital diameter, cephalic index, or calculated a head circumference, it can be suggested from the following two observations: Socal et al.[12] stated that although there was slowing of twin biparietal diameter growth, the newborn twin head circumferences were comparable to singleton gestations. Persson and Grennert[15] found in 80% of cases that the twin in vertex presentation (with the head in the pelvis) had a consistently larger biparietal diameter measurement. Since the larger fetus should

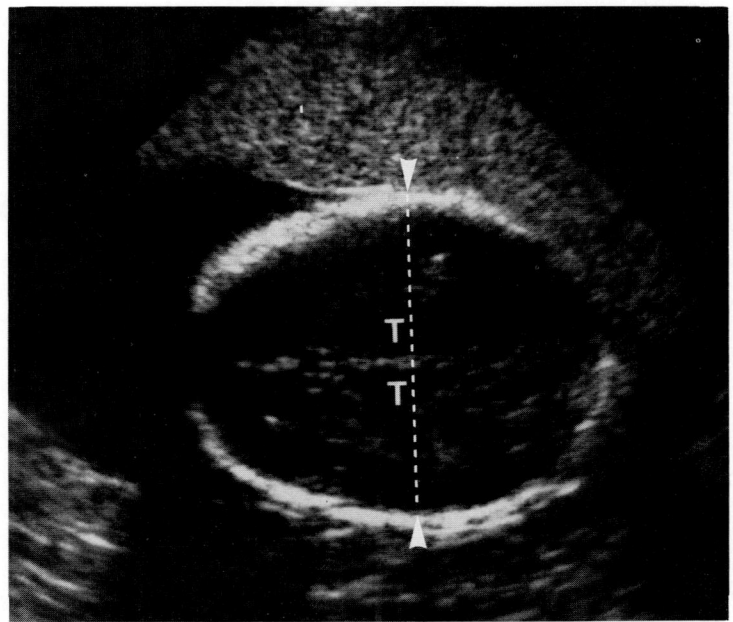

FIG 10–2.
The biparietal diameter measurement is taken in transaxial view with the thalamus *(T)* or midbrain in the midline. The measurement *(arrowheads* and *dotted line)* is taken from leading edge (outer margin) to leading edge (inner margin).

TABLE 10–1.
Fetal Measurements in Twin Gestations*†

Gestational Age, wk	Biparietal Diameter, mm		Abdominal Circumference, mm	
	Predicted Mean	Range From 5th to 95th Percentile	Predicted Mean	Range From 5th to 95th Percentile
27	69	61–78	236	202–273
28	74	66–82	239	185–293
29	74	66–82	249	199–299
30	74	64–84	253	215–291
31	78	68–88	269	231–307
32	79	71–87	272	236–308
33	81	73–89	271	229–313
34	82	76–88	289	251–327
35	84	76–92	296	262–330
36	85	79–91	298	266–330
37	85	79–91	292	240–344

*From Grumbach K, Coleman BG, Arger PH, et al: Twin and singleton growth patterns compared using ultrasound. *Radiology* 1986; 158:237–241. Used by permission.
†Data obtained on 103 twin pairs.

be randomly placed in either the lower or upper part of the uterus, the detection of most of the "larger" heads in the lower uterine segment implies that different head shapes, rather than true differences in head size, are responsible for the discrepancies in the biparietal diameter.

When discrepancies do exist, however, there is also disagreement about the value of divergent biparietal diameters in establishing the diagnosis of growth retardation. The authors of four articles[13, 16, 20, 21] thought that if a discrepancy between the two biparietal diameters was either more than 5 mm or 5%[16] or increased by ≥3 mm over at least a two-week period, growth retardation should be suggested. Using these criteria, 2 series[13, 20] detected 53% and 77% of growth retarded fetuses. Authors of three other articles, however, thought that the biparietal diameter difference alone was not enough to permit the detection of growth retardation in twins, since, on occasion, both fetuses could be growth retarded, thus invalidating the differences in the biparietal diameters.[8, 17, 18] One of the articles[8] found that even when a 5-mm or more difference existed between the biparietal diameters, the weight difference of the infants at birth was only infrequently 25% or greater. The other 2,[17, 18] without showing tables or graphs concluded that the biparietal diameter growth was not adequate for detection of growth retardation. Nevertheless, although perhaps not accurate in all cases, twin gestations do share the same environment. A discrepancy of greater than 5 mm or an increasing discrepancy between the biparietal diameters cannot be taken casually but should be judged as a warning of potential growth retardation in the smaller twins or for a twin-twin transfusion syndrome in both.

Evaluation of the fetal body in twin gestations has been reported in 4 articles.[12, 18, 19, 22] Secher et al.[22] measured the twin abdominal diameters and found them to grow normally throughout gestation. Socol et al.[12] and Grumbach et al.,[19] however, found the abdominal circumference to decrease slightly in the latter part of the third trimester. Nevertheless, the curves for normal singleton and twin gestations overlapped at 2 SD, even at term. Neilson[18] determined the product of the crown-rump length and the trunk area of twins at 34 to 36 weeks. Using static scans, the long axis of the fetus was measured from the top of the head to the bottom of the urinary bladder, and the abdominal area measurement was taken at the level of the liver. In a prospective study, this product detected all 15 of 21 twin pairs that were small-for-dates with a 22% false positive rate. A follow-up study by Neilson[23] similarly detected all 19 small-for-date twin fetuses of the 62 studied. Of the additional 43 babies that were normal at birth, there were 11 falsely predicted to be small-for-gestational age. While this work has a high degree of accuracy, it is oversensitive and further work will be necessary prior to its routine use. A table of abdominal circumference is included as a reminder of the slightly different growth of twins[19] (Fig 10–3; see Table 10–1). The mean numbers, when compared to the abdominal circumferences of singleton gestations, showed a decrease in abdominal growth after 32 weeks, somewhat similar to but less in degree than the decrease in the biparietal diameter. The standard deviation is relatively large because of the small number of cases in the series.

It would therefore seem that all twin parameters should decrease after the mid-third trimester. If so, this would be consistent with the newborn findings that twin gestations are smaller than singleton gestations. Surprisingly, Grumbach et al.[19] found that the femur length remained normal, equal to that of singleton gestational measurements, until the end of their study at 37 weeks (Fig 10–4). While this work needs further corroboration, it implies that the twin fetal parameters may not be smaller in the late third trimester. Instead, the femur may be normal, because it is the only major parameter which is not distorted by the crowding of the enlarging twins. It is therefore recommended, based on this work,[19] that, when there are discrepancies in the head and body measurements of either twin, the femur length be used to date the pregnancy and evaluate appropriate growth.

Articles on aborted fetuses[24] and on live newborn infants[1, 2, 25] have shown that in the first and second trimester the fetal weights of twins closely approximates those of singleton gestations (similar to the biparietal diameter findings). After approximately 27 weeks, the weights of twin gestations decreased in relation to singleton twin gestations, an effect which was more pronounced in monochorionic than in dichorionic twins. Asymmetric growth retardation usually occurs after 34 weeks. A discrepancy of at least 15%, and more likely 25%, in body weight between the two fetuses strongly suggests that the smaller of the two is growth retarded.[21, 26]

Two articles have evaluated fetal weight in twin gestations.[27, 28] Relatively small series of twin gestations were analyzed, 35[27] and 43[28] twin pairs. One article[27] used a weight chart based on biparietal and abdominal circumference. A curvilinear growth was detected, and the values were presented in number and graph form with a 2 SD range. In the third trimester there was a slowing in fetal weight gain caused by slowing in the biparietal diameter growth. The abdominal circumference growth remained constant, and the weights of the

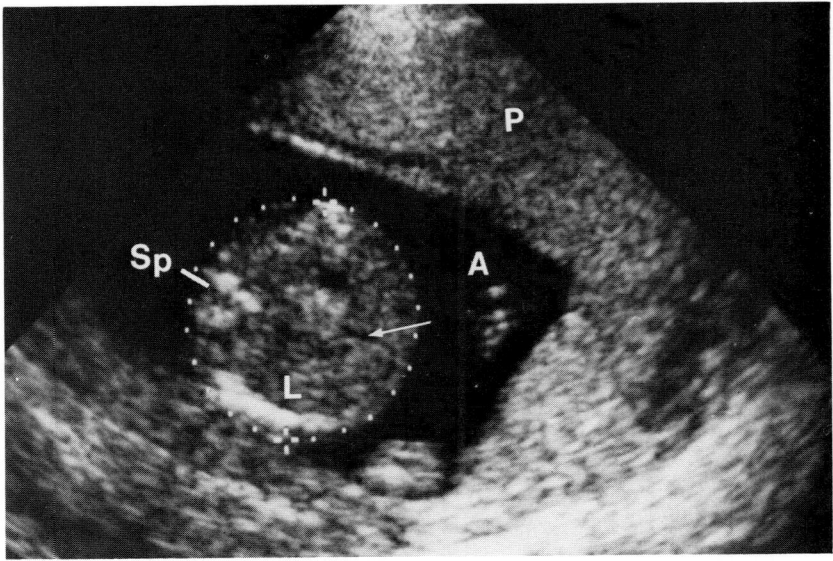

FIG 10–3.
Abdominal circumference. Transaxial image of the upper abdomen at the region of the liver *(L)*. The umbilical portion of the left portal vein *(arrow)* is situated within the liver in the midline. The circumference is traced with a digitizer or map reader *(dotted line)* or can be calculated from an equation. *P* indicates placenta; *Sp,* spine; *A,* amniotic fluid.

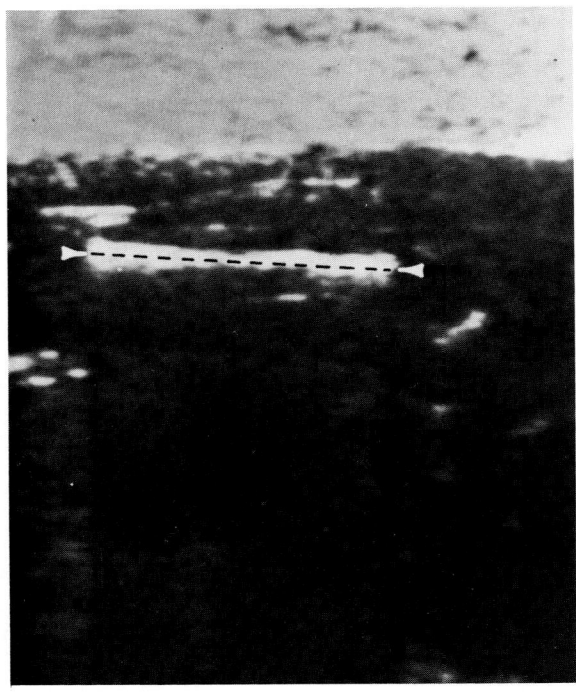

FIG 10–4.
Femur length measurement. The long axis of the hyperechoic femoral shaft is measured *(arrowheads and dotted line)*, disregarding the hypoechoic nonossified epiphyseal cartilages.

twins remained close. The other study[28] evaluated twin fetal weights using the biparietal diameter, abdominal circumference, and femur lengths. While no numbers were given, this article found that fetal weight was the most sensitive predictor of discordant fetal growth, particularly caused by an abdominal circumference difference of 20 mm or more.

While the weights of twin gestations were not significantly different at 2 SD from singleton gestations, the mean numbers are smaller for twin than for singleton gestations.[27] While it is important that this work be substantiated, a table is recommended to give the reader an understanding of expected fetal weight in twins[27] (Table 10–2). The weight is calculated using the biparietal diameter (see Fig 10–2) and abdominal circumference (see Fig 10–3) from the weight table[29] discussed in the chapter on fetal weight.

TABLE 10–2.
Estimated Fetal Weight in Twin Pregnancies*†

Gestational Age, wk	Weight, gm				
	Percentile				
	5th	25th	50th	75th	95th
16	132	141	154	189	207
17	173	194	215	239	249
18	214	248	276	289	291
19	223	253	300	333	412
20	232	259	324	378	534
21	275	355	432	482	705
22	319	452	540	586	876
23	347	497	598	684	880
24	376	543	656	783	885
25	549	677	793	916	1,118
26	722	812	931	1,049	1,352
27	755	978	1,087	1,193	1,563
28	789	1,145	1,244	1,337	1,774
29	900	1,266	1,395	1,509	1,883
30	1,011	1,387	1,546	1,682	1,992
31	1,198	1,532	1,693	1,875	2,392
32	1,385	1,677	1,840	2,068	2,793
33	1,491	1,771	2,032	2,334	3,000
34	1,597	1,866	2,224	2,601	3,208
35	1,703	2,093	2,427	2,716	3,336
36	1,809	2,321	2,631	2,832	3,465
37	2,239	2,540	2,824	3,035	3,679
38	2,669	2,760	3,017	3,239	3,894

*From Yarkoni S, Reece EA, Holford T, et al: Estimated fetal weight in the evaluation of growth in twin gestations: A prospective longitudinal study. *Obstet Gynecol* 1987; 69:636–639. Used by permission.
†Weight calculated from formula by Shepard MJ, Richards VA, Berkowitz RL, et al: An evaluation of two equations for predicting fetal weight by ultrasound. *Am J Obstet Gynecol* 1982; 142:42–54.

REFERENCES

1. Guttmacher AF, Kohl SG: The fetus of multiple gestations. *Obstet Gynecol* 1985; 12:528–541.
2. Gruenwald R: Growth of the human fetus: II. Abnormal growth in twins and infants of mothers with diabetes, hypertension, or isoimmunization. *Am J Obstet Gynecol* 1966; 94:1120–1132.
3. Tamura RK, Sabbagha RE, Pan WH, et al: Ultrasonic fetal abdominal circumference: Comparison of direct versus calculated measurement. *Obstet Gynecol* 1986; 67:833–835.
4. Naeye RL, Tafari N, Judge D, et al: Twins: Causes of perinatal death in 12 United States cities and one African city. *Am J Obstet Gynecol* 1978; 131:267–272.
5. Mahony BS, Filly RA, Callen PW: Amnionicity and chorionicity in twin pregnancies: Prediction using ultrasound. *Radiology* 1985; 155:205–209.
6. Barss VA, Benacerraf BR, Frigoletto FD Jr: Ultrasonographic determination of chorion type in twin gestation. *Obstet Gynecol* 1985; 66:779–783.

7. Hertzberg BS, Kurtz AB, Choi HY, et al: Significance of membrane thickness in the sonographic evaluation of twin gestations. *AJR* 1987; 148:151–153.
8. Erkkola R, Ala-Mello S, Piiroinen O, et al: Growth discordancy in twin pregnancies: A risk factor not detected by measurements of biparietal diameter. *Obstet Gynecol* 1985; 66:203–206.
9. Leveno KJ, Santos-Ramos R, Duenhoelter JH, et al: Sonar cephalometry in twins: A table of biparietal diameters for normal twin fetuses and a comparison with singletons. *Am J Obstet Gynecol* 1979; 135:727–730.
10. Divers WA, Hemsell DL: The use of ultrasound in multiple gestations. *Obstet Gynecol* 53:500–504.
11. Gottlicher S, Madjaric J, Krone HA: Der Biparietale Durchmesser des Fetalen Kopfes bei Zwillingen und Einlingen im Berlauf der Schwagerschaft. Eine Vergleichende Studie. *Geburtshilfe Frauenheilkd* 1977: 37:762–767.
12. Socol ML, Tamura RK, Sabbagha RE, et al: Diminished biparietal diameter and abdominal circumference growth in twins. *Obstet Gynecol* 1984; 64:235–238.
13. Houlton MCC: Divergent biparietal diameter growth rates in twin pregnancies. *Obstet Gynecol* 1977; 49:542–545.
14. Grennert L, Persson PH, Genser F: Intrauterine growth of twins judged by BPD measurements. *Acta Obstet Gynecol Scand [Suppl]* 1978; 78:28–32.
15. Persson PH, Grennert L: The intrauterine growth of the biparietal diameter of twins. *Acta Genet Med Gemellol (Roma)* 1979; 28:273–277.
16. Crane JF, Tomich PG, Kopta M: Ultrasonic growth patterns in normal and discordant twins. *Obstet Gynecol* 1980; 55:678–683.
17. Schneider L, Bessis, R, Tabaste JL, et al: Foetal twin biometry. *Acta Genet Med Gemellol (Roma)* 1979; 28:299–301.
18. Neilson JP: Detection of the small-for-dates twin fetus by ultrasound. *Br J Obstet Gynaecol* 1981; 88:27–32.
19. Grumbach K, Coleman BG, Arger PH, et al: Twin and singleton growth patterns compared using US[1]. *Radiology* 1986; 158:237–241.
20. Houlton MCC, Marivate M, Philpott RH: The prediction of fetal growth retardation in twin pregnancy. *Br J Obstet Gynaecol* 1981; 88:264–273.
21. Haney AF, Crenshaw MC, Dempsey PJ: Significance of biparietal diameter differences between twins. *Obstet Gynecol* 1978; 51(5):609–613.
22. Secher NF, Kaern J, Hansen PK: Intrauterine growth in twin pregnancies: Prediction of fetal growth retardation. *Obstet Gynecol* 1985; 66:63–67.
23. Neilson JP: Detection of the small-for-gestational age twin fetus by a two stage ultrasound examination schedule. *Acta Genet Med Gemellol (Roma)* 1982; 31:235–240.
24. Iffy L, Lavenhar MA, Jakobovits A, et al: The rate of early intrauterine growth in twin gestation. *Am J Obstet Gynecol* 1983; 146:970–972.
25. Naeye RL, Benirschke K, Hagstrom JWC, et al: Intrauterine growth of twins as estimated from liveborn birth-weight data. *Pediatrics* 1966; 37:409–416.
26. O'Brien WF, Knuppel RA, Scerbo JC, et al: Birth weight in twins: An analysis of discordancy and growth retardation. *Obstet Gynecol* 1986; 67:483–486.
27. Yarkoni S, Reece EA, Holford T, et al: Estimated fetal weight in the evaluation of growth in twin gestations: A prospective longitudinal study. *Obstet Gynecol* 1987; 69:636–639.
28. Storlazzi E, Vintzileos AM, Campbell WA, et al: Ultrasonic diagnosis of discordant fetal growth in twin gestations. *Obstet Gynecol* 1987; 69:363–367.
29. Shepard MJ, Richards VA, Berkowitz RL, et al: An evaluation of two equations for predicting fetal weight by ultrasound. *Am J Obstet Gynecol* 1982; 142:42–54.

Index

A

Abdomen, fetal
  area of, 71, 73–74
  to chest, comparison of, 131–133
  circumference of, 66–67, 69–71, 72–73
    fetal weight and, 148, 151, 152–171
    in twin gestations, 206, 207
  diameter of, 64–65, 68
  to femur, comparison of, 133–136
  and head, comparison of, 125–131
Adrenal glands, fetal, 86–88
Age, fetal
  multiple parameter, 137, 138, 139, 140–141
  sonographic, growth-adjusted, 142
Amniotic fluid, amount of, 187–190
Anechoic space in fetal kidney, 89, 91
Arms, fetal, 115–116
Atria
  fetal, 81, 82
  of fetal lateral ventricles, evaluation of, 40–42

B

Biparietal diameter (BPD), 22–27
  abdominal diameter and, 125–128
  area-corrected, for unusual head shape, 32
  cerebellar dimensions and, 51, 53–54
  femoral length and, 131, 132, 133
  fetal weight and, 147–148, 152–164, 165
  in first trimester, crown-rump length and, 14–15, 16–17
  in gestational age prediction, 25
  in hydrocephalus diagnosis, 27
  instrumentation errors in, 24–25
  in interval growth analysis, 142–143, 144–146
  long bone length and, 104, 105, 110, 111, 113
  observational errors in, 22–23
  range tables for, 27, 28–29
  technical factors in, 23–24
  total uterine volume and, 184
  in twin gestations, 203–206
Bladder, urinary, fetal, 93–94

Blood vessels, umbilical, number and size of, 191
Body volume, fetal, 74
Bowel, fetal, 95

C

Cardiac measurements, fetal, 77–83
Cephalic index (CI) in transaxial head shape computation, 29–32
Cerebellar dimensions, fetal, 51, 52, 53–54
Cervix, evaluation of, 193–196
Chest, fetal, to abdomen, comparison of, 131–133
Cisterns, subarachnoid, fetal, 51–52, 54, 55
Clavicle, fetal, 115
Congenital anomalies, abnormal first trimester growth and, 15–16
Cord, umbilical, length and width of, 190–192
Crown-rump length
  in first trimester, 12–17
    biparietal diameters and, 14–15, 16–17
    congenital anomalies and, 15–16
    real-time scanning for, 12, 14, 15
    uncorrected regression analysis in, 12–13
  and trunk area, product of, 138, 141

D

Diabetes mellitus
  abdominal circumference of fetus in, 71
  biparietal diameter and, 26
  crown-rump length and, 15
Dichorionic twins, 203
Dizygotic twins, 202
Dysplasia, skeletal, fetal femoral length and, 103

E

Endovaginal imaging for gestational sac measurement, 3–4, 8–9

Ethnic differences in biparital diameter, 26–27
Extremity, fetal, 95–114
Eyeball, fetal, evaluation of, 44–45, 46

F

Femur, fetal
   to abdomen, comparison of, 133–136
   to head, comparison of, 131, 132, 133, 134
   length of, 96–97, 98, 99, 105–109
     errors in, 100–103
     fetal weight and, 149, 151, 167–171
     gestational age and, 99–100
     interval growth of, 146
     in twin gestations, 206–207
Fetal body measurements, 63–116
   abdominal area in, 71, 73–74
   abdominal circumference in, 66–71, 72–73
   abdominal diameter in, 64–66
   of adrenal glands, 86–88
   body volume in, 74
   of bowel, 95
   of clavicle, 115
   of extremities, 95–114
   fetal weight and, 148
   and head measurements, combined, 125–171 (*see also* Fetal head measurements and body measurements, combined)
   of heart, 77–83
   of kidneys, 88–91
   of liver, 83–85
   of organs, 77–95
   of soft tissues, 115–116
   of spleen, 85–86
   thoracic area in, 64
   thoracic circumference in, 63–64
   thoracic diameter in, 63
   total fetal length in, 74–75
   total fetal volumes in, 74
   of urinary bladder, 93–94
Fetal head measurement(s), 22–55
   biparietal diameter as, 22–29
   and body measurements, combined, 125–171
     for fetal measurement comparisons, 125–136 (*see also* Fetal measurement comparisons)
     for interval growth analysis, 141–146
     multiple parameters in, 137–141
     weight and, 146–171 (*see also* Weight, fetal)
   cerebellar dimensions in, 51, 52, 53–54
   head area in, 35
   head circumference in, 32–34, 36–37
   head volume in, 35
   ocular dimensions in, 44–45, 46
   orbital dimensions in, 45–51
   subarachnoid cisterns in, 51–52, 54, 55
   unusual head shape and, 29–32
   ventricular size in, 38–44 (*see also* Ventricle(s), fetal)
Fetal measurement comparisons, 125–136
   of chest to abdomen, 131–133
   of femur
     to abdomen, 133–136
     to head, 131, 132, 133, 134
   to head to abdomen, 125–131
Fetus
   growth of, mathematical models of, 199
   length of, total, 74–75
   volumes of, total, 74–75
   weight of, 146–171 (*see also* Weight, fetal)
Fibula, fetal, length of, 98–99, 113
First trimester measurements, 1–19
   of crown-rump length, 12–17
   of gestational sac, 3–10
   of trunk circumference, 19
   of uterine length, 2
Fluid, amniotic, amount of, 187–190
Foot, fetal, gestational age and, 110
Fronto-occipital diameter (FOD), 29

G

Gestational age
   abdominal area and, 71, 73
   abdominal circumference and, 69–71, 72–73
   abdominal diameter and, 64, 66, 68
   biparietal diameter and, 25
   body volumes and, 74
   femoral length and, 99–100, 105, 110
   fibular length and, 113
   foot length and, 110
   globe diameter and, 46
   head area and, 35
   head circumference and, 33–34
   liver dimensions and, 85
   orbital diameter and, 48–51
   radial length and, 111
   renal dimensions and, 89–90, 92
   thoracic area and, 64
   thoracic circumference and, 63–64
   thoracic diameter and, 63
   tibial length and, 113, 114
   total uterine volume and, 185

ulnar length and, 111, 112
Gestational sac
　growth rate for, interval growth analysis and, 143–144
　measurement of, in first trimester, 3–10
　　tables for, 4, 10
Gestations
　multiple, 201–209
　twin, 202–208
Glands, adrenal, fetal, 86–88
Globe, fetal, evaluation of, 44–45, 46
Growth, fetal
　interval, analysis of, 141–146
　mathematical models of, 199
　retardation of
　　fetal femoral length and, 103–104
　　intrauterine, evaluation of, head and abdominal circumference ratio in, 129–130
Growth-adjusted sonographic age (GASA), 142

H

Head, fetal
　and abdomen, comparison of, 125–131
　area of, 35
　circumference of, 32–34, 36–37
　to femur, comparison of, 131, 132, 133, 134
　measurements of, 22–25 (*see also* Fetal head measurements)
　shape of, unusual, fetal head measurements in, 29–32
　volume of, calculation of, 35
Heart, fetal measurements of, 77–83
Humerus, length of, 97–98, 100, 101, 105–109
Hydrocephalus, diagnosis of, biparietal diameter in, 27
Hydrops, fetal, liver size and growth in, 84

I

Interval growth analysis, 141–146
Interventricular septum, fetal, 80–81
Intrauterine growth retardation, fetal femoral length and, 103–104
Isoimmunization, Rh, umbilical vein size and, 192
Isoimmunized fetuses, liver size and growth in, 84

K

Kidneys, fetal, 88–91

L

Large-for-gestational-age (LGA) fetus
　complications of, 147
　detection of, femur to abdomen ratio in, 133–135
Lasix challenge test for fetal kidney dysfunction, 94
Lateral ventricles
　atria of, evaluation of, 40–42
　evaluation of, 38–43
Leg, fetal, 115–116
Length, crown-rump in first trimester, 12–17 (*see also* Crown-rump length in first trimester)
Liver, fetal, 83–85
Long bones, fetal, 95–110
Low-birth-weight infants, complications of, 146–147

M

Macrosomic fetus, detection of, femur to abdomen ratio in, 133–135
Mathematical growth models, 199
Microcephaly, evaluation of, head and abdominal diameters in, 128
M-mode recording for fetal heart evaluation, 78–79
Monochorionic twins, 202–203
Monozygotic twins, 202
Multiple parameter fetal age, 137, 138, 139, 140–141

N

Neck, fetal, 115–116

O

Ocular dimensions, fetal, 44–45, 46
Oligohydramnios, complications of, 187
Orbital dimensions, fetal, 45–51
　outer, measurement of
　　reasons for, 46–47
　　tables for, 47, 48–51
　　technical difficulties in, 46, 47
Ossification centers, gestational age and, 110

P

Placenta, weight and thickness of, 182–186
Polyhydramnios, complications of, 187
Pyelectasis, 89, 91

R

Racial differences in biparietal diameter, 26–27
Radius, fetal, length of, 98, 111
Real-time scanning
   for crown-rump length, 12, 14, 15
   for fetal heart orientation, 78
Rh isoimmunization, umbilical vein size and, 192

S

Sac, gestational
   growth rate for, interval growth analysis and, 143–144
   measurement of, in first trimester, 3–10
      tables for, 4, 10
Second/third trimester measurements, 21–200
   for fetal body, 63–116
   of fetal head, 22–55 (see also Fetal head measurement(s)
   and body, combined, 125–171
   mathematical growth models of, 199
   of uterus, 181–196
Sickle cell trait (HbAS), fetal femoral length and, 103–104
Skeletal dysplasia, fetal femoral length and, 103
Small-for-gestational-age (SGA) fetus
   complications of, 146–147
   detection of, femur to abdomen ratio in, 135
Soft tissues, fetal, 115–116
Spleen, fetal, 85–86
Subarachnoid cisterns, fetal, 51–52, 54, 55

T

Third ventricle, fetal, evaluation of, 43–44
Thorax, fetal
   area of, 64
   circumference of, 63–64
   diameter of, 63
Tibia, fetal, length of, 98, 113–114
Total intrauterine volume (TIUV), 181
Total uterine volume (TUV), 181–182, 183, 184, 185
Trunk circumference in first trimester, 19

Twin gestations, 202–208
   estimated fetal weight in, 209t

U

Ulna, fetal, length of, 98, 99, 111–112
Umbilical blood vessels, number and size of, 191
Umbilical cord, length and width of, 190–192
Umbilical vein, size of, Rh isoimmunization and, 192
Urinary bladder, fetal, 93–94
Uterus
   length of, in first trimester, 2
   measurements of, 181–194
      of amniotic fluid, 187–190
      of cervix, 193–194
      of placenta, 182–186
      of umbilical cord, 190–192
      of umbilical vein, 190–192
      volume, 181–182, 183, 184, 185

V

Vein, umbilical, size of, Rh isoimmunization and, 192
Ventricle(s)
   cardiac, fetal, dimensions of, analysis of, 80
   fetal
      enlarged, diagnosis of, 44
      lateral
         atria of, evaluation of, 40–42
         evaluation of, 38–43
      size of, evaluation of, 38–44
      third, evaluation of, 43–44
Very-low-birth-weight infants, complications of, 146–147

W

Weight, fetal, 146–171
   abnormal, complications of, 146–147
   equation with three variables for, 166
   estimated, in twin pregnancy(ies), 209t
   pregnancy outcome and, 147
   tables for, 151
      based on biparietal diameter and abdominal circumference, 152–165
      estimated, based on abdominal circumference, 166
      and femur length, 168–171
   in twin gestations, 207–209
   variations in evaluation of, 149–151